Immunomodulation
BY BACTERIA AND THEIR PRODUCTS

Immunomodulation
BY BACTERIA AND THEIR PRODUCTS

Edited by
Herman Friedman, Thomas W. Klein,
and
Andor Szentivanyi

University of South Florida
Tampa, Florida

PLENUM PRESS • NEW YORK AND LONDON

Library of Congress Cataloging in Publication Data
Main entry under title:

Immunomodulation by bacteria and their products.

"Based on the proceedings of a conference on Immunomodulation by Bacteria and Their Products, held on November 18-20, 1979, in Tampa, Florida."

Bibliography: p.

Includes index.

1. Immune response—Regulation—Congresses. 2. Microbial metabolites—Physiological effect—Congresses. 3. Adjuvants, Immunological—Congresses. I. Friedman, Herman, 1931- . II. Klein, Thomas W. III. Szentivanyi, Andor [DNLM: 1. Antibody formation—Congresses. 2. Immunity, Cellular—Congresses. 3. Bacteria—Immunology—Congresses. Bacteria—Immunology—Congresses. 4. Lymphocytes—Immunology—Congresses. QW 568 I336 1979]

QR186.I469 616.07'9 81-17888

ISBN-13: 978-1-4684-4117-8 e-ISBN-13: 978-1-4684-4115-4 AACR2

DOI: 10.1007/978-1-4684-4115-4

Based on the proceedings of a conference on Immunomodulation by Bacteria and Their Products held on November 18-20, 1979, in Tampa, Florida

Softcover reprint of the hardcover 1st edition 1981

A Division of Plenum Publishing Corporation
233 Spring Street, New York, N.Y. 10013

PREFACE

It is almost axiomatic that an explosive increase in knowledge and interest concerning host immune defense mechanisms and the immune response system in general is occurring. Many new developments are evident at the interphase between the areas of immunology, infectious diseases, and host defenses to microorganisms. It is now widely recognized that a functioning host immune defense system consists of a variety of lymphoid cells. These include effector and affector cells consisting of both B and T cells and their progeny. Mononuclear phagocytes which are widely distributed throughout the body are also intimately involved in these processes. These cells are involved not only in the clearance of particulate matter including bacteria, viruses and fungi, but also presumably in host defense against neoplasia. Among the many triumphs of the biological revolution over the past decade or so is the rapidly developing understanding of how these cells and their products, including antibody, lymphokines, monokines, etc., function and interact.

It is now recognized that although the immune defense system is involved in defense against infectious agents, it is also now becoming quite clear that many infectious agents, including bacteria, viruses and fungi, as well as their products, can interact with the immune response system. For example, it has been long recognized that many of the "adjuvants" which enhance the immune responses in nonspecific ways are derived from microorganisms. Microbial products have marked effects on the immume response system. In this regard, many microorganisms and their products have been shown to depress immune response. Such depression has been associated with effects on specific cell classes, including B and T cells, as well as macrophages. On the other hand, microbial infections are associated with immunoderegulation in that enhanced antibody or cell mediated immune response may occur. Much enhancement may be often associated with autoimmune phenomena as well as polyclonal activation of a variety of lymphoid cells.

The general topic of how microbial agents interact with the immune response system, both in enhancing or suppressing responsiveness, has not been reviewed in detail previously. Thus, it was felt of value to gather together at one time investigators studying a variety of parameters associated with microbial infection and immune responses. This volume summarizes in a number of chapters the newer knowledge concerning immunomodulation by microorganisms. Dr. Arthur Johnson, one of the first investigators in the area of microbial adjuvants, reviews historical developments and some of the background information concerning microbial adjuvants and immune responses. The role of microbial agents in augmenting or affecting macrophage-lymphocyte interactions is discussed by Dr. Joost Oppenheim from the National Institutes of Health. Biochemical aspects of microbial interactions with the immune system is discussed by Dr. Richard Winchurch, who describes affects of bacterial products on cyclic nucleotide metabolism of lymphocytes.

It is now widely recognized that immune response genes and genetic controls are quite important in regulation of a wide variety of immune responses, both in man and experimental animals. The genetic control of resistance to Salmonella typhimurium infection is discussed by Dr. Allison O'Brien and colleagues in terms of modern aspects of genetics. The effects of gram positive bacteria and their components, including streptococci, on modulating immunity and affecting T lymphocytes are discussed. In addition, the almost classic observation of how pneumococcal polysaccharide affects immune responses, especially as it relates to suppressor T cell activity, is discussed in detail. The effects of staphylococcal cell wall products on immune responses is discussed by Dr. Roman Dziarski. The effects of teichoic acids and peptidoglycan from these organisms are reviewed and form the basis of an understanding of the role of these substances in modulating immune responses.

Corynebacterium parvum and the Mycobacteria such as BCG have been utilized as immunomodulators as well as adjuvants for cancer immunotherapy. Immunomodulation by Corynebacterium is discussed by Dr. A. Ghaffar. Dr. Louis Chedid, of the Institut Pasteur, discusses immunomodulation by BCG and synthetic bacterial-like adjuvants.

Lipopolysaccharides have been studied for many years in terms of their affects on the immune response system. Immunostimulation by LPS and its derivatives, including nontoxic polysaccharides, are discussed in two chapters. The effects of endotoxins on macrophages and lymphocytes are also discussed. In addition, a chapter concerning salmonella vaccines and the possibility that LPS contaminating components such as ribosomes are involved in adjuvantic activity is also presented. Immunomodulation by bacterial cell walls and components is discussed in detail by the group led by Dr. S. Kotani from Japan. The effects of pertussis in inducing immunomodulation are also presented.

It appears clear that the broad list of topics discussed in this volume focuses attention on what is now understood concerning the molecular and cellular basis of immune modulation by bacteria and their products. It certainly appears unique that bioscientists from many disciplines, including microbiology, immunology, biochemistry, and infectious diseases have focused their interest and attention on the exciting area of microorganisms and immunity. It is anticipated that publication of this series of papers by experts in the field will stimulate additional areas of investigative work which should be explored in the future.

H. Friedman
T. W. Klein
A. Szentivanyi

CONTENTS

MICROBIAL ADJUVANTS AND IMMUNE RESPONSIVENESS

Arthur G. Johnson

Department of Medical Microbiology/Immunology
School of Medicine, University of Minnesota
Duluth, MN 55812

My concern with immunomodulation began in 1952 as a member of a research team headed by Dr. Maurice Landy at Walter Reed Army Medical Center. Our objective was to purify the two known immunogenic components of typhoid vaccine, the Vi and O antigens, such that effective immunogenicity might be retained with elimination of the well known toxicity of the whole organism vaccine in use at that time. The Vi antigen turned out to be an aminogalactouronic acid which was highly effective in mouse protection tests, and presented no problem with regard to toxicity. In purifying the O antigen, we started with the Voivin product and with the expertise of our two biochemists, Drs. Marion Webster and Jerry Sagin, and through ammonium sulfate precipitations in the presence of high concentrations of sodium chloride we ended up with a product with only 0.6% nitrogen of which 0.4% was attributable to hexosamine (49). Such lipopolysaccharides (LPS) proved to be very active as antigens, but were much less protective than the Vi. They also exhibited potent endotoxic activity with extraordinary, diverse properties (30, 31).

As part of the spin-off of that effort resulting in the availability of purified bacterial components, we tested the lipopolysaccharide for any contribution it might be making to the previously observed adjuvant action of mixed vaccines which employed Gram negative bacteria as one of their constituents (18). Thus, inclusion of Hemophilis pertussis vaccine with diphtheria and tetanus toxoid had been found to result in higher antitoxin titers than when each toxoid was injected singularly. Accordingly, we designed a simple experiment in which one group of rabbits received egg albumin alone, an antigen to which the antibody response could be measured with analytical precision, and a second group received this antigen plus as little as five micrograms of the purified endotoxin. Eighteen hours after setting up the sera for analysis by the quantitative precipitin reaction, all the tubes containing antigen added to serum from rabbits receiving egg albumin alone were completely clear, but those from animals receiving the few micrograms of endotoxin along with the antigen contained large amounts of precipitate. Similar results were obtained when using diphtheria toxoid as antigen. The rest is history (24), and the extraordinary modulation of the immune response by this bacterial component, which is found in nearly all Gram negative bacteria, is under study in many laboratories.

What then should be our concerns in our pursuit of the mechanisms by which these and other bacterial products affect the immune response. In my opinion the following are important questions to be answered:

1. Are any toxic manifestations of the adjuvant required for its action? This was one of the obvious early thrusts for the endotoxin, and indirect studies suggested the answer to be in the affirmative (24). Later investigations however, have shown that LPS preparations with greatly diminished toxicity retained a significant portion of their capacity to enhance antibody formation (26, 43) as well as non-specific immunity (9). Accordingly, full scale toxicity studies of these endotoxoids should be conducted to determine possible application to veterinary and/or human medicine. Also, dose response titrations are imperative to rule out the enhancement being due to a portion of the endotoxin preparation escaping detoxification. In addition, the marked variation of responsiveness of different animal species to LPS is well documented and should be taken into account in experimental designs and interpretations. Man and the rabbit appear to be uniquely susceptible to its actions.

2. What is the chemical definition of the ligand responsible for enhancement of antibody synthesis to unrelated antigens? Most of the evidence to date implicates the lipid moiety of the LPS as influential in this respect (11), although certain polysaccharide preparations recently have been shown to elevate murine PFC (4). Perhaps, different mechanisms are involved. Nevertheless, although the lipid moiety free of polysaccharide, designated lipid A, is a potent adjuvant, the preparations in use are heterogenous mixtures (10) and we have no knowledge of the actual structure which initiates this activity. An important consideration would be whether the chemical moiety responsible for stimulation of antibody formation is different from those associated with the various toxic manifestations. Direct approaches to these questions are now feasible with the newer knowledge of the structure and composition of these fascinating molecules (40). Covalent linkage of defined adjuvant structures of minimum molecular weight to antigens may prove to be the most effective way in the future to stimulate high levels of specific immunity.

3. A third question lies in the cellular target and the nature of the receptor receiving the stimulatory action of LPS. With the large background of data unravelling the complexities of the immune system now available, sophisticated ideas as to where and how the endotoxin and other adjuvants affect the complex series of events leading to stimulation of the immune response will be evident in the following chapters. However, when the B cell polyclonal activation property of LPS was described (38), it logically was assumed that this direct mitogenicity explained the enhancement of antibody synthesis by increasing the numbers of B cells reacting to antigen. In keeping with this were our early morphological characterizations of the adjuvant effect, wherein the major change resulting from endotoxin stimulation was a marked increase in the number and size of germinal centers, now known to be comprised mainly of B cells (46, 47).

Yet, provocative evidence exists that the adjuvant action of this bacterial product may be mediated through the T cell and/or macrophage compartment with the increased B cell antibody production simply reflecting the heightened accessory cell stimulation. For example, a number of investigators have shown independently that the enhancing action of LPS in vivo and in vitro is dependent on the presence of T cells (2, 3, 28). In addition, effects on the composition of thymic tissue in endotoxin treated animals have been reported. Rowlands et al. in 1965 showed that 3 days after an i.v. injection of endotoxin into CBA mice a decrease in thymus weight to a minimum of 1/3 to 1/4 normalcy occurred (41). Normal thymus architecture was not restored until days 10-14. McMaster and Franzl also reported a dose dependent decrease induced by endotoxin in the weight of the thymus, with the normal average volume of 100 mg dropping to 30-40 mg two days after injection (33). Perhaps this endotoxin induced atrophy of the thymus may reflect "flushing out" or peripheralization of immunocompetent T cells. However, Moatamed, Karnovsky and Unanue observed a marked reduction in peripheral T cell zones of the spleens of a number of different strains of mice one day following injection of LPS, which resembled that seen in neonatally thymectomized mice (37). Increased graft vs host activity exerted by thymus cells removed from mice given endotoxin i.p. four days previously as compared to normal controls has been recorded by Uccini et al. (45). An enhancing effect of LPS on the helper activity of thymus cells also was found by them. Thus, thymus cells removed 4 days after an i.p. injection of LPS caused an approximate two fold rise in PFC/spleen when transferred to X-irradiated recipient syngeneic mice. Associated with both of these parameters was once again a decrease in thymus weight incited by the LPS treatment, i.e. from 1-80 μg elicited a dose related inverse relationship between the log of thymus weight and log PFC.

Implication of T cells in the adjuvant action of LPS has been solidified very recently by the elegant studies of McGhee at al. (32).

These investigators designed co-culture experiments between purified cell populations from the unique mouse strain C3H/HeJ which is not susceptible to the adjuvant action of endotoxin, and its genetically compatible, susceptible counterpart, the C3H/HeN strain. In order for the adjuvant action to be expressed, they found both the macrophage and the T cell needed to be derived from the endotoxin-sensitive C3H/HeN strain. Thus, their results offered convincing evidence that adjuvanticity is not mediated through a direct action on B cells.

A second member of the T cell compartment, the T suppressor cell, also can be activated by the LPS. When LPS injection preceded the antigen by several days, suppression of the immune response was readily induced (19). Preliminary evidence using co-culture experiments and spleen cells from the endotoxin resistant C3H/HeJ strain of mice suggested that purified T cells from the suppressed mice have the capacity to transfer the suppression to normal, syngeneic spleen cell populations (Molde and Johnson, unpublished experiments).

As a matter of fact, this broad capability of stimulating many different cell types, paradoxically is emerging as a major problem with regard to the practical application of adjuvants. This appears to be particularly true in the case of the endotoxins as cited above, where both enhancement and suppression of the immune response can be induced depending on the time of exposure to antigen relative to endotoxin administration. Also, multiple antibodies with different binding characteristics and biologic potentials are enhanced (38). Consequently, it is an important challenge to find the conditions needed to direct these adjuvants to cellular targets and/or receptors such that a response with only the specific desired function is elicited.

With regard to the nature of the cellular receptor through which the LPS exerts its initial stimulus, nothing is known. What complicates this problem and is not generally appreciated is that the endotoxin molecule binds to the surface of many cells and tissues (e.g. red blood cells, polymorphonuclear leukocytes, lymphocytes, macrophages, platelets, capillary endothelium (6, 16, 42). In addition, the minute microgram and nanogram quantities which elicit many of its activities make meaningful tracer experiments in vivo practically impossible. A different approach which may prove more feasible has been that of Adye and Springer who have isolated glycerophosphatides from human platelets and leukocytes which will bind endotoxin (1). Although an antiserum specific for the LPS receptor on murine B cells has been reported (14, 15) confirmation has not been readily forthcoming (48).

4. Is the adjuvant action mediated through release of endogenous helper factors or other lymphokines? In our studies of the adjuvant action of endotoxins, we observed repeatedly that the LPS triggering action was exerted early and was ineffective if given only hours after

antigen (29). A smudging of lymphocyte staining in splenic sections obtained within hours from endotoxin treated rabbits appeared to correlate with this (47). Consequently, we formulated the hypothesis that a rapid cytotoxic action of endotoxin was exerted on lymphocytes releasing host nucleic acids, which in a trephocytic fashion were stimulatory to immunocompetent cells in the vicinity. Support for this hypothesis was gained with our demonstration that homologous and heterologous nucleic acids also non-specifically stimulated antibody formation (35). Indeed, nuclease derived oligonucleotides also proved to be active (25), and when synthetic polynucleotide complexes were found by Braun and Nakano to be potent adjuvants, analysis of this phenomenon was facilitated greatly (8). This was confirmed by us and characterized in depth by both of our groups (7, 23). An entirely different rationale, i.e.that these synthetic polynucleotides might mimic the structure in viruses responsible for interferon induction, resulted in further broadening of their immunomodulatory properties. Thus, Field, et al (17) documented the capacity of synthetic polyinosinic-polycytidylic acid complexes, as well as native double stranded nucleic acids, to elevate interferon levels in animals.

One of these synthetic nucleotide complexes, polyadenylic-polyuridylic acid (poly A:U) proved to be an effective, nontoxic stimulator of the T cell compartment (21). A remarkable effect was exerted on low numbers of thymocytes such that it took only 5 x 10^4 cells incubated with poly A:U to achieve the same helper effect seen with 10^6 normal thymocytes in passive transfer experiments (13). No mitogenic effect could be measured on exposure of thymocytes to poly A:U, and the numbers of such cells were not increased (20). Rather, the evidence favored the hypothesis that the homoribopolymers restored the deficient immune response of thymectomized or anti-thymocyte treated mice by increasing the function of each residual cell (5). Thus, it was found that thymocytes incubated with poly A:U for as short a time as 10 minutes, and cultured for an additional 6 hr after removal of the polynucleotide by washing, secreted into the culture fluids a factor(s) which was capable of restoring the deficient immune response of the very young (1 week) and aging (1-2 years) mice. T cytotoxic cells were stimulated also by this adjuvant (22), as well as T suppressor cells when given 1-2 days prior to antigen (39).

The evidence to date tends to suggest that the adjuvant action of the synthetic polynucleotides is distinct from that exerted by the LPS. Consequently, the original hypothesis suggesting that LPS acted by releasing endogenous factors of a nucleic acid nature may need to be modified. There is no question that endotoxin releases endogenous host factors, but they appear to be mostly protein in nature and possess properties different from the polynucleotides.

Several well characterized endogenous mediators might be implicated in the various effects of the LPS on the immune response. These have been described in detail in a recent international conference on endotoxin induced mediators (34). Lymphocyte activating factor (LAF) can be released by endotoxin from human mononuclear cells (44) as well as mouse macrophage cell lines (36). It appears to be a single polypeptide chain of molecular weight 12-16,000 daltons which activates and induces proliferation of thymus derived lymphocytes (36). A second, termed tumor necrosis serum (TNS) induced by LPS in mice previously sensitized to BCG or *Corynebacterium parvum*, will substitute for helper T cells, cause differentiation of B cells and induce non-specific natural killer cells (12). The immunoregulator molecule, interferon also is readily induced by LPS (27). Any or all of these logically could be expected to participate in the enhancement of the immune system characteristic of the endotoxin. As one can perceive, the problem is not whether mediators affecting the immune response can be induced by endotoxin, but the conditions under which factors can be selectively induced to act on specific functions.

5. *What is the significance to the microorganism of its immune modulation capabilities?* Hidden in this interesting teleological question in the implication that those strains of microorganisms with the capability of increasing antibody and cell mediated immunity should be the least virulent, and generally incapable of maintaining an infective state. This suicidal characteristic might contribute to the lack of virulence of the rough as compared to smooth Gram negative bacteria. One would assume the stimulatory ligands were much more "available" and active in the rough state. On the other hand, the adjuvant action on suppressor cells by some microorganisms should favor establishment of the organism in the host. However, the kinetics of such development would rarely be of sufficient rapidity to offset the opsonic effect of pre-existing antibody, etc. Nevertheless, the capacity to incite suppressor cells may prove to be an important factor contributing to chronic infections.

6. *Lastly, the question of safety tests for the practical utilization of adjuvants is raised.* Beside the standard battery of testing needed for any product prior to use in human beings, additional precautions need to be defined with respect to adjuvants and possible excess or undesired stimulation of the immune system. Antigen-antibody complex disease, autoimmunity, tumor enhancing antibody, unwarranted immunosuppression, and multiple myeloma are all conditions needing consideration prior to advocating the use of these potent immune adjuvants.

In view of this, it may be that the time is ripe for greater effort to be expended in identification and isolation of the endogenous mediators rather than continued characterization of microbial products. The inherent specificity in the isolated mediator and the greater control over side effects and excess stimulation may be dividends balancing the difficulty in isolating such trace substances.

REFERENCES

1. Adye, J. C., and Springer, G. F., 1977, Binding of endotoxin (LPS) by glycerophosphatides from human platelets and leukocytes. Naturwissenschaften 64: 150.

2. Allison, A. C., and Davies, A. T. S., 1972, Requirements of thymus dependent lymphocytes for potentiation by adjuvants of anytibody formation. Nature 233: 330.

3. Armerding, D., and Katz, D. H., 1974, Activation of T and B lymphocyte in vitro. I. Regulatory influence of bacterial lipopolysaccharide (LPS) on specific T cell helper function. J. Exp. Med. 139: 24.

4. Behling, U. H., and Nowotny, A., 1977, Immune adjuvancy of lipopolysaccharide and a nontoxic hydrolytic product demonstrating oscillating effects with time. J. Immunol. 118: 1905.

5. Bick, P. H., and Johnson, A. G., 1977, Poly A:U-induced secretion of T lymphocyte helper factors. Scand. J. Immunol. 6: 1133.

6. Braude, A. I., Carey, F. J., Sutherland, D., and Zalesky, M., 1955, Studies with radioactive endotoxin. II. Correlation of physiologic effects with distribution of radioactivity in rabbits injected with lethal doses of E. coli endotoxin labelled with radioactive sodium chromate. J. Clin. Invest. 34: 858.

7. Braun, W., Ishizuka, M., Yajima, Y., Webb, D., and Winchurch, R., 1971, Spectrum and mode of action of poly A:U in the stimulation of immune responses, in: "Biological Effects of Polynucleotides", R. F. Beers and W. Braun, ed., Springer-Verlag, NY, pp. 139.

8. Braun, W., and Nakano, M., 1967, Antibody formation: stimulation by polyadenylic and polycytidylic acids. SCIENCE 157: 819.

9. Chedid, L., Audibert, F., Bona, C., Damais, C., Parant, F., and Parant, M., 1975, Biological activities of endotoxins detoxified by alkylation. Infect. Immun. 12: 712.

10. Chen, C. H., Johnson, A. G., Kasai, N., Key, B. A., Levin, J., and Nowotny, A., 1973, Heterogeneity and biological activity of endotoxin glycolipid from Salmonella minnesota R595, J. Inf. Dis. 1285: 35.

11. Chiller, J. M., Skidmore, B. J., Morrison, D. C., and Weigle, W. O., 1973, Relationship of the structure of bacterial lipopolysaccharide to its function in mitogenesis and adjuvanticity. Proc. Natl. Acad. Sci. 70: 2129.

12. Chun, M., Pasanen, V., Hammerling, U., Hammerling, G. F., and Hoffman, M. K., 1979, Tumor necrosis serum induces a serologically distinct population of NK cells. J. Exp. Med. 150: 426.

13. Cone, R. E., and Johnson, A. G., 1971, Regulation of the immune system by snythetic polynucleotides. III. Action on antigen reactive cells of thymus origin. J. Exp. Med. 133: 649.

14. Coutinlu, A., Forni, L., and Watanabe, T., 1978, Genetic and functional characterization of an antiserum to the lipid A specific triggering receptor on murine B lymphocytes. Eur. J. Immunol. 8: 63.

15. Coutinlu, A., Meo, A., and Watanabe, T., 1977, Independent segregation of two functional markers expressed on the same B cell subset in the mouse: the Mls determinants and the LPS receptors. Scand. J. Immunol. 6: 1005.

16. Cremer, N., and Watson, D. W., 1957, Influence of stress on distribution of endotoxin in RES determined by fluorescein antibody technic. Proc. Soc. Exp. Biol. Med. 95: 510.

17. Field, A. K., Tytell, A. A., Lampson, G. P., and Hilleman, M. R., 1967, Inducers of interferon and host resistance. II. Multistranded synthetic polynucleotide complexes. Proc. Natl. Acad. Sci. 58: 1004.

18. Fleming, D. S., Greenberg, L., and Beith, E. M., 1948, The use of combined antigens in the immunization of infants. Canad. Med. Assoc. J. 59: 101.

19. Haas, G. P., Johnson, A. G., and Nowotny, A., 1978, Suppression of the immune response in C3H/HeJ mice by protein free lipopolysaccharides. J. Exp. Med. 148: 1081.

20. Han, I. H., and Johnson, A. G., 1975, The mitogenic activity of polyadenylicpolyuridylic acid complexes. Ann. N.Y. Acad. Sci. 249: 370.

21. Johnson, A. G., 1976, The adjuvant action of synthetic polynucleotides on the immune response, in: "Immune RNA", E. P. Cohen, ed., Cleveland: CRC Press, Inc., Cleveland, OH, pp. 17.

22. Johnson, A. G., 1979, Modulation of the immune system by synthetic polynucleotides, in: "Seminars in Immunopathology". P. Miescher, ed., New York: Springer-Verlag.

23. Johnson, A. G., Cone, R. E., Friedman, H. M., Han, I. H., Johnson, H. G., Schmidtke, J. R., and Stout, R. D., 1971, Stimulation of the immune system by homopolyribonucleotides, in: "Biological Effects of Polynucleotides", R. F. Beers and W. Braun, ed. New York: Springer-Verlag, pp. 157.

24. Johnson, A. G., Gaines, S., and Landy, M., 1956, Studies on the O antigen of Salmonella typhosa. V. Enhancement of antibody response to protein antigens by the purified lipopolysaccharide, J. Exp. Med. 103: 225.

25. Johnson, A. G., and Hoekstra, G., 1967, Acceleration of the primary antibody response, in: "Ontogeny of Immunity", R. T. Smith, R. A. Good, P. A. Miescher, ed. Gainesville: University of Florida Press, pp. 187.

26. Johnson, A. G., and Nowotny, A., 1964, Relationship of structure to function in bacterial O antigens. III. Biological properties of endotoxoids. J. Bact. 87: 809.

27. Johnson, H. M., and Baron, S., 1976, The nature of the suppressive effect of interferon and interferon inducers on the in vitro immune response, Cell. Immunol. 25: 106.

28. Kagnoff, M. F., Billings, P., and Cohn, M., 1974, Functional characteristics of Peyers patch lymphoid cells. II. Lipopolysaccharide is thymus dependent. J. Exp. Med. 139: 407.

29. Kind, P. D., and Johnson, A. G., 1949, Studies on the adjuvant action of bacterial endotoxins. I. Time limitation of enhancing effect and restoration of antibody formation in X-irradiated rabbits, J. Immunol 82: 415.

30. Landy, M., and Johnson, A. G., 1955, Studies on the O antigen of Salmonella typhosa. IV. Endotoxic properties of the purified antigen, Proc. Soc. Exp. Biol. Med. 90: 57.

31. Landy, M., Johnson, A. G., Webster, M. E., and Sagin, J. F., 1955, Studies on the O antigen of Salmonella typhosa. II. Immunological properties of the purified antigen, J. Immunol. 74: 466.

32. McGee, J. R., Farrar, J. J., Michalek, S. M., Mergenhagen S.E., and Rosenstreich, D. L., 1979, Cellular requirements for lipopolysaccharide adjuvanticity. A role for both T lymphocytes and macrophages for in vivo responses to particulate mitogens.

J. Exp. Med. 148: 793.

33. McMaster, P. D., and Franzl, R. E., 1968, The primary immune responses of lymphoid tissues accompanying the enhancement or complete suppression of antibody formation by a bacterial endotoxin. J. Exp. Med. 127: 1109.

34. Mergenhagen, S., Berry, L. J., and Rosenstreich, D., 1979, ASM Conference on endogenous mediators in host responses to bacterial endotoxins.

35. Merritt, K., and Johnson, A. G., 1965, Studies on the adjuvant action of bacterial endotoxins. IV. Enhancement of antibody formation by nucleic acids. J. Immunol. 94: 416.

36. Mizel, S. B., 1979, Physiochemical characterization of lymphocyte activating factor (LAF). J. Immunol. 122: 2167.

37. Moatamed, F., Karnowsky, M. J., and Unanue, E. R., 1975, Early cellular responses to mitogens and adjuvants in the mouse spleen. Lab. Invest. 32: 303.

38. Moller, G., ed. 1972, Lymphocyte activation by mitogens. Transpl. Rev. 11.

39. Morris, C. K., and Johnson, A. G., 1978, Regulation of the immune system by synthetic polynucleotides. VII. Suppression induced by pre-treatment with poly A:U. Cell. Immunol. 39: 345.

40. Reitschel, E. H., 1976, Absolute configuration of 3-hydroxy fatty acids present in lipopolysaccharides from various bacterial groups. Eur. J. Biochem. 64: 423.

41. Rowlands, D. T., Claman, H. T., and Kind, P. D., 1965, The effect of endotoxin on the thymus of young mice. Am. J. Path. 46: 165.

42. Rubenstein, H. S., Fine, J., and Coons, A. H., 1962. Localization of endotoxin in the walls of the peripheral vascular system during lethal endotoxemia. Proc. Soc. Exp. Biol. Med. 111: 458.

43. Schenck, J. R., Hargie, M. P., Brown, M. S., Ebert, D. S., Yoo, A. L., and McIntire, F. C., 1969, The enhancement of antibody formation by Escherichia coli lipopolysaccharide and detoxified derivative. J. Immunol. 102: 1411.

44. Togawa, A., Oppenheim, J. J., and Mizel, J. B., 1979, Characterization of lymphocyte activating factor (LAF) produced by human mononuclear cells: Biochemical relationship of high

and low molecular weight forms of LAF. J. Immunol. 122: 2112.

45. Uccini, S., Ruco, L., Saravito, G., Aderini, L., Doria, G., and Barani, C. D., 1976, Cell selection in the thymus of mice treated with Escherichia coli lipopolysaccharide (LPS). Adv. Exp. Med. Biol. 66: 95.

46. Ward, P. A., Abell, M. R., and Johnson, A. G., 1961, Studies on the adjuvant action of bacterial endotoxins on antibody formation. IV. Histologic study of cortisone treated rabbits. Am. J. Path. 38: 189.

47. Ward, P. A., Johnson, A. G., and Abell, M. R., 1959, Studies on the adjuvant action of bacterial endotoxins on antibody formation. III. Histologic response of the rabbit spleen to a single injection of a purified protein antigen. J. Exp. Med. 109: 463.

48. Watson, J., 1979, in ASM Conference on Endotoxin Mediators. (in press).

49. Webster, M. E., Sagin, J. F., Landy, M., and Johnson, A. G., 1955, Studies on the O antigen of Salmonella typhosa. I. Purification of the antigen. J. Immunol. 74: 455.

BI-DIRECTIONAL MACROPHAGE-LYMPHOCYTE INTERACTIONS MODULATE IMMUNE RESPONSES

J. J. Oppenheim, P. S. Steeg and R. N. Moore

NIH, NIDR, Bethesda, MD 20205

The activation of macrophages and lymphocytes is initiated by exogenous stimuli which often are bacterial in origin. Some of the most potent activating agents are bacterial endotoxin lipopolysaccharide (LPS), antigenic bacterial components and exotoxins. Macrophages and lymphocytes in turn modulate each other's level of activation through cell contact and/or mediator dependent mechanisms. For example, some macrophage products suppress lymphocyte proliferation and antibody production. These include thymidine, arginase, prostaglandins and oxygen metabolites, as will be discussed by Dr. Hoffeld (8). Conversely, interferon produced by lymphocytes may have suppressive effects on the activity of macrophages (9). In addition, macrophages and lymphocytes stimulate each other in many ways. In this presentation, we will discuss the multiplicity of endogenous pathways by which lymphocytes and macrophages mutually augment each other's reactions in their effort to eliminate bacteria or other non-self antigens.

It is generally accepted that viable macrophages are absolutely necessary as accessory cells for the activation of thymic derived (T) lymphocytes. This includes T cell proliferation, the production of lymphokines and the induction of T cell anti-dependent antibody production in response to antigenic or mitogenic stimuli. Thus, macrophages play a vital role in the inductive phase of the immune response, as well as acting as effector cells that phagocytose and digest the exogenous stimulant.

Macrophages are much more effective in activating syngeneic than allogeneic T lymphocytes. Studies of congenic mice have revealed that this is because Ia identity at the major histocompatibility locus (MHC) is required for optimal "antigen presentation" by macrophages to lymphocytes (17). Not all macrophages express Ia antigens and only the Ia bearing subpopulations of macrophages are actually capable of performing the "antigen presentation" function (3). Consequently, murine Kupffer cells, alveolar and splenic macrophages which are 60% Ia+ are more effective as accessory cells than peritoneal exudate cells (PEC) which include only 5-10% Ia+ macrophages (16). Conversely, the residual Ia- macrophages that survive treatment with cytotoxic anti-Ia antiserum in the presence of complement are not capable of the accessory antigen presentation function. These findings may be explained by the proposal that an antigen can be recognized as a non-self consituent and activates lymphocytes only if it somehow distorts or modifies the configuration of macrophage self (Ia) antigens (20).

Macrophages also synthesize and secrete polypeptide mediator(s) that have multiple biological effects on lymphocytes. The most thoroughly studied "monokine" is called Lymphocyte Activating Factor (LAF) or Interleukin I (IL-1). LAF is produced by Ia- as well as Ia+ macrophages (C. Cowing and J. J. Oppenheim, unpublished observation) and by macrophage cell lines (14). All of the innumerable stimulants which are known to activate macrophages also increase macrophage LAF production (14). LAF is a 12,000-16,000 MW single polypeptide chain that is resistant to trypsin but sensitive to pronase digestion (11). Murine LAF has been purified to a relatively high degree by sequential ammonium sulfate fractionation, DEAE cellulose, sephacryl S200 and phenyl sepharose chromatography followed by electrophoresis on 10% discontinuous polyacrylamide gels. Nanogram amounts of LAF with 20,000 fold increases in activity and 4-7% yield have been obtained. Isoelectrofocusing of this material on 7.5% polyacrylamide gels (pH 4-6) yields a single protein band at pI 5.6 (11). Thus, LAF like other mediators is biologically active at concentrations below the nanogram level.

Monokines have a multiplicity of biological effects (Table 1):

1. LAF is directly mitogenic for peanut agglutinin nonagglutinable (PNA-) and cortisone resistant murine thymocyte subpopulation (15).

2. LAF synergizes with another stimulant such as phytohemagglutinin (PHA) to become mitogenic for PNA+ and to enhance the responses of PNA-thymocytes. It can only augment the peripheralized T lymphoproliferative response to antigens and mitogens. LAF cannot restore the proliferative response of lymphocytes that have been completely depleted of antigen-presenting accessory macrophages (15). Thus LAF serves as an augmenting rather than as an initiating signal for peripheralized lymphocytes (15).

3. LAF promotes antibody production by macrophage depleted B lymphocytes to T cell dependent antigens. LAF has been found to be

TABLE I

Macrophage-Lymphocyte Interaction

A. Cell Contact (IR) Dependent

B. Macrophage Mediator Effects

1. Lymphocyte Activating Factor (LAF = IL-1)
   a) Mitogenic for PNA-Mouse Thymocytes
   b) Enhances Lectin Mitogenicity for PNA+ and PNA- Thymocytes and Lymphocytes
   c) Enhances Antibody Production (BAF)
   d) Replaces Macrophages Needed for Induction of Cytotoxic T Lymphocytes
   d) Replaces Macrophages Needed for Induction of Lymphokine (IL-2) Production

2. Thymocyte Differentiation Factor (TDF=LAF)
   a) TDF Decreases Il and Increases H-2 Expression
   b) LAF Increased Lyt-1 and Decreased Lyt-2 Expression
   c) An Unknown Monokine Increases Ia and Antigen Binding by Lymphocytes
   d) LAF Increases Stable E-Rosette-forming Lymphocytes

3. Genetically Restricted Factor (GRF)
   a) Induces Antigen Specific Antibody Production

4. Interferon
   a) Suppresses Lymphocyte Proliferation
   b) Inhibits Antibody Production and Delayed Hypersensitivity
   c) Enhances H-2 Expression on Lymphocytes
   d) Promotes Natural Killer Cell Functions

chromatographically inseparable from a "monokine" with the same activities, called B cell activating factor (BAF) (19).

4. LAF replaces the requirement for macrophages in the induction of cytotoxic T lymphocytes (5).

5. LAF can stimulate monocyte depleted lymphocytes to produce a lymphokine called IL-2 which in turn promotes lymphocyte proliferation and differentiation. IL-2 may actually be responsible for the enhancing effect of LAF on antibody production and T killer cell development (6).

6. LAF or related macrophage mediators promote lymphocyte differentiation: (a) LAF has been shown to promote the development of stable E rosette formation by peripheral lymphocytes (A.

Ben-Zvi, S. Mizel and J. J. Oppenheim, unpublished observations). (b) An uncharacterized factor present in supernatants of murine adherent peritoneal cells has been reported to promote the expression of lymphocyte Ia antigens and antigen binding receptors (10). (c) Supernatants of murine adherent cells are also said to contain a thymocyte differentiation factor (TDF) which chromatographs in the 30,000-50,000 MW range (1). TDF reduces the expression of T1 but promotes the expression of H-2 antigens on thymocytes. (d) LAF induces a sub-population of small thymocytes to express more Lyt - 1 antigen (15).

7. Parenthetically, it should be mentioned that LAF also contributes to inflammatory reactions through its biological effects on non-lymphoid cells (a) LAF is chromatographically inseparable from endogenous pyrogen (18). LAF, therefore, is involved in the generation of the prostaglandins that stimulate the hypothalamic fever center. (b) LAF also stimulates a synovial fibroblast in arthritic joints to elaborate prostaglandins and collagenase (12) and may thus promote inflammatory reactions.

8. Another product of macrophages that promotes antibody production has geen reported to be a genetically restricted factor (GRF) (4). GRF is produced by antigen pulsed macrophage cultures. It appears to consist of a complex that includes an antigen binding receptor, and Ia antigen which accounts for its ability to stimulate only syngeneic antigen specific lymphocyte reactions.

9. Interferon, which can be made by macrophages, can suppress lymphocyte proliferation, antibody production and delayed type hypersensitivity, but also enhances the expression of H-2 antigens on cytotoxic T cells and promotes natural killer activities (7).

From the foregoing it is apparent that as macrophages are stimulated by bacterial invaders or other stimuli, they in turn recruit lymphocytes, activate them to proliferate and enhance their functional capacity to react to the stimulant.

Lymphocytes play a crucial role in regulating macrophage effector functions through contact and mediator dependent mechansims. The capacity of the macrophage to phagocytose and degrade foreign antigens, to be activated to differentiate and to synthesize and secrete a wide variety of enzymes, enable it to eliminate bacteria. Consequently, the macrophage serves as the central effector cell for lymphocyte dependent immunological reactions.

Activated lymphocytes can activate macrophages in a cell contact dependent manner. It has been reported that murine T lymphocytes sensitized to Listeria monocytogenes can, in conjunction with the bacterial antigen, activate macrophages to produce a "monokine" (1).

Neither the bacterial antigen nor the lymphocytes by themselves have any effect. The reaction exhibits antigen specificity since neither unsensitized lymphocytes nor unrelated antigen will activate the macrophages. The effect is not due to a mediator since separation of the sensitized lymphocytes and Listeria from the macrophages by a cell-impermeable membrane blocks the effect. The most intriguing observation is that only syngeneic lymphocytes which share the Ia subregion of the H-2 complex with the macrophages were effective in activating macrophages. This requirement for Ia region homology in cell contact dependent lymphocyte-macrophage interactions is the mirror image of the genetic restriction of macrophage-lymphocyte interactions. This suggests that the effects of such interactions may occur simultaneously and be bi-directional.

Macrophages also are the target cell for many of the lymphokines (2). Lymphocytes produce these mediators in response to infectious agents, antigens, or mitogens. Most of the mediators are immunologically nonspecific in their effects (Table 2).

(1) One of the biologically most important lymphokines is lymphocyte derived chemotactic factor (LDCF). It attracts macrophages along a concentration gradient of LDCF toward the site of lymphocyte activation. LDCF has been recovered from in vivo sites of inflammation. Antibody to LDCF decreases inflammatory reactions.

(2) The most thoroughly studied lymphokine is macrophage activating factor (MAF). Over a period of 48 - 72 hours MAF stimulates the metabolic activity, enzyme and mediator production, size, adhesion, capacity to spread, pinocytosis and phagocytosis of macrophages. MAF cannot be chromatographically separated from a migration inhibitory factory (MIF) activity which, in a 24 hour period, decreases the mobility and increases the adhesion of macrophages. Presumably, MIF/MAF activity may serve to retain macrophages at inflammatory sites and would promote their degradative functions.

TABLE II

Lymphocyte-Macrophage Interaction

A. Cell Contact (IR) Dependent

B. Lymphocyte Mediator Effects
1. Monocyte Chemotactic Factor (LDCF)
2. Macrophage Activating Factor (MAF)
3. Migration Inhibitory Factor (MIF=MAF)
4. Colony Stimulating Factor (CSF)
5. Interferon
6. Soluble Immune Response Suppressor (SIRS)
7. Cytophilic Antibody
8. Ia Inducing Factor

(3) Another lymphokine, colony stimulating factor (CSF), this is elaborated by activated lymphocytes induces bone marrow stem cell precursors to proliferate and differentiate into monocytes. In addition, it has recently become apparent that CSF can further promote the growth and also the activation of peripheral monocytes (13).

(4) In response to bacterial antigens, activated lymphocytes can also produce an "immune" interferon (Type II), which has relatively weak anti-viral but considerable anti-proliferative and immunosuppressive effects. The effects of interferon on macrophages are controversial. It has been reported to activate macrophages (2), but this may be attributable to contamination by MAF. Conversely, there is a recent report that interferon may have "deactivating" effects on macrophages (9).

(5) Suppressor lymphocytes when activated by Concanavalin A produce a soluble immune response suppressor (SIRS) (2). This lymphokine inhibits B cell antibody production and proliferation. Paradoxically, it can only act in the presence of viable macrophages. Its immunosuppressive effects are mediated in some unknown manner by activated macrophages.

(6) Cytophilic antibodies are B lymphocyte products that play a crucial role in controlling macrophage function. Their Fc ends absorb onto macrophage Fc receptors and this anchorage selectively facilitates the phagocytosis of antigens recognized by the antibody combining sites. Cytophilic antibodies thus endow the macrophage with the capacity to differentiate between antigenic and nonantigenic stimuli.

(7) Finally, we would like to present one recent experimental result that adds another link to the reverberating consanguineous lymphocyte-macrophage interactions. We postulated that lymphocytes may influence the capacity of macrophages to present antigen by regulating their Ia expression. We, therefore, tested the effect of a variety of stimulants on the expression of Ia by cultured macrophages. We observed that adherent PEC which were usually more than 90% Ia negative, when incubated with supernatants of Concanavalin-A activated murine spleen cells become progressively more susceptible to killing by cytotoxic anti-Ia antibodies in the presence of complement (Table 3). After five to nine days of incubation with the lymphokine containing supernatant, the vast majority of PEC macrophages were Ia positive. Thus a nonspecific mediator can induce an immunogenetically restricted MHC product. In contrast, control supernatants reconstituted with Concanavalin A, a potent exogenous stimulant, namely LPS, and CSF with macrophage activating effects (13) had no signficant effect. Although both the lymphokine which induces macrophage Ia expression and the functional import of induced macrophage Ia remain to be established, these findings further

TABLE III

Effect of Supernatants of Concanavalin A Stimulated Spleen Cells On the Expression of Ia Antigens by Peritoneal Exudate Cells

Dilution of Supernatant	N	Mean Cytotoxicity Index ± S.E.M.*: Supernatant of Concanavalin A Stimulated DBA/2 Spleen Cells**	Mean Cytotoxicity Index ± S.E.M.*: Supernatant of Unstimulated DBA/2 Spleen Cells Supplemented with Concanavalin A
1:4	2	86.2 ± 6.7	9.1 ± 7.7
1:8	2	75.4 ± 1.1	3.1 ± 3.1
1:16	2	71.8 ± 4.0	0
1:32	2	58.1 ± 10.6	0
1:64	2	50.3 ± 4.3	N.D.***
1:128	2	31.4 ± 16.4	N.D.
None	8	2.5 ± 1.5	

$$\text{*Cytotoxicity} = \frac{\text{\% cytotoxicity (antibody + complement) \% cytoxicity (complement) x 100}}{\text{100 - \% Cytotoxicity (complement)}}$$

** C_3H/HeN peritoneal exudate cells incubated in McCoys 5A enriched medium for seven days. Supernatants prepared using DBA/2 spleen cells.

*** Not done.

illustrate the mutually amplifying effects of lymphocyte induction of macrophage Ia and presumably antigen presentation capacity.

In conclusion, bacterial invaders are potent initiators of a multiplicity of amplifying immunomodulating signals which are cell contact and/or mediator dependent. These signals rapidly promote lymphocyte and macrophage proliferation and differentiation and thus enable these cells to rapidly eliminate invading organisms.

ACKNOWLEDGEMENT

We are grateful to Drs. J. T. Hoffeld and Julie Sando for critiquing the manuscript and for the secretarial assistance of Mrs. Elizabeth Oppenheim and Mrs. Carol Oesch.

REFERENCES

1. Beller, D. I., Farr, A. G., and Unanue, E. R., 1978, Regulation of lymphocyte proliferation and differentiation by macrophages. Fed. Proc. 37: 91.

2. Cohen, S., Pick, E., and Oppenheim, J. J., 1979, The Biology of the lymphokines. Pub. Acad. Press. NY.

3. Cowing, C., Pincus, S. H., Sachs, D. H., and Dickler, H. B., 1978, A subpopulation of adherent accessory cells bearing both I_A and I_E or I_C subregion antigens is required for antigen-specific murine T lymphocyte proliferation. J. Immunol. 121: 1680.

4. Erb, P., Feldmann, M., and Hogg, N., 1976, The role of macrophages in the generation of T helper cells. IV. Nature of GRF. Eur. J. Immunol. 6: 369.

5. Farrar, W. L., Mizel, S. B., and Farrar, J. J., 1979, Initiation of alloantigen-specific cytotoxic T lymphocyte responses by LAF. Fed. Proc. 38: 1006.

6. Farrar, J. J., Mizel, S. B., Fuller-Bonar, J., Hilfiker, M. L., and Farrar, W. G., 1979, LPS-mediated adjuvanticity, effect of LPS on the production of T cell growth factor (IL-2). Microbiol. ASM Washington, D. C., in press.

7. Gresser, I., Demaeyer-Guignard, J., Tovey, M. G., and Demaeyer, E., 1979, Electrophoretically pure mouse interferon exerts multiple biological effects. PNAS 76: 5308.

8. Hoffeld, J. T., Metzger, Z., and Oppenheim, J. J., 1980, Role of activated macrophage superoxide anions and hydrogen peroxide in immune suppression. This volume (in press).

9. Lee, S. H. S., and Epstein, L. B., 1979, Reversible inhibition by interferon of the maturation of human peripheral blood monocytes to macrophages. Cell. Immunol., in press.

10. Lonai, P., and Steinman, L., 1977, Physiological regulation of antigen binding to T cells: role for a soluble macrophage factor and of interferon of the maturation of human peripheral blood monocytes to macrophages. Cell. Immunol., in press.

11. Mizel, S. B., 1980, Lymphocyte activating factor (Interleukin-1): A possible mediator of endotoxin adjuvanticity, in: Microbiol. in press.

12. Mizel, S. B., Dayer, J. M., Krane, S. S. M., and Mergenhagen, S. E., 1980, Stimulation of rheumatoid synovial cell collagenase and prostaglandin production by partially purified LAF. PNAS, submitted.

13. Moore, R. N., Oppenheim, J. J., Farrar, J. J., Carter, C. S., Waheed, A., and Shadduck, R. K., 1980, Macrophage activation by CSF: Stimulation of LAF (IL-1) Production. Nature (submitted).

14. Oppenheim, J. J., Mizel, S. B., and Meltzer, M. S., 1979, Biological effects of lymphocyte and macrophage derived mitogenic amplication factors. in: "Biology of the Lymphokines", S. Cohen, E. Pick and J. J. Oppenheim, ed. Academic Press.

15. Oppenheim, J. J., Moore, R., Melig-Meyling, F. M. G.,Togawa, A., Wahl, S., Mathieson, B. F., Dougherty, S., and Carter, C., 1979, Role of cytokine and endotoxin induced monokines in lymphocyte proliferation, differentiation and immunoglobulin production, in: "Regulatory Role of Macrophages in Immunity", E. R. Unanue and A. S. Rosenthal, ed. Acad. Press, in press.

16. Rogoff, T. M., and Lipsky, P. E., 1979, Characterization of isolated guinea pig Kupffer cells: accessory cell function in mitogen-induced T lymphocyte activation. J. Immunol. 123: 1920.

17. Rosenthal, A. S., 1978, Determinant selection and macrophage function in genetic control of the immune response. Immunol. Rev. 40: 136.

18. Rosenwasser, L. J., Dinarello, C. A., and Rosenthal, A. S., 1979, Adherent cell function in murine T lymphocyte antigen recognition. IV. Enhancement of murine T cell antigen recognition by human leukocytic pyrogen. J. Exp. Med. 150: 709.

19. Wood, D. D., 1979, Purification and properties of human B cell-activating factor. J. Immunol. 123: 2395.

20. Zinkernagel, R. M., Callahan, G. N., Althage, A., Cooper, S., Klein, P. A., and Klein, J., 1978, On the thymus in the differentiation of H-2 self-recognition by T cells: evidence for dual recognition. J. Exp. Med. 147: 882.

THE INFLUENCE OF BACTERIAL PRODUCTS ON CYCLIC NUCLEOTIDE METABOLISM OF LYMPHOCYTES

Richard A. Winchurch

Department of Surgery, Baltimore Firefighters Research Laboratory, Johns Hopkins University School of Medicine at Baltimore City Hospitals, Baltimore, MD 21224

A wide variety of bacteria and bacterial products have been shown to influence the immune system. This arsenal of bacterial immunomodulating agents is of diverse origin and includes mycobacteria and their products, *Corynebacterium parvum*, *Bordetella pertussis*, gram negative lipopolysaccharides (LPS), the enterotoxins from *Vibrio cholera* and streptococcal products. Specific effects elicited by many of these substances will be discussed in detail elsewhere in this volume. The present discussion will be confined to two of these materials, LPS and *Vibrio cholera* enterotoxin and will be directed toward possible mechanisms by which these substances are able to mediate both positive and negative effects on the immune system.

REGULATORY EFFECTS OF LPS AND CHOLERA TOXIN ON IMMUNITY

The adjuvant effects of LPS and cholera toxin have been reviewed extensively. Briefly summarized, LPS has been shown to enhance antibody responses to erythrocyte antigens (14, 15), soluble proteins (23) and a monovalent hapten (31). These adjuvant effects have been manifested *in vivo* as well as *in vitro* systems (25). It has been shown further that LPS can exert its immunoenhancing potential *in vitro* by stimulating IgM antibody synthesis to SRBC in lymphocytes from congenitally athymic nude mice as well as in cells from normal mice depleted of T cell function (28). These findings imply that LPS may act by either substituting for T helper activity or at least by amplifying very low levels of T cell help. The concept that LPS can substitute for T cell help is supported by the finding that coupling with LPS can render an antigen T independent (21). It has been recently proposed that LPS adjuvant properties may be related in some cases to its ability to act on B cells synergistically with factors derived from T cells,thymus replacing factors (TRF), and that the adjuvanticity of LPS may be due to a conversion of B cells to a state in which they are more responsive to TRF (13). The requirement for T cell function in some manifestations of LPS-induced adjuvanticity is further supported by the finding that LPS is able to stimulate *in vivo* T dependent IgG secondary responses to the synthetic antigen (T, G) A-L (22). LPS, in addition to its adjuvanticity can also stimulate mitogenicity in B lymphocytes (26) but not in T cells (1). Despite this fact, LPS appears to bind to both T and B lymphocytes (2). Furthermore, LPS, when given without antigen, is able to stimulate polyclonal antibody formation and this effect may be related to its mitogenic effects on B cells (5). Additional studies have also shown that LPS is able to prevent the induction of immunologic tolerance (10). While LPS can act as an immune adjuvant, it has also been reported that, under certain conditions, it can inhibit immune responses. Generally, inhibition is observed when LPS is administered before antigenic challenge *in vivo* (32) or when cells have been preincubated with LPS *in vitro* prior to exposure to an antigen (27).

Cholera enterotoxin, like gram negative lipopolysaccharides, can also influence immune systems. It has been shown that cholera toxin enhances the generation of hemolysin-forming cells to sheep red cells when administered at the same time as antigen (4, 24). Cholera toxin has also been shown to stimulate secondary antibody responses to keyhole limpet hemocyanin (KLH) in rabbit lymphocytes *in vitro* if the toxin is administered within 24 hours of antigen (6). Enhancement of immunity by cholera toxin appears to be both dose and time dependent. When given at the same time as antigen, lower doses of toxin appear to be enhancing while higher doses actually inhibit antibody responses (6). Similarly, the addition of the toxin to cell cultures at or near the time of antigen presentation is stimulatory while later additions appear to be inhibitory. Pretreatment of animals with cholera toxin one to seven days before injection of antigen results in a depression of antibody responses (19) and pretreatment of lymphocytes *in vitro* with cholera toxin results in a depression of some manifestations of cell-mediated immunity (Winchurch et al., unpublished). Unlike LPS, cholera toxin does not appear to be mitogenic for either T or B lymphocytes and does stimulate polyclonal antibody formation.

THE INDUCTION OF IMMUNE SUPPRESSION BY BACTERIAL PRODUCTS

Several years ago, we observed that the administration of *S. Marcescens* LPS to 3 day old mice could depress humoral immune responses (37). In these studies, LPS was administered with or without erythrocyte antigens and the early hemolysin-forming response was measured. The results showed that when either LPS or sheep erythrocytes were injected alone, there was no apparent effect.

At least, no antibody-forming cells appeared in the spleens after treatment. However, when the two were given together, a very early anti-sheep hemolysin response resulted. When animals treated with LPS or antigen at three days of age were challenged with sheep erythrocytes four weeks later, those mice which received both LPS and antigen again gave a good response. As expected, those mice which received sheep erythrocytes alone responded poorly but, surprisingly, those mice which received LPS alone also responded poorly. The poor responses in the antigen-treated group could be explained on the basis of the tolerizing effect of antigen but the diminished reactivity in the LPS-treated group was an enigma. At the time, we knew nothing of suppressor cell activity. More recent studies have confirmed and extended these findings and have shown that perinatal injection of LPS (3 days after birth) results in a diminished response to erythrocyte antigens in vitro four weeks later (Table 1). Moreover, when cells from mice which received the LPS as newborns were mixed in Mishell-Dutton cultures with normal splenic lymphocytes, a suppression of the normal antibody response was observed. Both the depression of responsiveness and the generation of suppressor activity were dose dependent (Table 2). Using an LPS derived from E. coli 0127:B8 which contains relatively low percentages of Lipid A, neonatal injection of 5 micrograms depressed responses in the LPS-treated mice marginally and did not suppress the response of normal cell responses. In fact, cells derived from low dose-treated mice enhanced normal responses. Doses of 10 and 15 micrograms depressed responses significantly in the LPS-treated group and were suppressive of normal responses as well.

TABLE I

Suppressive Effects of Neonatal Injection of 5 μg LPS (055:B5) on Normal Adult In Vitro Antibody Responses

Group	Cultures containing cells from C57 Bl/6	Average Number of PFC/10^6 cells (+ S.E.) 4 weeks after treatment of newborn: Expected	Observed
I	Adult C57 Bl/6 (control)	-	565 ± 48
II	4-week old C57 Bl/6 (control)	-	329 ± 24
III	4-week old C 57 Bl/6 (LPS-treated)	-	192 ± 11
IV	Adult C57 Bl/6 (control) + 4-week old C57 Bl/6 (control)	447	425 ± 34
V	Adult C57 Bl/6 (control) + 4-week old C57 Bl/6 (LPS-treated)	379	291 ± 54

TABLE II

Dose-Dependent Suppression of Antibody Responses Following Neonatal Injections of LPS 0127:B8

Treatment at 3 Days	In Vitro PFC/10^6 Cells ± S.E. at 4 Weeks In Cultures Containing Cells from			
	LPS-Treated C57 Bl/6 Mice	LPS-Treated C57 Bl/6 Mice + Normal Control C57 Bl/6 Mice		
		Expected	Observed	Δ PFC (%)
5 μg LPS	200 ± 23	315	478 ± 77	+ 52
10 μg LPS	75 ± 21	304	224 ± 37	- 26
15 μg LPS	26 ± 7	661	519 ± 36	- 21

The treatment of cells from LPS-injected mice with adsorbed rabbit anti-mouse brain antisera plus complement does not abrogate suppression of normal responses. Thus the cell type programmed for suppressor activity by neonatal injection of LPS is probably not a T lymphocyte. This finding agrees with the results obtained by Hoffman and his colleagues as well as those obtained by Persson who showed that LPS can induce a population of suppressor B cells (16, 27). The injection of adult mice with LPS also results in a profound depression of immunity and in the generation of a population of cells capable of suppressing normal immune responses (Table 3). In these experiments, animals were injected with 100 micrograms of LPS and at varying intervals after injection animals were sacrificed and splenic lymphocytes were set in Mishell-Dutton cultures either alone or in the presence of normal, untreated lymphocytes. The data show a profound suppression in the capacity of LPS-treated mice to respond to erythrocyte antigens for at least two weeks after injection. Restoration of responsiveness in this population occurs beginning around two weeks and the responses in these cells are completely restored at one month after injection. Co-culture of cells from LPS-treated animals with normal lymphocytes indicates that the cells from LPS-treated mice are capable of suppressing normal immune responses for up to three weeks after injection of LPS.

CYCLIC NUCLEOTIDES AND IMMUNE SUPPRESSION

The demonstration that LPS can enhance immunity under some conditions and activate suppressor cells when given under other con-

TABLE III

In Vitro Antibody Responses in Adult C57 Bl/6 Mice Injected with 100 μg LPS

		PFC/10^6 Cells ± S.E. in Cultures in Cultures Set on Day After Injection				
		2	7	15	22	30
C57 Bl/6 Control		630 ± 9	891 ± 73	1057 ± 65	1184 ± 48	1142 ± 28
C57 Bl/6 LPS-Treated		21 ± 7	50 ± 6	304 ± 17	782 ± 45	1042 ± 54
C57 Bl/6 Control	Observed	210 ±22	279 ±23	485 ± 27	727 ± 18	1209 ± 23
C57 Bl/6 LPS-Treated	Expected	326	470	681	983	1092

ditions raised the possibility of whether the adjuvanticity and suppressor-inducing properties of LPS were due to qualitatively similar, but quantitatively different effects on the metabolism of lymphocytes. It has been shown that higher doses of LPS as well as high concentrations of other polyclonal B cells mitogens can stimulate increases in intracellular cyclic AMP (33). It has also been reported that, in lymphocytes, LPS can activate epinephrine-sensitive adenyl cyclase, the enzyme responsible for the generation of intracellular cyclic AMP (3). The concentrations of LPS and other polyclonal B cell activators which elevate cyclic AMP are supraoptimal for mitogen activity (33). Mitogenically optimal doses have little effect on cyclic AMP levels but increased cyclic GMP levels. The lack of correlation between the mitogenic and cyclic AMP-stimulating doses of B cell mitogens supports the premise that elevations in intracellular cyclic AMP are not necessarily associated with the proliferative response in lymphocytes. Several independent studies have essentially confirmed these findings (8, 9, 29). On the other hand, it has been shown that cyclic GMP stimulates lymphocyte proliferation (35) and that elevations in intracellular cyclic GMP are associated with lymphocyte proliferative responses (11). Although cyclic AMP is not associated with a proliferative stimulus, the question remains as to whether or not it is associated with any aspect of lymphocyte activation.

Vibrio cholera enterotoxin is a potent stimulator of adenyl cyclase activity and lymphocytes treated with cholera toxin generate large increases in intracellular cyclic AMP (8). It has been demonstrated that lymphocytes from animals pretreated with cholera toxin were also deficient in their ability to respond in vitro to erythrocyte antigens and that cells from these animals suppressed normal lymphocyte responses (19). However, the suppressive effects of cholera toxin in vivo may be due to an indirect mechanism effected by hormonal changes in the toxin-treated animals. If the suppressive effects of LPS in our antibody-forming system were directly related to cyclic nucleotide-mediated events, then pretreatment of normal lymphocytes with cholera toxin in vitro should also result in the generation of suppressor activity. We tested this hypothesis by pretreating lymphocytes in vitro with varying doses of cholera toxin for 24 hours, washing these cells and adding them to normal lymphocytes in mixed lymphocyte cultures. In some of these experiments, we took advantage of the observations of Metzler, et al (20), who observed that stimulator F_1 lymphocytes were capable of suppressing responder parental lymphocytes in vitro. The data in Table 4 indicate that preincubation of F_1 cells with concentrations of 10 or 1 micrograms per ml of cholera toxin resulted in a suppression of the MLC responses of parental strain responder lymphocytes. At concentrations of 0.1 micrograms per ml the suppressive effect was diminished and at concentrations of 0.01 micrograms per ml there was no suppressive effect. Similar suppressive effects were obtained when cells identical to responder lymphocytes were pre-incubated in vitro with cholera toxin and added back to mixed lymphocyte cultures. Cyclic AMP itself is able to suppress the proliferative responses of lymphocytes in vitro but the suppression observed in our system is not likely to be due to the release of cyclic AMP from the toxin-pretreated cells since the total accumulation of cyclic AMP from these cells should not exceed 10^{-6}M. Exogenous cyclic AMP added to MLC cultures at a concentration of 10^{-6} M is not suppressive. In fact, suppressive concentrations are often stimulatory (Table 5). Thus the effects of LPS and cholera toxin could be due to cyclic AMP-mediated activation of suppressor lymphocytes.

THE ROLE OF CYCLIC NUCLEOTIDES IN THE REGULATION OF IMMUNE RESPONSES BY BACTERIAL PRODUCTS

Data currently available indicates that cyclic AMP and cyclic GMP influence different functions in the sequence of cellular events following lymphocyte activation. Although convincing data have been reported which show that cyclic AMP inhibits cell-mediated immunity, particularly effector functions such as lymphocyte-mediated cytotoxicity (12) and in vitro cellular proliferation, other data support the concept that cyclic AMP can also play a more positive role. For example, it has been shown that lymphocyte activation is accompanied by early, but transient, increases in intracellular levels of cyclic AMP (17, 30) and that agents which facilitate this increase are

TABLE IV

Suppressive Effects of Cholera Toxin-Treated C57 Bl/6 Cells (B6) and BDF_1 Cells on C57 Bl/6 MLC Responses, CPM ± S.E.

		Cholera Toxin Concentration μg/ml				
		None	10	1	10^{-2}	10^{-4}
	B6 Responder + Toxin-Treated B6-M*	7,365 ±216	4,309 ±218	4,406 ±310	8,093 ±344	7,950 ±105
Experiment 1	B6 Responder + Toxin-Treated B6-M* + BDF_1 Stimulator	18,963 ±599	8,433 ±649	7,957 ±277	14,528 ±943	15,697 ±423
Experiment 2	B6 Responder Alone	7,443 ±271	--	--	--	--
	B6 Responder + Toxin-Treated BDF_1-M Stimulator	15,999 ±747	5,690 ±199	11,800 ±589	15,532 ±354	15,614 ±744
	Δ CPM	8,556 ±795	-1,753 ±336	4,357 ±648	8,089 ±446	8,171 ±792

*Cells pre-incubated with cholera toxin on 24 hours, washed and treated with mitomycin C.

TABLE V

Inhibition of C57 B1/6 (B6) MLC Responses by Exogenous Cyclic AMP, CPM ± S.E.

	Concentration of Cyclic AMP (M)				
	None	10^{-7}	10^{-6}	10^{-5}	10^{-4}
B6 Responder	12,828	12,470	9,524	9,932	10,309
	± 168	± 602	± 227	± 588	± 396
B6 Responder + BDF_1 Stimulator*	17,742	18,443	17,756	15,334	12,034
	±1632	± 273	±1387	± 459	± 787
Δ CPM	4,914	5,973	8,232	5,402	1,725
	±1640	± 661	±1402	± 746	± 881

*Mitomycin Treated.

immunoenhancing (18). It has also been shown that early activation of lymphocyte cyclic AMP results in the phosphorylation of nuclear histones and other non-histone proteins (7, 17, 34). Histone phosphorylation is thought to be associated with derepression of the genome and indicative of the earliest events in the activation of a cell. Increases in intracellular cyclic GMP are also immunoenhancing and this activity is probably related to the fact that cyclic GMP facilitates lymphocyte proliferation. Cyclic GMP itself is mitogenic for lymphocytes in a manner somewhat similar to that of bacterial LPS (36) but cyclic GMP produces no effects on protein phosphorylation (34). The probable role for cyclic AMP in immune processes is as an early mediator of lymphocyte activation. Cyclic GMP, on the other hand, functions later in the cycle of events following cell activation and appears to be associated with the clonal expansion of populations of activated lymphocytes. Bacterial products which can both enhance and suppress immune processes may act by producing quantitatively different effects on lymphocyte cyclic nucleotide metabolism or by producing these effects in distinct subpopulations of lymphocytes. Thus the adjuvant properties of substances such as LPS might be explained on the basis of their effects on cyclic GMP levels. Concentrations of LPS which augment increases in intracellular cyclic GMP would enhance immunity by facilitating the clonal expansion of antigen-activated lymphocytes. In contrast, the enhancing effects of low concentrations of cholera toxin may be related to its ability to stimulate transient increases in cyclic AMP and thus to facilitate the activation of antigen-primed cells. The suppressive effects of both LPS and cholera toxin may be related to their effects on cyclic AMP. Since it appears that cyclic AMP is involved in the early activation of immune lymphocytes, it is an equally likely possibility that it may also be involved in the activation of suppressor lymphocytes. In this case, however, activation could result from higher concentrations of LPS or cholera toxin or from administration prior to antigen presentation and might also involve a different lymphocyte subpopulation i.e., suppressor cell precursors. High doses of LPS are poorly mitogenic *in vitro* and are known to stimulate increases in intracellular cyclic AMP. Cells from LPS-treated animals can suppress normal immune responses several weeks after treatment and lymphocytes preincubated *in vitro* with cholera toxin are also suppressive. This suppression cannot be explained on the basis of a cyclic AMP-induced inhibition of cell proliferation but can be explained on the basis of a cyclic AMP-mediated induction of suppressor cell activity.

REFERENCES

1. Andersson, J., Möller, G., and Sjöberg, O., 1972, Selective induction of DNA synthesis in T and B lymphocyte cells. *Immunol.* 4: 381.

2. Andersson, J., Sjöberg, O., and Möller, G., 1972, Transplant Rev. 11, 131.

3. Bitensky, M. W., Gorman, R. E., and Thomas, L., 1971, Selective stimulation of Epinephrine-Responsive Adenyl Cyclase in mice by endotoxin, Proc. Soc. Exp. Biol. Med. 138: 773.

4. Chisari, F. V., Northrup, R. S., and Chen, L. C., 1974, The modulating effect of cholera enterotoxin on the immune response K. J. Immunol. 113: 729.

5. Continho, A., Gronowicz, E., Bullock, W. W., and Möller, G., 1974, Mechanism of a thymus-independent immunocyte triggering. Mitogenic activation of B cells results in specific immune responses. J. Exp. Med. 139: 74.

6. Cook, R. G., Stavitsky, A. B., and Schoenberg, M. D., 1975, Regulation of the in vitro early anamnestic antibody response by exogenous cholera entertoxin and cyclic AMP. J. Immunol. 114: 426.

7. Cross, M., and Ord, M., 1971, Changes in histone phosphorylation and early metabolic events in pig lymphocyte cultures transformed by phytohemagglutinin and 6-N, 2'-o-Dibutyryladenosine 3'-5'-cyclic monophosphate Biochem. J. 124: 241.

8. DeRubertis, F. R., Zenser, T. V., Adler, W. H., and Hudson, T., 1974, Role of cyclic adenosine 3'-5' monophosphate in lymphocyte mitogenesis. J. Immunol. 113: 151.

9. Estes, G., Solomon, S. S., and Norton, W. C., 1971. Inhibition of lymphocyte stimulation by cyclic and non-cyclic nucleotides. J. Immunol. 101: 1489.

10. Golub, E. S., Weigle, W. O., 1967, Studies on the induction of immunologic unresponsiveness. ᵀ. Effects of endotoxin and phytohemagglutinin. J. Immunol. 98: 1241.

11. Haddox, J. K., Furcht, L. T., Gentry, S. R., et al. 1976, Periodate induced increases in cyclic GMP in mouse and guinea pig splenic cells in association with mitogenesis. Nature. 262: 146.

12. Henney, C. S., Bourne, H. R., and Lichtenstein, L. M., 1977, The role of cyclic 3'-5' Adenosine monophosphate in the specific cytolytic activity of lymphocytes. J. Immunol. 6: 1526.

13. Jacobs, D., 1979, Synergy between T cell-replacing factor and bacterial lipopolysaccharide (LPS) in the primary antibody response in vitro: A model for lipopolysaccharide adjuvant action. J. Immunol. 122: 1421.

14. Johnson, A. G., Gaines, S., and Landy, M., 1956, Studies on the O antigen of Salmonella typhosa. V. Enhancement of antibody response to protein antigen by purified lipopolysaccharide. J. Exp. Med. 103: 225.

15. Jones, M. M., and Kind, P. D., 1972, Enhancing effects of bacterial endotoxins on bone marrow cells in the immune response to SRB. J. Immunol. 108: 1453.

16. Koenig, S., and Hoffmann, M. K., 1979, Bacterial lipopolysaccharide activates suppressor B lymphocytes. Proc. Natl. Acad. Sci. USA, 76: 4608.

17. Kishimoto, T., Nishizawa, Y., Kikutani, H., and Yamanura, Y., 1977, Biphasic effect of cyclic AMP on IgG production and on the changes of non-histone nuclear proteins induced with anti-immunoglobulin and enhancing soluble factor. J. Immunol. 118: 2027.

18. Kook, A., and Trainin, N., 1975, The control exerted by thymic hormone (THF) on cellular cAMP levels and immune reactivity of spleen cells in the MLC Assay. J. Immunol. 115: 8.

19. Lyons, S. F., and Friedman, H., 1978, Differential effects of cholera toxin pre-treatment on in vitro immunocyte responses. Proc. Soc. Exp. Biol. Med. 157: 631.

20. Metzler, C. M., Kostyk, T. G., and Gershon, R. K., 1976, Mixed lymphocyte reactions: Augmentation by drugs that inhibit stimulator cell protein synthesis. J. Immunol. 117: 1295.

21. Möller, G., Anderson, J., and Sjöberg, O., 1972, Lipopolysacchardies can convert heterologous red cells into thymus-independent antigens. Cell. Immunol. 4: 416.

22. Ness, D. B., Smith, S., Talcott, J. A., and Grumet, F. C., 1976, T cell requirements for the e xpression of the lipopolysaccharide adjuvant effect in vivo: Evidence for a T cell dependent and a T cell independent mode of action. Eur. J. Immunol. 6: 650.

23. Neter, E., 1969, Endotoxins and the immune response. Curr. Top. Microbiol. Immunol. 47: 92.

24. Northrup, R. S., and Fanci, A. S., 1972, Adjuvant effect of cholera enterotoxin on the immune response of the mouse to sheep red blood cells. J. Infec. Dis. 125: 672.

25. Ortiz-Ortiz, L., and Jaroslow, B. N., 1970, Enhancement by the adjuvant endotoxin of an immune response induced in vitro. Immunol. 19: 387.

26. Peavy, D. L., Adler, W. H., and Smith, R. T., 1970, The mitogenic effects of endotoxin and staphylococcal enterotoxin B on mouse spleen cells and human peripheral blood lymphocytes, J. Immunol. 105: 1453.

27. Persson, O., 1977, Lipopolysaccharide-induced suppression of the primary immune response to a thymus-dependent antigen. J. Immunol. 118: 789.

28. Sjöberg, O., Andersson, J., and Möller, G., 1972, Lipopolysaccharide can substitute for helper cells in the antibody response *in vitro*, Eur. J. Immunol. 2: 326.

29. Smith, J. W., Steiner, A. L., and Parker, C. W., 1971, Human lymphocyte metabolism. Effects of cyclic and non-cyclic nucleotides on stimulation by phytohemagglutinin. J. Clin. Invest. 50: 442.

30. Teh, H. S., and Paetkau, V., 1974, Biphasic effect of cyclic AMP on an immune response, Nature. 250: 505.

31. Trenkner, E., 1974, The use of allogenic T lymphocytes and bacterial lipopolysaccharide to induce immune responses to monovalent haptens *in vitro*, J. Immunol. 113: 918.

32. Uchiyama, T., and Jacobs, D., 1978, Modulation of immune response by bacterial lipopolysaccharide (LPS): Multifocal effects of LPS-induced suppression of the primary antibody response to a T dependent antigen, J. Immunol. 121: 2340.

33. Watson, J., 1976, The involvement of cyclic nucleotide metabolism in the initiation of lymphocyte proliferation induced by mitogens, J. Immunol. 117: 1656.

34. Wedner, H. J., and Parker, C. W., 1975, Protein phosphorylation in human peripheral lymphocytes - Stimulation by phytohemagglutinin and N^6 Monobutyryl cyclic AMP, Biochem. Biophys. Res. Comm. 62: 808.

35. Weinstein, Y., Chambers, D. A., Bourne, H. R., and Melmon, K. L., 1974, Cyclic GMP stimulates lymphocyte nucleic acid synthesis, Nature. 251: 352.

36. Weinstein, Y., Segal, S., and Melmon, K. L., 1975, Specific mitogenic activity of 8-Br-Guanosine 3', 5'-Monophosphate (Br-cyclic GMP) on B lymphocytes, J. Immunol. 115: 112.

37. Winchurch, R., and Braun, W., 1969, Antibody Formation: Premature initiation by endotoxin or synthetic polynucleotides in newborn mice. Nature. 223: 843.

GENETIC CONTROL OF MURINE RESISTANCE TO SALMONELLA TYPHIMURIUM INFECTION

Alison D. O'Brien[1], David L. Rosenstreich[2], and Irwin Scher[3]

Departments of Microbiology[1] and Medicine[3],
Uniformed Services University of the Health Sciences
Bethesda, MD 20014
The Laboratory of Microbiology and Immunology[2]
National Institutes of Dental Research, National Institutes of Health, Bethesda, MD 20254
The Department of Immunology[3]
Naval Medical Research Institute, Bethesda, MD 20014

Mice infected with *Salmonella typhimurium* develop a disease which is similar in its pathogenesis to typhoid fever (42). This facultative intracellular organism multiplies in the phagocytic cells of the murine reticuloendothelial cell system, and unrestricted bacterial growth results in death of the host. However, mice of various inbred strains differ in response to *S. typhimurium* infection. Some strains of mice invariably succumb to infection with $<$ 10 organisms, whereas other strains survive challenge doses of $\geq 10^4$ bacteria (21, 24). Webster, Schott and Gowen (9, 34, 39-41) were the first to recognize that this differential susceptibility was genetically regulated, and they subsequently developed salmonella-susceptible and resistant mouse strains (39). Although their pioneering work was performed in the 1930's, the delineation of the genes involved in resistance to murine typhoid occurred only recently.

Current evidence indicates that at least three distinct genetic loci influence the susceptibility of mice to *S. typhimurium* infection. These loci have been designated Ity, Lps^d, and xid. The distribution of these loci among inbred strains of mice varies considerably. The primary regulator of resistance appears to be the Ity gene, and resistant and susceptible alleles of it are distributed widely throughout inbred mouse strains. In contrast, Lps^d and xid are mutant alleles which render only a few strains of mice salmonella-susceptible. In this report, we will discuss the genetic analyses which have led to the identification of these three loci. We will also summarize the information that has been obtained from several laboratories on the mechanisms by which these genes govern the murine response to salmonellosis.

THE Ity LOCUS

Robson and Vas (24) and Plant and Glynn (21) were the first workers to categorize inbred strains of mice as innately resistant or susceptible to murine typhoid. Although there were differences in the LD_{50} of S. typhimurium for strains reported as resistant by these two groups of investigators, such variance is expected when different challenge routes of inoculation are used. Indeed, our own observations taken together with those of other researchers indicate that the degree of resistance (LD_{50}) is directly related to the route of infection (24, 40). Overall, mice are most susceptible to intraperitoneal challenge and least susceptible to oral inoculation with salmonellae. Nonetheless, the relative susceptibility to S. typhimurium of various mouse strains is generally consistent, regardless of the method of challenge. A summary of the responses of some inbred strains of mice to S. typhimurium is shown in Table 1.

In addition to classifying mice as sensitive (s) or resistant (r), Plant and Glynn also examined the genetic basis for resistance by testing the F_1, F_2, and backcross generations from matings of CBA (r) and BALB/c (s) mice (21). They found that resistance in these crosses was controlled by a single, dominant, autosomal gene that was not linked to the H-2 locus (21). These investigators subsequently named the locus which controlled the response to infection Ity (for immunity to typhimurium), and they called the susceptible allele Ity^s, and the dominant resistant allele Ity^r (22). More recently, in an elegant series of linkage studies performed with salmonella-susceptible and resistant hybrid populations, these same investigators analyzed the association between resistance and the expression of phenotypic markers encoded by genes present on different chromosomes (23). The results demonstrated a close linkage between Ity and the chromosome 1 color-coat marker, leaden (ln). We have also located Ity on chromosome 1 by an analysis of the pattern of salmonella-susceptibility among 21 recombinant inbred (RI) mouse strains (O'Brien, A. D., D. L. Rosenstreich, and B. A. Taylor; manuscript in preparation). RI strains are a useful tool for determining the chromosomal position of a gene (2). They are produced by inbreeding the F_2 progeny from two inbred progenitor strains. Since these new inbred strains contain a random assortment of genes from each parent, the strains can be phenotyped for all the genetic differences carried by the original progenitors. By an assessment of the distribution of these phenotypic traits and the pattern of salmonella resistance (for example) among the strains, linkage of a new locus to a chromosomal marker can be established.

TABLE I

RESPONSE OF VARIOUS INBRED STRAINS OF MICE TO S. tymphimurium INFECTION

STRAIN	REFERENCE
	Salmonella-susceptible[a]
BSVS	39, 40, Personal Obs.
DBA/1	24
BALB/c	10, 18, 21, 24
C57BL/6	10, 18, 21, 24
B10.D2	10, 24
C3H/HeJ	17, 24, 36
CBA/N	18
	Salmonella-resistant[b]
C3H/He	24
C3H/HeN	17
C3H/St	17
C3H/Bi	17
CBA	10, 21
CBA/Ca	18
BRVR	39, 40, Personal Obs.
A/J	10, 24
A/HeN	Personal Obs.
SWR/J	Personal Obs.
DBA/2[c]	10, 18, 21, 24
C57L[c]	23, Personal Obs.

[a] Susceptible = $LD_{50} < 2 \times 10^1$ s.c., i.v., or i.p.

[b] Resistant = $LD_{50} \geq 1 \times 10^3$ s.c., i.v., or i.p.

[c] These mice are resistant when infected s.c. but respond intermediately when challenged i.p.

The mechanism whereby the Ity locus controls resistance to salmonellae is unknown. However, it has been suggested by several investigators that Ity may control the initial rate of multiplication of the bacterium in the hepatic and splenic macrophages of the mouse (10, 11, 21, 23, 24). This hypothesis is based on several lines of evidence. First, five days after challenge with a single dose of S. typhimurium, the number of bacteria in the spleens and livers of salmonella-susceptible (Ity^s/Ity^s) mice is significantly greater than in the organs of salmonella-resistant (Ity^r/Ity^r or Ity^r/Ity^s) mice (10, 21). Furthermore, mice which exhibit this rapid net growth rate in the RES usually die early (< 10 days) after i.p., i.v., or s.c. infection, regardless of the challenge dose (24). Secondly, Maier and Oels showed that the microbicidal capacity of macrophages from BRVR mice (*S. typhimuium*-resistant) was greater than the killing activity of macrophages from BSVS mice (*S. typhimurium* susceptible) (14). Although the Ity types of the mice used in their study have not been directly tested, it is probable that BSVS mice carry the same salmonella susceptibility gene(s) as do C57BL/6 mice (Ity^s/Ity^s) since F_1 hybrids derived from the two strains remain salmonella-susceptible (O'Brien, A. D., and D. L. Rosenstreich, unpublished data). Thirdly, treatment with silica, an agent which selectively inactivates macrophages, can convert a salmonella-resistant mouse to a susceptible one (19).

THE Lps LOCUS

The response of mice to lipopolysaccharide (LPS) is controlled by a chromosome-4 gene, Lps (37). A mutant allele of the endotoxin gene, Lps^d (for defective LPS response), is carried by C3H/HeJ and C57BL/10/ScCr, whereas all other inbred strains have the normal allele, Lps^n (16, 37). Lps^d mice are poorly responsive to all the known biological effects of endotoxin, including lethality (35), non-specific resistance to infection (4), and antibody production (38). The abnormal LPS phenotype is expressed in many different types of cells, such as B cells (7), T cells (8, 13), macrophages (25, 27), and fibroblasts (28). Furthermore, the Lps^d allele confers a defect in macrophage activation that is not related to the exogenous administration of LPS; macrophages from Lps^d mice are poorly tumoricidal *in vitro* (27) and cannot be stimulated by the lymphokine MIF (28).

LPS-unresponsive C3H/HeJ mice are also highly susceptible to *S. typhimurium* infection (24, 36). The available evidence, as summarized below, indicates that this susceptibility is conferred by the Lps^d allele. Genetic analyses were performed in our laboratory to characterize the gene(s) responsible for the susceptibility of C3H/HeJ mice to murine typhoid and to assess the influence of Lps^d on this sensitivity to infection (17). First, we compared the salmonella-susceptibility of C3H/HeJ mice to other C3H substrains to determine whether their response to challenge is unique among genetically related animals. The LD_{50} of *S. typhimurium* strain TML (6) was < 2 for C3H/HeJ mice when the bacterium was administered i.p., s.c., or i.v. In contrast, the LD_{50} of *S. typhimurium* for LPS-responsive C3H/HeN, C3H/Bi, and C3H/St mice was $\geq 2 \times 10^3$. Moreover, deaths of the C3H/HeJ mice after infection appeared to follow uncontrolled multiplication of the bacterium in the RES of these animals, whereas the mean number of organisms per spleen of

C3H/St mice was maintained at a relatively low level. Thus, the Lps^d C3H/HeJ mouse is exquisitely sensitive to murine typhoid, in contrast to other C3H substrains which are Lps^n.

Further studies revealed that the gene(s) which confers salmonella susceptibility on C3H/HeJ mice is distinct from both of the other genes known to render mice sensitive to this bacterial challenge. The F_1 progeny derived from crosses of C3H/HeJ mice with the highly susceptible C57BL/6J strain (Ity^s/Ity^s) were resistant ($LD_{50} \geq 8 \times 10^3$) which indicated that gene complementation had occurred and that the C3H/HeJ susceptibility gene is distinct from Ity^s. Furthermore, since both (C3H/HeJ x C3H/HeN) F_1 males and females were equally resistant to murine typhoid ($LD_{50} \geq 8 \times 10^3$), the X-linked susceptibility gene (xid) plays no apparent role in the response of C3H/HeJ mice to *S. typhimurium*.

Taken together, these findings suggested that the susceptibility of C3H/HeJ mice to *S. typhimurium* might be due to expression of Lps^d. To test this hypothesis, a backcross linkage analysis was performed using the progeny derived from C3H/HeJ and (C3H/HeJ x C37BL/6J)F_1 parents. The results of such experiments revealed a close correlation between the phenotypic expression of Lps^d (defective LPS-induced B cell mitogenesis *in vitro*) and salmonella susceptibility, since 13/14 LPS-unresponsive mice succumbed to infection whereas only 2/13 LPS-responsive animals died. The susceptibility of backcross mice was also closely linked to another chromosome-4 locus, Mup-1^a. These data locate the C3H/H3J *S. thyphimurium* susceptibility gene on chromosome 4 and provide evidence that this gene is either closely linked or identical to Lps^d.

At present, one can only speculate on the mechanisms of Lps^d-controlled susceptibility to murine typhoid. Nonetheless, since functional macrophages are a requisite for resistance to salmonella infection (19) and since so much evidence has accumulated which demonstrates a profound defect in the macrophages of Lps^d mice (25, 27), it is reasonable to presume that the salmonella-susceptibility of C3H/HeJ mice is a reflection of this cellular defect. Several experiments performed in our laboratory not only support this suggestion, but also show that the phenotypic expression of Lps^d resembles that of Ity^s. First, like Ity^s mice, C3H/HeJ mice are unable to control the growth of *S. typhimurium* in the spleen, and they generally die early after infection (17). In addition, as is the case with Ity^s mice (24), C3H/HeJ mice cannot be protected by standard vaccines or by passive transfer of immune serum but can be protected by the adoptive transfer of bone marrow cells from the syngeneic LPS-responsive C3H/HeN strain (O'Brien, A. D. and D. L. Rosenstreich; manuscript in preparation). Similarly, Hormaeche showed that the phenotype of Ity^s (early, rapid growth of *S. typhimurium* in the spleen) could be changed by adoptive transfer of bone marrow from Ity^r animals (12).

Although Lps^d and Ity^s mice are phenotypically salmonella-susceptible, major differences in the expression of Lps^d and Ity^s must exist since gene complementation occurs among the progeny of mice of these genotypes (17). The macrophage defect caused by Ity^s appears to be less generalized than that of Lps^d, since macrophages from these mice are normally tumoricidal in vitro and respond to lymphokines. Studies are in progress to compare both the phagocytic and microbicidal capacities of Lps^d and Ity^s macrophages.

THE xid LOCUS

Antibody production by mice is controlled by a number of genes which are located on different chromosomes. A mutation in one of these genes has been identified in the CBA/N strain of mice (1, 31). The X-linked recessive allele carried by these animals (CBA/N male and female mice and F_1 male mice derived from a CBA/N female parent) is called xid for X-linked immunodeficiency (3). Such mice make poor or absent antibody responses to both thymic-independent (1, 31, 33) and thymic-dependent (14, 30) antigens, and they have low serum IgM and IgG_3 levels (1, 20). The xid allele also results in the absence of a mature or late-developing subpopulation of B lymphocytes (5, 32). In contrast, the T-cell (14, 29) and macrophage (26) functions of xid mice appear to be normal.

We investigated the effect of this selective B-cell defect on the susceptibility of mice to S. typhimurium (18). The LD_{50} of S. typhimurium for CBA/N mice was 1000-fold less than for the immunologically normal histocompatible, CBA/CaHN strain. Genetic analysis revealed that, like the immune defect, the susceptibility of CBA/N mice to S. typhimurium is X-linked. Immune-defective F_1 male mice derived from crosses between CBA/N and immunologically normal strains were susceptible to S. typhimurium ($LD_{50} \leq 20$), whereas immunologically normal F_1 males and females derived from these matings were resistant ($LD_{50} \geq 5 \times 10^3$).

To assess the role of xid in the S. typhimurium-susceptibility of B-cell defective mice, a linkage analysis was performed. Backcross and F_2 parents derived from CBA/N and DBA/2N strains were phenotyped for the immune defect by quantitation of their serum IgM levels. The frequency of mice with low serum IgM levels was close to the expected frequency. The mice were then challenged with S. typhimurium. Although no formal linkage between the expression of xid and salmonella-susceptibility was established, 93% of mice (52/56) with low serum IgM levels died. In contrast, only 22/50 (44%) of mice with normal serum IgM levels succumbed to infection. Furthermore, the death of 44% of F_2 and backcross mice with normal serum IgM levels was similar to the incidence of deaths among immunologically normal F_1 female control mice. Based on these findings, we feel that the B-lymphocyte defect conferred by the expression of xid renders mice salmonella-susceptible. Two important observations support this suggestion. First, passive administration of mouse anti-salmonella serum markedly increases the resistance of immune-defective mice to infection (O'Brien, A.D., I. Scher, and E. S. Metcalf; manuscript in preparation). Secondly, mice which express the xid allele die relatively late in the course of infection (18). This finding is consistent with the hypothesis that early resistance is macrophage-dependent while antibodies are required for later control of infection.

DISCUSSION

The following model of the genetic control of murine resistance to S. typhimurium infection is proposed based on the experiments described in this communication. The host response to murine typhoid can be divided into two stages, early (< 10 days post-challenge) and late (> 10 days post-challenge). The capacity of the macrophage to control the net multiplication of salmonellae early in the infectious process is a requisite for survival of the mouse. Both Ity and Lps^d appear to regulate the microbicidal capacity of these phagocytes at this early stage. The mechanisms by which Lps^d and Ity control macrophage-salmonellae interactions are not known, but the products of these genes must differ since the progeny of salmonella-susceptible Ity^s and Lps^d mice are salmonella-resistant. Only mice which are LPS-responsive (Lps^n/Lps^n or Lps^d/Lps^n) and carry the Ity^r allele (Ity^r/Ity^r or Ity^r/Ity^s) are able to keep the multiplication of S. typhimurium in their RES cells in check; LPS-unresponsive (Lps^d/Lps^d) or Ity^s/Ity^s animals are unable to do so, and they die within 10 days of challenge. If the genetic constitution of a mouse allows it to survive the early phase of infection, it will begin to form anti-S. typhimurium antibodies (O'Brien, A. D., I. Scher, and E. S. Metcalf; manuscript in preparation). The importance of specific antibody in the second phase of the infectious process is illustrated both by the late deaths of antibody-defective xid mice and by the capacity of such mice to survive infection if they are given immune serum. The role antibody plays in the eventual elimination of salmonella from infected animals is not known. Perhaps anti-salmonellae antibodies serve as opsonins or perhaps, in the presence of complement, they are bactericidial. In either case, both antibody and microbicidal macrophages are required for an animal to survive S. typhimurium infection. Furthermore, if any one of the three alleles (Lps^d, Ity^s, or xid) which affect these functions are expressed by the host, the animal will die. A summary of the data which led to this conclusion is shown in Table 2.

Although investigations performed in this and other laboratories have delineated genes which control the murine response to salmonellosis, we do not know how these genes regulate the host responses at the cellular level. Thus, future work in this laboratory will focus on identification of the products of the salmonella-response genes. If

TABLE II

Influence of Ity, Lps, and xid on the Response of Inbred Mice to S. typhimurium

Strain	Presumptive Genotype Ity	Lps	xid[a]	Salmonella Phenotype[b]
C57Bl/6 ♂ or ♀	s/s	n/n	xy or xx	Sus
BALB/c ♂ or ♀	s/s	n/n	xy or xx	Sus
C3H/HeN ♂ or ♀	r/r	n/n	xy or xx	Res
C3H/HeJ ♂ or ♀	r/r[c]	d/d	xy or xx	Sus
(C3H/HeJ x C57BL/6)F_1 ♂ or ♀	r/s	d/n	xy or xx	Res
(C3H/HeJ x C3H/H3N)F_1 ♂ or ♀	r/r	d/n	xy or xx	Res
CBA/N ♂ or ♀	r/r[d]	n/n	x*y or x*x*	Sus
(CBA/N x BALB/c)F_1 ♂	r/s	n/n	x*y	Sus
(CBA/N x BALB/c)F_1 ♀	r/s	n/n	x*x	Res

[a] Male mice which express xid will be designated x*y. Female mice which express or carry xid will be designated x*x* or x*x, respectively.

[b] The susceptible (sus) and resistant (res) S. typhimurium phenotypes are taken from references 17 and 18.

[c] Evidence that S. typhimurium-susceptible C3H/HeJ mice are Ity^r/Ity^r is given in reference 17.

[d] Evidence that S. typhimurium-susceptible CBA/N mice are Ity^r/Ity^r is tiven in reference 18.

the search for these gene products is successful, we should be able to more clearly define those events required for survival of the host.

REFERENCES

1. Ambaugh, D. F., Hansen, C. T., Prescott, B., Strashak, P. W., Bartold, D. R., and Baker, P., 1972, Genetic control of the antibody response to type III pneumococcal polysaccharide in mice. J. Exp. Med. 136: 931.

2. Bailey, D. W., 1971, Recombinant-inbred strains, an aid to finding identity, linkage, and function of histocompatibility and other genes. Transplantation 11: 325.

3. Berning, A., Eicher, E., Paul, W. E., and Scher, I., 1978, Mapping the X-linked immune deficiency gene of CBA/N mice. Fed. Proc. 37: 1396.

4. Chedid, L., Parant, M., Damais, C., Parant, F., Juy, D., and Galelli, A., 1976, Failure of endotoxin to increase non-specific resistance to infection of lipopolysaccharide low-responder mice. Infect. Immun. 13: 722.

5. Finkelman, F. D., Smith, A. H., Scher, I., and Paul, W. E., 1975, Abnormal ratio of membrane immunoglobin classes in mice with an X0linked B-lymphocyte defect. J. Exp. Med. 142: 1316.

6. Gianella, R. A., Broitman, S. A., and Zamcheck, N. Z., 1971, Salmonella enteritis: fulmanent diarrhea in and effects on the small intestine. Am. J. Dig. Dis. 16: 1007.

7. Glode, M. S., Scher, I., Osborne, B., and Rosenstreich, D. L., 1976, Cellular mechanisms of endotoxin unresponsiveness in C3H/HeJ mice. J. Immunol. 116: 454.

8. Goodman, M. G., and Weigle, W. O., 1979, T-cell regulation of polyclonal B-cell responsiveness. I. Helper effects of T cells. J. Immunol. 122: 2548.

9. Gowen, J. W., and Schott, R. G., 1933, A genetic rechnique for differentiating between acquired and genetic immunity. Am. J. Hyg. 18: 688.

10. Hormaeche, C. E., 1979, Natural resistance to Salmonella typhimurium in different inbred mouse strains. Immunology. 37: 311.

11. Hormaeche, C. E., 1979, Genetics of natural resistance to salmonellae in mice. Immunology. 37: 319.

12. Hormaeche, C. E., 1979, The natural resistance of radiation chimeras to S. typhimurium C5. Immunology. 37: 329.

13. Koenig, S., Hoffman, M. K., and Thomas, L., 1977, Induction of phenotypic lymphocyte differentiation in LPS unresponsive mice by an LPS-induced serum factor and by lipid-A-associated protein. J. Immunol. 118: 1910.

14. Janeway, C. A., and Barthold, D. R., 1975, An analysis of the defective response of CBA/N mice to T-dependent antigens. J.

Immunol. 115: 898.

15. Maier, I., and Oels, H. C., 1972, Role of the macrophage in natural resistance to salmonellosis in mice. Infect. Immun. 6: 438.

16. McAdam, K. P. W. J., and Ryan, J. L., 1978, C57BL/10CR mice: nonresponders to activation by the lipid A moiety of bacterial lipopolysaccharide. J. Immunol. 120: 249.

17. O'Brien, A. D., Rosenstreich, D. L., Scher, I., Campbell, G. H., MacDermott, R. P., and Formal, S. B., 1979, Genetic control of susceptibility to Salmonella typhimurium in mice: role of the Lps gene. J. Immunol. In press.

18. O'Brien, A. D., Scher, Campbell, G. H., MacDermott, R. P., and Formal, S. B., 1979, Susceptibility of CBA/N mice to infection with Salmonella typhimurium: influence of the X-linked gene controlling B lymphocyte function. J. Immunol. 123: 720.

19. O'Brien, A. D., Scher, I., and Formal, S. B., 1979, Effect of silica on the innate resistance of inbred mice to Salmonella typhimurium infection. Infect. Immun. 25: 513.

20. Perlmutter, R. M., Nahn, M., Stein, K. E., Slack, J., Zitron, I,., Paul, W. E., and Davie, J. M., 1979. Immunoglobulin subclass-specific immunodeficiency in mice with an X-linked B-lymphocyte defect. J. Exp. Med. 149: 993.

21. Plant, J., and Glynn, A. A., 1976, Genetics of resistance to infection with Salmonella typhimurium in mice. J. Infect. Dis. 133: 72.

22. Plant, J., and Glynn, A. A., 1977, In Mouse News Letter, Vol. 57, p. 38. Jackson Laboratory Bar Harbor, ME.

23. Plant, J., and Glynn, A. A., 1979, Locating salmonella resistance gene on mouse chromosome 1. Clin. Exp. Immunol. 37: 1.

24. Robson, G. G., and Vas, S. J., 1972, Resistance of inbred mice to Salmonella typhimurium. J. Infect. Dis. 126: 378.

25. Rosenstreich, D. L., Vogel, S. N., Jacques, A. R., Wahl, L.M., and Oppenheim, J. J., 1978, Macrophage sensitivity to endotoxin: genetic control by a single condominant gene. J. Immunol. 121: 1664.

26. Rosenstreich, D. L., Vogel, S. N., Jacques, A., Wahl, L. M., Scher, I., and Mergenhagen, S. E., 1978, Differential endo-

toxin: genetic control by a single condominant gene. J. Immunol. 121: 685.

27. Ruco, L., and Meltzer, M. S., 1978, Defective tumoricidal capacity of macrophages from C3H/HeJ mice. J. Immunol. 120: 329.

28. Ryan, J. L., and McAdam, K. P. W. J., 1977. Genetic unresponsiveness of murine fibroblasts to bacterial endotoxin. Nature. 269: 153.

29. Scher, I., Ahmed, A., Strong, D. M., Steinburg, A. D., and Paul, W. E., 1975, X-Linked B-lymphocyte immune defect in CBA/NH mice. I. Studies of the function and composition of spleen cells. J. Exp. Med. 141: 788.

30. Scher, I., Berning, A. K., and Asofsky, R., 1979, X-linked B lymphocyte defect in CBA/N mice. IV. Cellular and environmental influences on the thymus dependent IgG anti-sheep red blood cell response. J. Immunol. 123: 477.

31. Scher, I., Franz, M. M., and Steinburg, A. D., 1973. The genetics of the immune response to a synthetic double-stranded RNA in a mutant CBA mouse strain. J. Immunol. 110: 1396.

32. Scher, I., Sharrow, S. O., and Paul, W. E., 1976, X-linked B-lymphocyte defect in CBA/N mice. III. Abnormal development of B-lymphocyte populations defined by their density of surface immunoglobin. J. Exp. Med. 144: 507.

33. Scher, I., Steinberg, A. D., Berning, A. K., and Paul, W. E., 1975, X-linked B-lymphocyte immune defect in CBA/N mice. II. Studies of the mechanisms underlying the immune defect. J. Exp. Med. 142: 637.

34. Schott, R. G., 1932, The inheritance of Salmonella aertrycke in various strains of mice. Genetics. 17: 203.

35. Sultzer, B. M., 1968, Genetic control of leucocyte responses to endotoxin. Nature. (London) 219: 1253.

36. VonJeney, N., Gunther, E., and Jann, K., 1977, Mitogenic stimulation of murine spleen cells: relation to susceptibility to Salmonella infection. Infect. Immun. 15: 26.

37. Watson, J., Kelly, K., Largen, M., and Taylor, B. A., 1978, The genetic mapping of a defective LPS response gene. J. Immunol. 120: 422.

38. Watson, J., and Riblet, 1974, Genetic control of responses to bacterial lipopolysaccharides in mice. J. Exp. Med. 140: 1147.

39. Webster, L. T., 1933, Inherited and acquired factors in resistance to infection. I. Development of resistant and susceptible lines of mice through selective breeding. J. Exp. Med. 57: 793.

40. Webster, L. T., 1933, Inherited and acquired factors in resistance to infection. II. A comparison of mice inherently resistant or susceptible to Bacillus enteritidis with respect to fertility, weight, and susceptibility to various routes and types of infection. J. Exp. Med. 57: 819.

41. Webster, L. T., 1937, Inheritance of resistance of mice to enteric bacterial and neurotropic virus infections. J. Exp. Med. 65: 261.

42. Wilson, G. S., and Miles, A., 1975, Salmonella. In Topley and Wilson's "Principles of Bacteriology and Immunity" Vol. I, p. 939. Williams and Wilkins Company, Baltimore, MD.

EFFECTS OF STREPTOCOCCAL COMPONENTS ON IMMUNITY*

John H. Schwab, Dena L. Toffaletti and Roger R. Brown

Department of Bacteriology and Immunology
University of North Carolina Medical School
Chapel Hill, NC 27514

INTRODUCTION

The group A streptococcus is an example of a bacterial cell from which several, apparently antagonistic, immunomodulating activities have been isolated (5, 6, 7, 8, 9, 10). The substances we have studied are derived from the cell envelope. We have reported that the peptidoglycan isolated from the cell wall contained the adjuvant activity associated with cells and cell walls (7). Many biological properties, which may be relevant to the immunopotentiating activity, have been described for peptidoglycan and the muramyl dipeptide moiety (1). We have been interested in the capacity of peptidoglycan to activate the alternative complement pathway (ACP), since complement can influence the immune system, especially macrophage activity (11). In our studies, peptidoglycan was the most potent activator of the ACP in human serum (5).

In addition to the immunopotentiating activity of peptidoglycan, we have also described the suppression of antibody response by extracts of group A streptococcal cells (8, 9). The IgG and IgM plaque forming cells (PFC) are suppressed in primary and secondary responses to sheep red blood cells (SRBC) in mice injected intraperitoneally or intravenously with streptococcal fractions 24 hr before the antigen. While antibody-forming cells are suppressed by injection of this cytoplasmic fraction of streptococcal cells, certain T cell functions are enhanced (3, 14). This paper summarizes recent studies on the isolation and activity of bacterial cell fractions which suppress antibody response and B cell functions.

* Supported by Research Grant AI 13464 from the National Institute of Allergy and Infectious Diseases.

MATERIALS AND METHODS

The membrane preparations were obtained from protoplasts of a group A, type 3 streptococcus by a method of Freimer (2) as modified by Schwab and Brown (13). Bacteria suspended in 11.5% NaCl were treated with the muralytic amidase from lysate of group C streptococci infected with bacteriophage. The resulting protoplasts were washed with high salt buffer and lysed in .01M PO_4 buffer, pH 7.3. The membranes were collected by differential centrifugation, treated with ribonuclease and stored at -20°C.

In order to isolate the immunosuppressant material, membranes are solubilized by treatment with trypsin (3X recrystallized, 10 μg/mg membrane protein, 4 hr, 37°C, 0.04 M phosphate buffer pH 7.8). After centrifugation at 12,000 x g for 30 min the supernatant is concentrated by lyophilization. It is then separated by filtration on Sephadex G-100. The fraction elutin just behind dextran blue (Fraction I) contains all activity and is dialyzed and lyophilized.

The measurement of immunosuppressive activity is as follows: groups containing 5 to 10 mice (female, 8 to 10 wks, strains 21 M4, C57, A/J or 40 N X 1) are injected intraperitoneally with varying concentrations diluted in phosphate-buffered saline, pH 7.2. Twenty-four hr later mice are injected intraperitoneally with 4 X 10^8 sheep red blood cells (SRBC). Four days later a spleen cell suspension is prepared, cells are counted in a Coulter Counter and the number of plaque forming cells (PFC) are counted by the Jerne technique. The data is analyzed by one-way analysis of variance and by rank-order analysis.

The measurement of stimulation of lymphoid cells by mitogens *in vitro* has been described in detail (14).

PURSUIT OF THE ISOLATION AND CHARACTERIZATION OF THE IMMUNOSUPPRESSANT ACTIVITY

The immunosuppressive activity is associated with the cell envelope prepared by osmotic disruption of protoplasts. At this time we do not know if the active material is a component of the cytoplasmic membrane or is only associated with preparations of this cell fraction.

The effect of the dose of membrane preparation upon the direct PFC response to SRBC antigen is shown in Fig. 1. With this preparation significant inhibition (79%, $p < .03$) was obtained with 20 μgm. There is a 25 to 50 fold increase in activity of membrane preparations compared to crude cell extracts (Table 1). Fig. 1 illustrates three features which are typical of the titration of a membrane preparation, as well as the fractions derived from it: (i) There is a maximum inhibition of PFC which can be achieved; with membrane

TABLE I

Purification of Immunosuppressant Factor from Group A Streptococcal Cells

Sample	50% Inhibition (μgm)	Increase in activity per μg	Protein recovery (%)
Crude cell extract	1000	1	-
Purified membrane suspension	40	25	100
Trypsin-soluble fraction	2.4	416	70
Sephadex G-100 Fraction I	0.02	50000	8

preparations this is 60 to 80%. (ii) This level of inhibition is obtained over a broad range of concentrations. (iii) Increasing the dose to a much higher concentration results in less suppression.

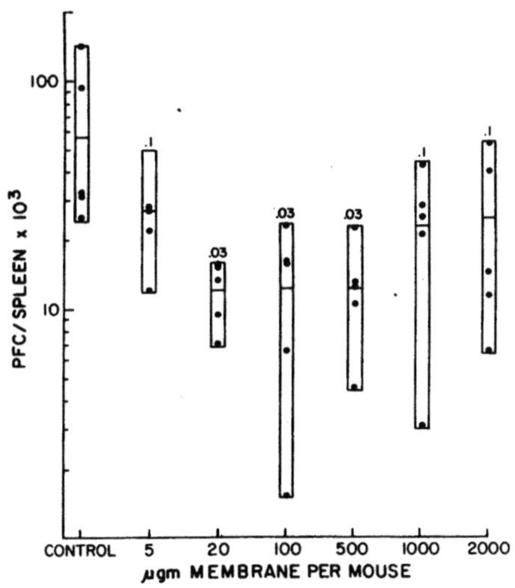

Fig. 1. Dose effect of protoplast membrane preparations on the number of antibody-producing cells (PFC) against SRBC. Female A/J mice 8 to 10 weeks old were injected i.p. with saline suspension of membrane preparation 24 hr before 4 x 10^8 SRBC were injected i.p. Spleen cells were collected 4 days later and direct PFC determined. Each point represents one mouse. Bars indicate the mean. Number above each column is the level of significance compared to control, calculated by one-way analysis of variance.

A significant enhancement of response with high doses is rarely observed. In contrast to membrane preparations and derived fractions, crude cell extracts can induce greater than 90% suppression (8). We interpret this to mean that there are several immunosuppressant factors in crude cell extracts with different mechanisms of action (12) which collectively can completely suppress the antibody response. As we pursue the isolation of one of these factors, the capacity to suppress all antibody response is limited.

In order to pursue the isolation of the active material several methods for solubilization of the membrane preparations, with retention of activity, have been tested. These include butanol, 3.0 M KCl, detergents, and enzymes. All of these methods solubilize some activity, but most consistent results are obtained by trypsin digestion (Table 2). The results recorded in Table 2 also indicate that the active factor is resistant to these enzymes, which were used in concentrations of 10 µg per mg substrate.

The trypsin-soluble fraction was further separated by gel filtration on sephadex G-100. As shown in Fig. 2, two major peaks were obtained, fraction I eluted just after the dextran blue marker and fraction II eluted behind trypsin (molecular weight 24,000). All of the activity is in fraction I which gives significant suppression of PFC in doses of 0.032 to 20 µg per mouse (Table 3). The only effect of fraction II is to induce enhancement of PFC at the highest concentration tested (Table 3).

TABLE II

Immunosuppressant Activity in the Supernatants of Membranes Solubilized by Enzyme Digestion

Treatment	Protein Solubilized %[a]	Dose (µg/mouse)	Direct PFC/10^6 Cells[b]	Inhibition(%)	P vs. Control
Control	-	0	437 ± 157	0	-
Trypsin	67	2	149 ± 85	66	< .007
		10	198 ± 71	55	< .01
Papain	43	2	162 ± 92	63	< .01
		10	200 ± 28	54	< .01
Lipase	17	2	134 ± 61	69	< .001
		10	184 ± 21	58	< .007

[a] 10 µg enzyme per 1 mg membrane, 4 hr, 37°C.

[b] Mean ± 1 SD, 5 mice per group.

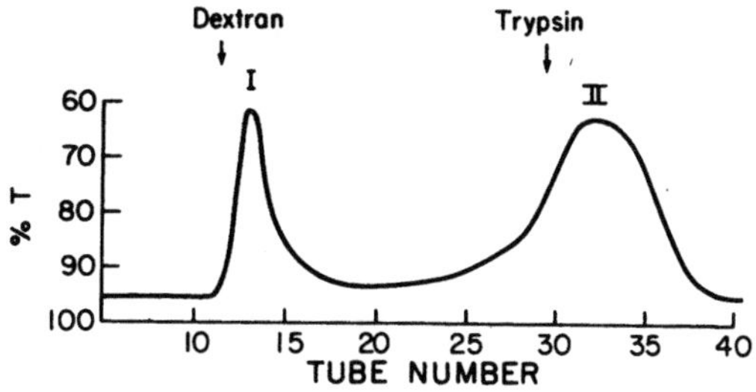

Fig. 2. Gel filtration on Sephadex G-100 of trypsin-soluble fraction of protoplast membrane preparation in 0.06 M phosphate buffer. Percent transmittance at 254 μm. Arrows indicate where dextran-blue 2000 and trypsin elute, relative to fractions I and II.

The relative activity of one membrane preparation, and the trypsin soluble and Sephadex G-100 fraction I preparations derived from it, are shown in Fig. 3. The pattern of the dose-response relationship is consistent in crude preparations and preparations of increasing purity. This suggests that the unusual dose effect is a characteristic of this factor. The increase in activity with separation is shown in Table 1. The large increase in activity is greater than could be expected from this limited purification process, and Sephadex fraction I is still heterogeneous. Therefore, part of the increased activity must reflect the separation of the immunosuppressant from an inhibitor or antagonist (i.e. an immunopotentiator).

The immunosuppressive activity of Sephadex fraction I is not effected by pronase or further treatment with trypsin (Table 4). It is also stable at 37°C for 4 hr (Table 4) and at 65°C for 20 min, but activity is lost at 80°C for 20 min (Table 5).

TABLE III

Comparison of Immunosuppression by Sephadex G-100 Fractions

Dose	Fraction I		Fraction II	
(μg/mouse)[a]	% of control	P vs control	% of Control	P vs Control
0	100	-	100	-
0.006	72	NS	-	-
0.03	30	.007	-	-
0.8	30	.005	109	NS
4.0	36	.01	118	NS
20.0	48	.03	56	NS
100.0	-	-	113	NS
500.0	-	-	223	.04

[a] Injected IP 24 hr before SRBC.

EFFECT OF MEMBRANE PREPARATIONS ON LYMPHOCYTE FUNCTIONS

Studies designed to identify the lymphoid cell populations affected by injection of mice with cytoplasmic fractions of group A streptococci are briefly summarized here. We have determined that bone marrow cell functions, such as hematopoiesis and the ability to synergize with normal T-cells, are suppressed (3). On the other hand, some T-cell functions such as stimulation by phytohemagglutinin (PHA), mixed lymphocyte culture, and synergism with bone marrow are unaffected or enhanced (3). To further define the murine B-cell population affected, we have investigated the effect of injection of protoplast membrane preparations upon the response of lymphoid cells to mitogens. Gronowicz and Coutinho (4) have shown that dextran sulfate (DS) stimulates immature B-cells and lipopolysaccharide (LPS) activates B-cells of intermediate to mature development. The mitogenic response of bone marrow cells to DS is selectively depressed by injection of mice with membrane preparations 24 or 72 hr (but not 12 hr) before collection of cells. The response of bone marrow cells to LPS, and spleen cells to DS and LPS is unaltered (14). Suppression of the response to DS *in vitro* is not mediated by Thy 1.2^+ T-cells or by adherent cells (14). Neither the Con A or PHA response of mouse bone marrow, spleen or thymus cells is altered by injection 24 hr before collection of lymphoid cells. Delayed hypersensitivity to SRBC, measured by foot pad swelling, is potentiated by injection of membranes 24 hr before sensitization with a high dose (4×10^8) of SRBC (14). The studies summarized above suggest that group A streptococcal membrane preparations preferentially suppress immature B-cells and enhance some T-cell functions.

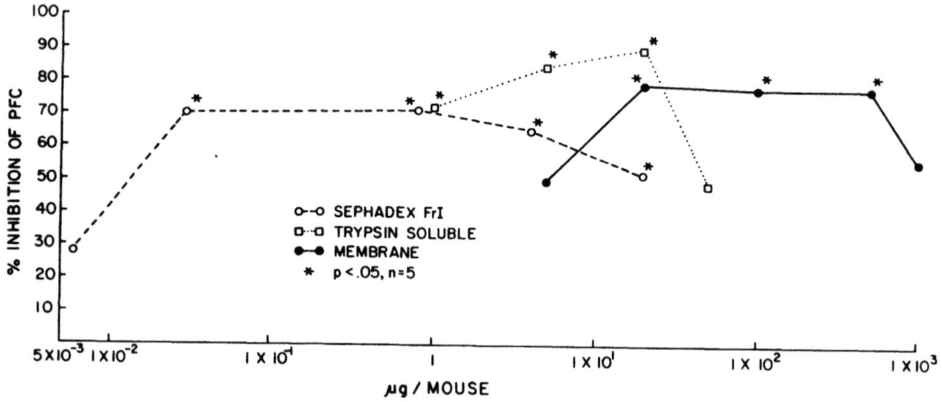

Fig. 3. Comparison of dose effect and relative immunosuppressant activity of a protoplast membrane preparation, the trypsin-soluble fraction, and the Sephadex G-100 fraction I.

TABLE IV

Effect of Pronase and Trypsin on Sephadex G-100 Fraction I

Treatment[a]	Dose (μg/mouse)	Direct PFC/Spleen[b]	% Inhibition	P vs Control
Control	0	330 ± 112	0	-
Incubation only	2.0	146 ± 33	56	<.008
	0.2	183 ± 97	45	<.05
	0.02	184 ± 96	45	<.05
Pronase	2.0	173 ± 84	48	<.04
	0.2	152 ± 32	54	<.01
	0.02	130 ± 70	61	<.01
Trypsin	0.02	145 ± 126	57	<.04
No Incubation	0.02	172 ± 89	48	<.04

[a] 10 μg enzyme per mg, 4 hr, 37°C

[b] Mean ± 1 SD x 10^3, 5 mice per group

It has been determined if the immunosuppressant factor separated from membrane preparations is responsivle for the effect of membrane preparations upon lymphocyte functions.

SUMMARY

1. An immunosuppressant obtained from group A streptococcal cells is associated with preparations of protoplast membranes.

2. Mice injected with membrane preparations display a depressed response of antibody-forming cells, a preferential suppression of immature bone marrow cells, and an enhancement of some T-cell functions.

3. A partially purified fraction has been isolated from the trypsin soluble fraction of the membrane preparation.

4. Antibody response can be suppressed by injection of mice with as little as 1 to 10 ng of this fraction.

5. The extremely low dose at which this factor is active after injection into an animal suggests that it functions either through the activation of an endogenous mediator or it mimics an endogenous mediator.

TABLE V

Effect of Heat on Immunosuppression by Sephadex Fraction I

Treatment	Dose (μg/mouse)	Direct PFC/Spleen[a]	Inhibition (%)	p
Control	0	330 ± 86	0	-
None	0.032	111 ± 52	66	.001
	4.0	139 ± 172	58	.05
Heated 65° 20 min	0.032	154 ± 70	53	.007
	4.0	151 ± 71	54	.007
Heated 80° 20 min	0.032	232 ± 74	30	NS
	4.0	335 ± 237	0	NS

[a] Mean ± 1 SD x 10^3, 5 mice per group.

REFERENCES

1. Azuma, I., Sugimura, K., Taniyama, T., Yamawaki, M., Yamamura, Y., Kusumoto, S., Okada, S., and Shiba, T., 1976, Adjuvant activity of mycobacterial fractions: adjuvant activity of synthetic N-acetylmuramyl-dipeptide and the related compounds. Infect. Immun. 14: 18.

2. Freimer, E. H., 1963, Studies of L forms and protoplasts of group A streptococci. II. Chemical and Immunological properties of the cell membrane. J. Exp. Med. 117: 377.

3. Gaumer, H. R., and Schwab, H. J., 1972, Differential susceptibility of mouse lymphocytes to an immunosuppressant from group A streptococci. Cellular Immunol. 4: 394.

4. Gronowicz, E., and Coutinho, A., 1974, Selective triggering of B cell subpopulations by mitogens. Eur. J. Immunol. 4: 771.

5. Greenblatt, J. J., Boackle, R. J., and Schwab, J. H., 1978, Activation of the alternate complement pathway by peptidoglycan from streptococcal cell wall. Infect. Immun. 19: 296.

6. Hanna, E. E., and Watson, D. W., 1973, Enhanced immune response after immunosuppression by streptococcal pyrogenic exotoxin Infect. Immun. 7: 1009.

7. Holton, J. B., and Schwab, J. W., 1966, Adjuvant properties of bacterial cell wall mucopeptides. J. Immunol. 96: 134.

8. Malakian, A., and Schwab, J. H., 1968. Immunosuppressant from group A streptococci. Sci. 159: 880.

9. Malakian, A., and Schwab, J. H., 1971, Biological characterization of an immunosuppressant from group A streptococci. J. Exp. Med. 134: 1253.

10. Miller, G. A., and Jackson, R. W., 1973, The effect of streptococcus pyogenes teichoic acid on the immune response of mice. J. Immunol. 110: 148.

11. Schorlemmer, H., Bitter -Suermann, D., and Allison, A. C., 1977, Complement activation by the alternate pathway and macrophage enzyme secretion in the pathogenesis of chronic inflammation. Immunol. 32: 939.

12. Schwab, J. H., 1974, Suppression of the immune response by microorganisms. Bact. Rev. 39: 121.

13. Schwab, J. H., and Brown, 1973, Heart autoantibodies in mice: genetic, bacterial and age determinants. J. Immunol. 111: 682.

14. Toffaletti, D. L., and Schwab, J. H., 1979, Modulation of lymphocyte functions by group A streptococcal membrane. Cellular Immunol. 42: 3.

MODULATION OF SUPPRESSOR T-CELLS BY STREPTOCOCCAL PYROGENIC EXOTOXIN

Edgar E. Hanna, Martha L. Hale and Michael L. Misfeldt

Laboratory of Molecular Genetics
National Institute of Child Health and Human Development
National Institutes of Health
Bethesda, MD 20205

ABSTRACT

The V-region gene repertoire which determines the qualitative nature of an organisms' antibody response is encoded in the genome of the immunoglobulin forming cells (B-lymphocytes) of the organism. Other cells such as thymus derived lymphocytes (T-cells) and macrophages appear to regulate or control the antibody responses of B-lymphocytes to many immunogens including trinitrophenylated rabbit erythrocytes (TNP-RE). Recently, we have been attempting to understand how this regulation is mediated at the cellular level. We have devised a model based on the observation that a toxic protein (SPE) which is elaborated by many Group A streptococci is capable of deregulating T-cell dependent antibody responses in mice. An in vitro cellular complementation system allowed us to perform reconstruction experiments in order to define the functions of isolated subpopulations of mouse spleen immunocytes, which include B-cells and macrophages obtained from NFR/nu nu mice and T-cells obtained from their +/nu littermates. Since these subpopulations of immunocytes are all required in order to generate a complete anti-TNP PFC response in Marbrook-type spleen cell cultures, we were able to test and to localize the susceptible target of SPE within the T-cell population. Subfractionation of the T-cell population into functional distinct subpopulations followed by demonstration of the unique T-cell surface markers on the cells which bound SPE allowed us to delineate the deregulating locus of SPE to native regulatory T-cells or to a normal suppressor T-cell subset.

INTRODUCTION

Modification of plaque-forming cells (PFC) and immunoglobulin

(Ig) responses to sheep erythrocytes (SE) or to trinitrophenylated rabbit erythrocytes (TNP-RE) with streptococcal pyrogenic exotoxin (SPE) in NFR/N mice has been documented (5, 8-11). In vivo or in vitro PFC responses to these T-cell-dependent immunogens are suppressed at 4-5 days after immunogen and SPE treatment. This is followed after 10-14 days by a delayed burst of PFC without further stimulation with immunogen. We have termed this effect a "deregulated response" (5, 8, 9). NFR athymic, T-cell deficient nude (nu/nu) mice do not exhibit a deregulated response, whereas their heterozygous (+/nu), T-cell sufficient littermates do exhibit the deregulated response. Gram negative endotoxin (Et or LPS), known B-cell polyclonal mitogens, do not induce the deregulated response, but may augment, rather than suppress, the early 4-5 day PFC response even in the nude (8). These observations suggested that SPE might affect T-cells preferentially. We were able to complement and increase the responses of nudes up to normal +/nu magnitudes by adoptive transfer of selected populations of +/nu littermate spleen cells. We have exploited this ability using reconstruction experiments in order to localize the cellular site of action of SPE. Our experiments test the effects of SPE on B-cells, T-cells and macrophages separately. The results indicated that the SPE generated deregulating effect was localized to regulatory T-cells (5, 8, 9). Our most recent experiments, some of which are highlighted in this report, investigated the effect of SPE on nylon wool column fractionated spleen T-lymphocyte subpopulations. We have utilized the complementation system as before (5) in order to further delineate the cellular site of action of SPE among the heterogeneous subpopulations of T-cells (1). The nylon wool fractionated cells were pooled according to their elution profiles and then assessed for their ability to complement nude PFC responses and for their ability to generate the SPE induced deregulation. The results indicate that SPE inhibits the function of normal suppressors and/or may deviate or drive multi-potential T-cells toward a delayed helper function.

MATERIALS AND METHODS

Mice

NFR/N nude (nu/nu) mice and their littermates (+/nu) were obtained from the Small Animal Section, Division of Research Services, NIH. The NFR/N mouse is an inbred substrain of the N:NIH mouse. These strains were derived and maintained as closed colonies here at NIH as detailed previously (4, 6).

Immunogens

Trinitrophenylated rabbit erythrocytes (TNP-RE) were prepared by the method of Rittenberg and Pratt (14). Prior to use, TNP-RE were washed and suspended in Hank's balanced salt solution (HBSS) without phenol red. All procedures were carried out under sterile conditions. Trinitrophenylated lipopolysaccharide (TNP-LPS) and dinitrophenylated ficoll (DNP-Ficoll) were gifts from Dr. Bruce Merchant, Bureau of Biologics, Food and Drug Administration, Bethesda, MD.

Spleen Cell Suspensions

Single cell suspensions were obtained as before (5, 8, 9). To obtain macrophage-depleted cell suspensions, an aliquot of the spleen cell suspension (SC) was incubated with 200 mg/ml of carbonyl iron (GAF Corporation, New York, NY) for 1 hr at 37C. The carbonyl iron was removed by a magnet and the resulting SC depleted of macrophages was washed in culture medium. Nylon wool column fractionation of the macrophage-depleted SC was performed essentially as described by Julius et al. (12) and modified by Handwerger and Schwartz (7). Briefly, nylon wool (Fenwal Labs., Deerfield, IL) was boiled in several changes of deionized glass distilled water, then dried in a 37C incubator overnight. Columns were loosely packed with 3 g of dry nylon wool in a 50 ml plastic syringe and equilibriated with Hank's balanced salt solution containing 5% heat inactivated fetal bovine serum (HBSS-FBS) at 37C for 15 min. Six ml of the SC at a cell density of 5×10^7 cells/ml were applied to the column. After incubating the columns at 37C for 45 min, Pool 1 cells were eluted first from the column with 37C HBSS-FBS in 5 ml samples to a total volume of 50 ml. An additional 25 ml of media was passed through the columns and discarded before the columns were shut off by use of a stopcock. Next, the top 3/4 of the nylon wool column was stirred gently with a pipette and Pool 2 cells were eluted from the column in 5 ml samples with HBSS-FBS at 4C to a total of 100 ml. The total yield of Pool 1 and Pool 2 cells was equal to approximately 50% of the total SC applied to the columns. In preliminary experiments the strongly adherent cells which were retained on the columns but could be squeezed off were found to be largely B cells and in subsequent experiments were left on the columns.

Spleen Cell Cultures

Spleen cells were cultured as detailed before in large Marbrook chambers (5, 8, 9). Briefly, spleen cells at a density of 3×10^7 cells in 1.0 ml of culture medium were seeded to Spectrapor dialysis membrane (Spectrum Medical Industries, Inc., Los Angeles, CA) of each inner Marbrook chamber. Twenty ml of media were added to the outer Marbrook chambers. The culture medium was a modified Eagle's medium (αMEM) (16) containing glutamine and supplemented with 15% fetal bovine serum of a pretested lot (Microbiological Associates, Bethesda, MD). Gentamicin at a concentration of 150 μg/ml was added as antibiotic. Cultures were immunized with 10^6 TNP-RE/culture, or 30 ng TNP-LPS/culture or 30 ng DNP-Ficoll/culture as was appropriate in particular experiments. Cultures were rocked continuously on a rocker platform at 5-7 cycles/min for a period of 5 or 10-12 days in a 37C incubator in an atmosphere of 7% oxygen, 10% carbon dioxide, 83% nitrogen and 100% relative humidity.

Cell Counting

Immunogen and spleen cell counts were performed electronically in the Autocytometer II (Fisher Scientific, Pittsburgh, PA).

Complementation Procedure

The procedure consisted of mixing nu/nu and +/nu spleen cell suspensions prior to seeding them into Marbrook cultures (5, 9). The cell density of the mixture was constant at 30 x 10^6 cells/culture. In experiments employing graded numbers of T-cells, additional reciprocal numbers of nude mouse spleen cells were added as filler cells to insure a total of 30 x 10^6 cells/culture.

Antisera

Characteristics of the antisera are described elsewhere (5, 9). Briefly, rabbit anti-mouse thymocyte antiserum (RAM-T) was prepared by hyper-immunizing New Zealand white rabbits with a mixture of sonicated neonatal BALB/c, C57Bl/6 and C3H/He mouse thymocytes. RAM-T consisted of a pool of two sera selected for their capacities to inhibit T-cell dependent PFC responses and was absorbed exhaustively with acetone-dried mouse liver powders, mouse erythrocytes, sheep erythrocytes and spleen cells from Type I, N:NIH nude mice (6).

Rabbit anti-mouse immunoglobulin antiserum (RAM-Ig) was prepared by the hyperimmunization of rabbits with a 1:1 mixture of early-bleed and late-bleed immune mouse immunoglobulins. The immunogen was a mixture of rabbit erythrocytes (RE) bound with mouse anti-RE antibodies which had been collected as early and late bleed antisera. The resulting antisera were selected on the basis of their capacities to inhibit PFC responses. The antisera selected were pooled and then absorbed with acetone-dried mouse liver powders, N:NIH mouse erythrocytes and sheep erythrocytes.

Mouse anti-Lyt1 (MA-Lyt-1) and anti-Lyt2 (MA-Lyt-2) antisera (1) were gifts of Drs. H. Cantor and F. W. Shen, Harvard Medical School, Boston, MA and the Sloan-Kettering Institute, New York, NY.

Horse anti-SPE-A, modified globulin (HA-SPE-A) (2) was a gift from Dr. D. W. Watson, University of Minnesota, Minneapolis.

Fluoresceinated F(ab')$_2$ fractions of goat anti-mouse IgG (Fl*-F(ab')$_2$GAM-IgG) and rodamine labeled F(ab')$_2$ fractions of rabbit anti-horse IgG (Rd*'F(ab')$_2$ RAH-IgG) and the respective unlabeled fractions were purchased from Cappel Laboratories, Cochranville, PA.

Streptococcal Pyrogenic Exotoxin (SPE)

Highly purified SPE (SPE-A) was a generous gift of Drs. P. M. Schlievert and D. W. Watson of the University of Minnesota Medical Center, Minneapolis. They have tailed the purification of SPE by preparative isoelectric focusing (2, 15). The toxin was tested in preliminary experiments and found to be active in our in vitro system over a dose range of 1.0 ng to 100 µg (unpublished observations). The dose used in this report was 5 µg/culture.

PFC Assays

Estimations of hapten-specific anti-TNP PFC responses to spleen cell cultures were done in agarose plates as before (5, 9). Trinitrophenylated sheep erythrocytes (TNP-SE), prepared by the method of Rittenberg and Pratt (14) were used as indicator target cells. Indicator target cells prepared in this way were used also to estimate the number of anti-TNP and the number of anti-DNP PFC raised against TNP-LPS and DNP-Ficoll.

Immunofluorescence

Indirect immunofluorescent staining of Pool 1 and Pool 2 cells was performed in order to localize the sites of binding of SPE and the location of membrane Lyt-1 and Lyt-2. Fluorescent cells were scored and photographed in the Leitz Ortholux II, consisting of the Ploem eliminator for vertical incident fluorescence excitation, and with the attached Leitz Orthomat-W automatic camera. Leitz filter systems H and K or M and N were used for the excitation of fluorescein and rhodamine stained cells respectively. Kodak Ektachrome-200 color slide film exposed and processed at ASA 400 was used to record fluorescence. The prints shown in this report were recorded on Kodak panchromatic film from the ektachrome slides. Immunofluorescent staining was by an indirect procedure. Thirty million Pool 1 or Pool 2 cells were incubated on ice with 25 µg of SPE-A in a volume of 1.0 ml for 3 hr on ice in modified Hank's balanced salt solution (without phenol red, with 24 mM HEPES buffer, with 0.2% sodium azide, with 1% heated fetal bovine serum) HBSS. The cells were next washed and resuspended in modified HBSS and incubated for 15 min on ice with HA-SPE-A (1:30 dilution) or MA-Lyt-1 (1:25 dilution) or MA-Lyt-2 (1:25 dilution) in reciprocal sequence (i.e. HA-SPE-A followed by either MA-Lyt-1 or MA-Lyt-2 or either of the latter applied first and then followed by HA-SPE-A). The cells were washed between each reagent exposure and finally resuspended and incubated on ice for a final 15 min in either a 1:30 dilution of Fl*-$F(ab')_2$ GAM-IgG and followed after washing by a 1:30 dilution of Rd*-$F(ab')_2$ RAH-IgG or the reverse order addition of these reagents. Fluorescence quenching controls using the appropriate unlabeled Ig reagents were carried out in parallel.

RESULTS AND DISCUSSION

It is now accepted by many laboratories that the qualitative aspects of an organism's antibody response is encoded within the V-region gene repertoire of B-cells. On the other hand, it is apparent that the expression of the V-region gene product of B-cells is regulated by other cells of the immune system. Regulatory cells which have been defined thus far are the macrophages and the positive helper and negative (suppressor) T-cells. The scope of the macrophage function appears to be to interact with antigen and in some way to present it in an optimal form to stimulate B-cells with the proper V-region product at their surfaces. The specificity of this event appears to be conferred by T-cells. Moreover, the exquisite specificity of T-cells relate also to their primary function within the scope of antibody formation, to the regulation of the expansion of B-cell clones following antigen stimulation.

We have been attempting to understand how this regulation is mediated at the cellular level. The observation that microorganisms have evolved mechanisms which may evade or even divert immune systems with which they interact, may suggest means toward a better understanding of the various regulatory mechanisms, i.e. and understanding of "deregulating" processes exerted by microorganisms may reveal useful clues to a better understanding of cellular regulatory mechanisms. In this respect, we have been exploiting the observation that a toxic protein elaborated by many strains of Group A streptococci is capable of strongly modulating the T-cell dependent antibody responses in mice and rabbits (5, 8-11). Early observations were that streptococcal pyrogenic exotoxin (SPE) can suppress the (4-5 day) primary peak PFC response (10). Equally exciting was the observation made later that following the event of suppression and without additional antigen exposure a late burst of antigen specific PFC could be observed to arise at about 10-12 days (5, 8, 9, 11). In order to attempt to understand the process of deregulation an <u>in vitro</u> system was developed which utilizes the T-cell dependence of PFC responses of NFR/N or NFR +/nu mice to the TNP-group of trinitrophenylated rabbit erythrocytes (TNP-RE). Moreover, NFR/nu nu mice do not display the deregulated effect of SPE. Thus we were provided a capacity to perform cellular complementation or reconstruction experiments <u>in vitro</u> by use of Marbrook-type PFC cultures (5, 9, 13). Spleens from nude mice were used as the source of immunocompetent B-cells and macrophages. Spleens from +/nu mice were used as the source of immunocytes rich in T-cells, thus completing the cellular requirements for a full anti-TNP PFC response in culture (Fig. 1).

Next, it was important to ascertain whether complemented cultures would be driven by SPE to generate a deregulated response (Fig. 2). It is summarized in Figure 2 also that indeed SPE could deregulate the PFC response of complemented cultures as well as and with a

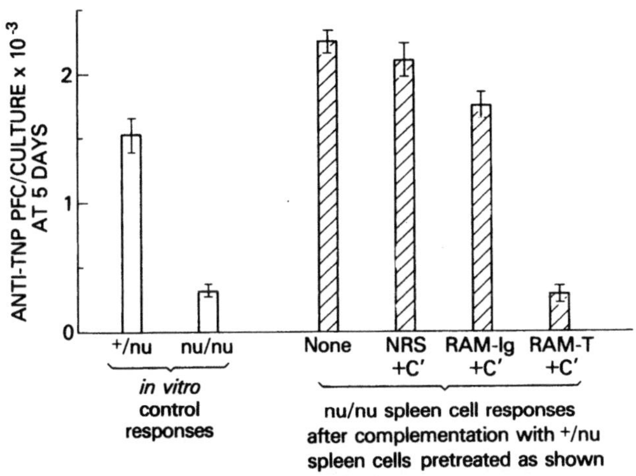

Fig. 1. Complementation of NFR nude mouse PFC responses to TNP-RE in vitro by admixture of 15 x 10^6 +/nu littermate splenocytes in Marbrook-type PFC cultures. Open bars, control PFC responses 5 days after initiation and immunization of cultures. Hatched bars, test PFC responses after none and various pretreatments of the +/nu splenocytes. NRS, normal rabbit serum. RAM-Ig, rabbit anti-mouse immunoglobulin antiserum. RAM-T, rabbit anti-mouse thymocyte antiserum. C', quinea pig serum complement. Each bar represents the means ± the standard errors for 4-5 cultures in a representative experiment.

similar magnitude as in the normal intact +/nu splenocyte cultures. Consistent with the model, nude splenocytes were not capable of generating a deregulated response after SPE exposure. This fact and the observation in Figure 1 that complementation can be inhibited by inactivation of T-cells but not by inactivation of donor B-cells, suggested that the deregulating effect of SPE was generated through a T-cell population.

Further support for the indication that deregulation was generated through T-cells was gained by the observation that PFC responses to T-cell independent immunogens were not affected similarly by SPE (Fig. 3). It was also important to ask what was the role of macrophages in the SPE induced deregulating effect. We observed that macrophages while required for a complete anti-TNP PFC response the SPE effect was not mediated through them (9). In fact, the macro-

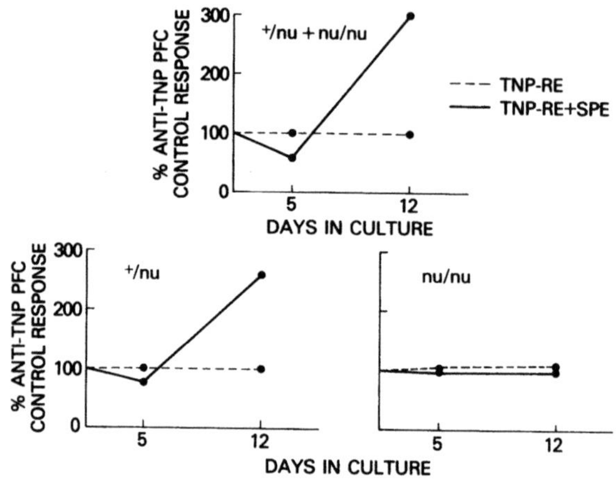

Fig. 2. Deregulation of the anti-TNP PFC responses of T-cell complemented nude mouse splenocytes in vitro by SPE. Lower left graph, +/nu SPE treated and untreated control responses. Lower right graph, nu/nu SPE treated and untreated control responses. Upper graph, nu/nu x +/nu mixture, SPE treated and untreated test responses. Cell density per culture was 3 x 10^7 splenocytes of each type. Percent control response is the percent of the untreated response to antigen alone as indicated by the broken lines in each graph.

phage function was not altered by SPE over a broad range of graded additions of SPE pretreated macrophages in cellular reconstruction and complementation experiments (unpublished work).

Experimental results to this point had localized the SPE induced effect to T-cells (5,9). The indications pointed toward a negative regulatory cell or a native suppressor since our source of immunocytes was usually unprimed mice (5, 8, 9). Figure 4 depicts some results from our current experiments in which we have attempted to delineate the subpopulation(s) of T-cells affected by SPE. Our approach was to fractionate the macrophage depleted donor splenocytes on nylon wool columns and to test the fractionated subpopulations of T-cells as targets of SPE. Cells which eluted similarly from the columns were pooled. Two dissimilar pools of T-cells were obtained on this basis. They were designated Pool 1 and Pool 2 as illustrated in Figure 4 (bottom half). The activities of Pool 1 and Pool 2 cells before their exposure to SPE are reported at the top half of Figure 4. The separated pools of mouse splenocytes were tested for their ability to complement T-cell deficient nude mouse spleen cell cultures up to the magnitude of +/nu PFC responsiveness. These experiments were performed by co-culturing 15 x 10^6 cells or

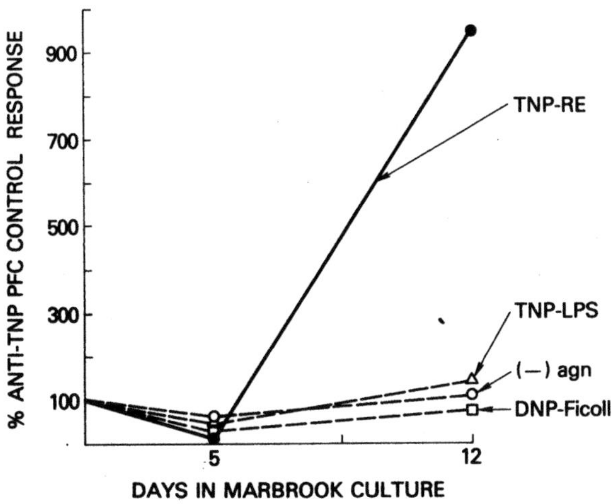

Fig. 3. Effect of SPE on the anti-TNP PFC responses of NFR/N splenocytes in vitro to TNP or DNP determinants when presented as T-cell independent immunogens. Control responses were the responses of cultures exposed to the respective immunogens alone and not exposed to SPE. The TNP-specific PFC responses at 5 days were 2993 ± 983, 1455 ± 120 and 1413 ± 89 respectively for TNP-RE (T-cell dependent) immunized cultures and for TNP-LPS and DNP-Ficoll (T cells independent) immunized cultures. Immunogen doses were given in the Materials and Methods section.

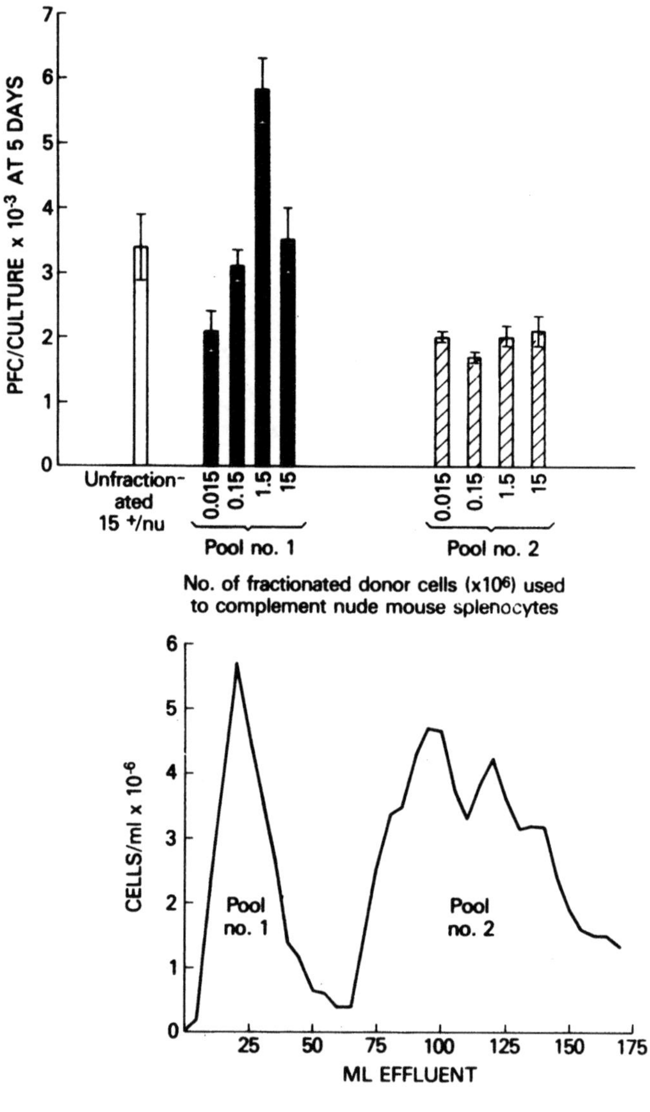

Fig. 4. Bottom. Elution profile of the nylon wool fractionation of macrophage depleted mouse splenocyte suspensions. A total of 3 x 10^8 splenocytes were applied to the column. Fractions of 5.0 ml were collected and pooled as indicated. Top. Complementation of the NFR/nude mouse anti-TNP PFC responses by the macrophage depleted nylon wool fractionated and pooled +/nu splenocytes represented in the bottom graph. The figure is self-explanatory and further detail is given in the Materials and Methods section.

log dilutions of this number of either pool with 15 x 10^6 nude mouse spleen cells in large Marbrook vessels. Figure 4 (top) characterizes the complementation achieved after the use of Pool 1 or Pool 2 cells. Results employing graded numbers of Pool 1 cells over a three log range showed that the optimal complementation was obtained with 1.5 x 10^6 Pool 1 cells. Pool 2 cells were incapable of complementing or they complemented very poorly as is shown in Figure 4. No difference was seen when the number of Pool 2 donor cells was varied. Pretreatment of either Pool 1 or Pool 2 donor cells with RAM-T and C' to establish their T-cell identity, markedly inhibited their ability to complement nude PFC responses. These results show that Pool 1 contains the major proportion of T-cells capable of complementing nude mouse PFC responses.

Since Pool 2 cells were incapable of complementing nude mouse PFC responses (see Figure 4), we asked the question whether Pool 2 cells could be native negative regulatory (suppressor) T-cells capable of suppressing the PFC response of cultures optimally complemented with Pool 1 cells. In order to investigate this question, we supplemented optimally complemented cultures (see Figure 4) with graded numbers of Pool 2 cells. The data from this experiment are shown in Figure 5.

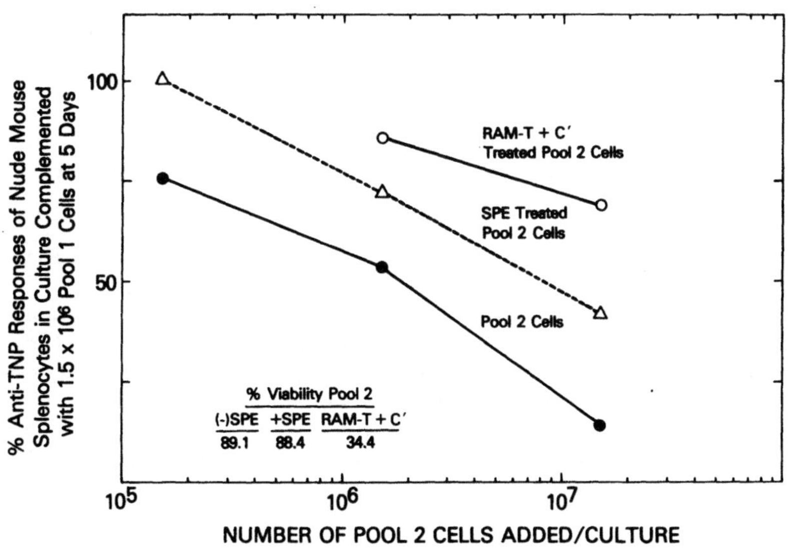

Fig. 5. Suppression of Pool 1 splenocyte complementation by the graded addition of Pool 2 splenocytes. Note that 1.5 x 10^6 Pool 1 cells was the optimal complementing cell number (see Figure 4). The data in the insert on percent viability was estimated by trypan blue dye exclusion tests. The points on the graph represent the means of two cultures in a single experiment performed.

The magnitude of the suppression by Pool 2 cells of the PFC responses of optimally complemented cultures increased progressively when 1.5 x 10^5, 1.5 x 10^6 and 1.5 x 10^7 Pool 2 cells respectively were added. This suppression by Pool 2 cells could be relieved by treatment of Pool 2 cells with SPE prior to their addition to the optimally complemented cultures. SPE treatment of Pool 2 cells relieved the suppression 24% to 28% for the increments of 1.5 x 10^5 to 1.5 x 10^7 Pool 2 cells respectively as compared with untreated Pool 2 cells. The relief of suppression by SPE treatment was not due to a cytolytic effect by SPE on Pool 2 cells as assessed by trypan blue viability studies. The viability of SPE treated and nontreated Pool 2 cells were not different, 88.4 ± 1.3% and 89.1 ± 1.7%, respectively, as shown in the inset of Figure 5. Whereas, the relief of suppression by RAM-T+C' treatment of Pool 2 cells was more likely due to a cytolytic effect on Pool 2 cells because the cell viability remaining after this treatment was very low (34.4 ± 3.9%). The ability of Pool 2 cells to suppress optimally complemented cultures progressively in proportion to the number of them added in the complementation test shows that Pool 2 is highly enriched in suppressor cells. This observation that Pool 2 cells are also highly enriched in cells which show positive immunofluorescence for the Lyt-2 differentiation antigen (see Fig. 6) suggests strongly that the suppressor cells are suppressor T-cells. Pool 1 T-cells were determined to be Lyt-1 cells by immunofluorescence. This is consistent with the literature which indicates that the cells which are least adherent to nylon wool and are Lyt-1^+ cells are helper T-cells (1, 7, 12, 17). Pool 2 cells were determined to be highly enriched in Lyt-2^+ cells by immunofluorescence (Fig. 6, C and D) and they were more adherent to nylon wool than Pool 1 cells. Because Pool 2 cells were suppressive by the complementation test as well, jointly these results are consistent with the literature to show that Pool 2 is rich in suppressor T-cells.

It was next important to ask to which T-cell subpopulation does SPE bind. Figure 6 shows by immunofluorescent staining, that SPE binds to both Pool 1 and Pool 2 T-cells. However, by comparison of the intensities of fluorescence on SPE-adsorbed Pool 1 cells which were double-stained for SPE and for Lyt-1 cell surface determinants approximately equal intensities were observed. But, comparison of the intensitives of fluorescence on SPE adsorbed Pool 2 cells which were double-stained for SPE and for the Lyt-2 cell surface determinants revealed that staining for Lyt-2 was partially blocked.

This suggests that SPE may bind closer to or in some order interfere with the binding of anti-Lyt-2 antibodies to the Lyt-2 surface determinant(s). Proof and the importance of this observation are under investigation.

Finally we have asked which subpopulation of T-cells is responsible

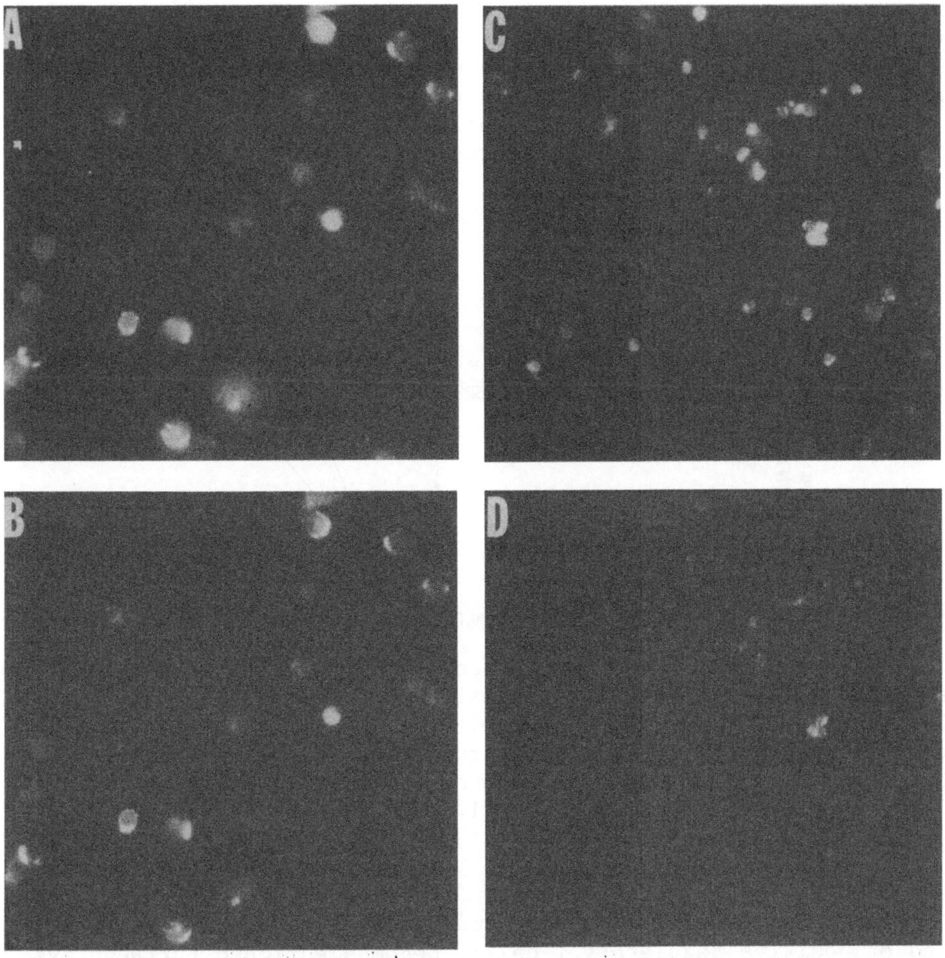

Fig. 6. Immunofluorescent staining for SPE and for the T-cell differentiation antigens Lyt-1 and Lyt-2 on SPE preadsorbed Pool 1 and Pool 2 cells. A, Pool 1 cells stained with and photographed for the rhodamine fluorochrome tag for SPE. B, the same field as A, double stained with and photographed for the fluorescein fluorochrome for Lyt-1. Note that A and B show approximately equal intensities of fluorescence. C, Pool 2 cells stained with and photographed for the rhodamine fluorochrome tag for SPE. D, The same field as C, double stained with and photographed for Lyt-2. Note that the intensity of fluorescence in C, for SPE is greater than that in D for the Lyt-2 antigen. Pool 1 and Pool 2 cells that were not preadsorbed with SPE showed equal intensities of fluorescence when stained for Lyt-1 and Lyt-2 (not shown). Refer to the Materials and Methods section for details and conditions of the procedures involved in this figure.

for the generation of the effect observed. The results depicted in Figure 7 show that Pool 2 cells generate the late burst of anti-TNP specific PFC which we have defined as a deregulated PFC response (8). Pool 1 cells were suppressed consistent with our very early observations (10) and as clearly delineated to T-helper cells by Cunningham and Watson more recently (3), but Pool 1 cells did not recover to generate a delayed primary peak increase in PFC.

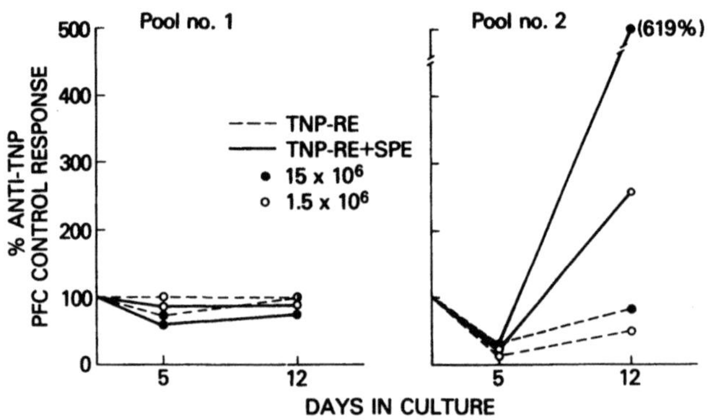

Fig. 7. Deregulation by SPE of the anti-TNP PFC responses of nude mouse splenocytes after optimal and supraoptimal complementation with fractionated +/nu Pool 1 or Pool 2 T-cells. The points on the graphs are for the means of four cultures in a representative experiment. The PFC control was the response of cultures complemented with the optimal number of Pool 1 cells (1.5 x 10^6). The Figure is otherwise self-explanatory.

The T-cell subpopulation contained in Pool 2, having been depleted of positive regulatory T-cells, becomes enriched for negative regulatory T-cells as observed in Figure 5. The negative regulatory T-cells in Pool 2 were able to inhibit the complementation of cultures supplemented with Pool 1 cells. Increasing log increments of Pool 2 cells when added to optimally complemented cultures, decreased the observed PFC proportionally. Treatment of Pool 2 cells with SPE relieved the suppression exerted by Pool 2 cells on the PFC responses of optimally complemented cultures. Thus, SPE shuts off the suppressor function of T-cells found in Pool 2.

Moreover, the SPE deregulating effect was also localized to a population of T-cells found in Pool 2 (Figure 8). Pool 2 may contain several subpopulations of T-cells as suggested by the polyphasic elution profile of Pool 2 (Figure 4). It is possible that the potentially distinct subpopulations of T-cells contained in Pool 2 are functionally diverse. Our results show that SPE inhibits the

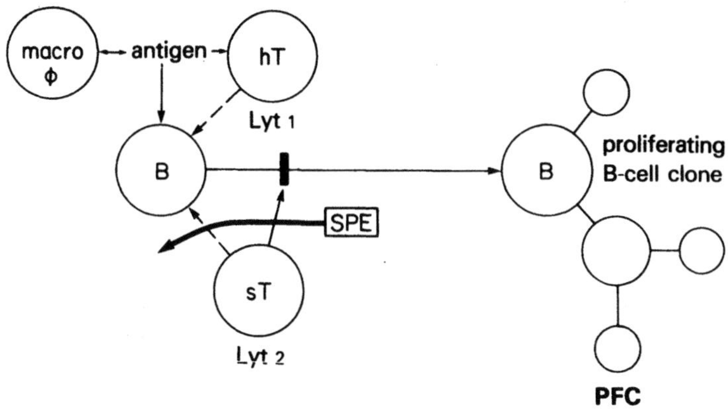

Fig. 8. Schema illustrating the site at which SPE initiates deregulation of the immune system as interpreted from the data to date. Macro Ø, macrophage. B, B-cell precursor and B-cell clone. hT, Helper T-cell phenotype. sT, Suppressor T-cell phenotype. Lyt-1, lymphocyte differentiation antigen characteristic of helper T-cells. Lyt-2, Lymphocyte differentiation antigen retained by suppressor T-cells. PFC, plaque forming cells (anti-TNP) by which the proliferating clone of B-cells was estimated. The schema shows that SPE shuts off the native negative regulatory (suppressor) T-cell. The Figure is otherwise self-explanatory.

function of the normal negative regulatory T-cells (suppressors) found in Pool 2. The late helper-like activity which is generated in Pool 2 could be explained if it could be demonstrated that SPE can drive multi-potential (precursor) T-cells toward a helper function. Alternatively, SPE could deviate the suppressor function of the suppressor cells toward a helper function after inhibiting their initial suppressing activity. Experiments to distinguish between these alternatives and to substantiate these hypotheses are progressing using the technique of cell fusion and construction of functional T-cell "hybridomas" within the T-cell pools. This technique would be expected to stablize distinct T-cell phenotypes.

ACKNOWLEDGEMENTS

We appreciate the cooperation of Dr. Carl Hansen and his staff, VRB, DRS, NIH in the development and breeding of the mice used in these experiments. We are grateful to Ms. Terri Broderick for expert secretarial assistance.

REFERENCES

1. Cantor, H., and Boyse, E. A., 1975, Functional subclasses of T lymphocytes bearing different Ly antigens. I. The generation of functionally distinct T-cell subclasses is a differentiative process independent of antigen. J. Exp. Med. 141: 1376.

2. Cunningham, C. M., Barsumian, E. L., and Watson, D. W., 1976. Further purification of group A streptococcal pyrogenic exotoxin and characterization of the purified toxin. Infect. Immun. 14: 767.

3. Cunningham, C. M., and Watson, D. W., 1978, Suppression of antibody response by group A streptococcal pyrogenic exotoxin and characterization of the cells involved. Infect. Immun. 19: 470.

4. Gershwin, M. E., Merchant, B., Gelfand, M. C., Vickers, J., Steinberg, A. D., and Hansen, C. T., 1975, The natural history and immunopathology of outbred athymic (nude) mice. Clinical Immunol. and Immunopath. 4:324.

5. Hale, M. L., and Hanna, E. E., 1976, Deregulation of mouse antibody-forming cells by streptococcal pyrogenic exotoxin. II. Modification of spleen T-cell-complemented nude mouse PFC responses. Cell. Immunol. 26: 168.

6. Hale, M. L., Hanna, E. E., and Hansen, C. T., 1976, Nude mice from homozygous nude parents show smaller PFC responses to sheep erythrocytes than nude mice from heterozygous mothers. Nature (London) 260: 44.

7. Handwerger, B. S., and Schwartz, R. H., 1974, Separation of murine lymphoid cells using nylon wool columns. Transplantation 18: 544.

8. Hanna, E. E., and Hale, M. L., 1975, Deregulation of mouse antibody-forming cells in vivo and in cell culture by streptococcal pyrogenic exotoxin. Infect. Immun. 11: 265.

9. Hanna, E. E., and Hale, M. L., 1976, Deregulation of mouse antibody-forming cells by a streptococcal exotoxin. A model study of the regulation of antibody formation by spleen cells, p. 309. In J. R. Battisto and J. W. Streilein (eds.),"Immuno-Aspects of the Spleen". Elsevier/North-Holland Biomedical Press, Amsterdam.

10. Hanna, E. E., and Watson, D. W., 1968, Host-parasite relationships among group A streptococci. IV. Suppression of antibody response by streptococcal pyrogenic exotoxin. J. Bacteriol.

95: 14.

11. Hanna, E. E., and Watson, D. W., 1973, Enhanced immune response after immunosuppression by streptococcal pyrogenic exotoxin. Infect. Immun. 7: 1009.

12. Julius, M. H., Simpson, E. and Herzenberg, L. A., 1973. A rapid method for the isolation of functional thymus-derived murine lymphocytes. Eur. J. Immunol. 3:645.

13. Marbrook, J., 1967, Primary immune response in cultures of spleen cells. Lancet ii: 1279.

14. Rittenberg, M. B., and Pratt, K. L., 1969, Antitrinitrophenyl (TNP) plaque assay. Primary response of Balb/c mice to soluble and particulate immunogen. Proc. Soc. Exp. Biol. Med. 132: 575.

15. Schlievert, P. M., Bettin, K. M., and Watson, D. W., 1977, Purification and characterization of group A streptococcal pyrogenic exotoxin type C. Infect. Immun. 16: 673.

16. Stanners, C. P., Eliceri, G. L., and Green, H., 1971, Two types of ribosomes in mouse-hamster hybrid cells. Nature (London) New Biol. 230: 52.

17. Tada, T., Takemori, T., Lkumura, K., Nonaka, M., and Tokuhisa, T., 1978, Two distinct types of helper T cells involved in the secondary antibody response. Independent and synergistic effects of Ia^- and Ia^+ helper T-cells. J. Exp. Med. 147: 446.

SPECIFICITY OF SUPPRESSOR T CELLS ACTIVATED DURING THE IMMUNE RESPONSE TO TYPE III PNEUMOCOCCAL POLYSACCHARIDE*

P. J. Baker[1], P. W. Stashak[1], D. F. Amsbaugh[1] and B. Prescott[2]

Laboratory of Microbial Immunity[1]
National Institute of Allergy and Infectious Diseases
National Institutes of Health
Bethesda, MD 20205

Biomedical Research Institute[2]
12111 Parklawn Drive
Rockville, MD 20852

ABSTRACT

Prior treatment (priming) with a single sub-immunogenic dose of Type III pneumococcal polysaccharide (SSS-III) greatly reduces the capacity of mice to make an antibody response to an optimally immunogenic dose of SSS-III; such unresponsiveness (low-dose paralysis) persists for several months after priming and is mediated by thymus-derived (T) suppressor cells. Priming with SSS-III does not influence the magnitude of the antibody response to serologically unrelated antigens, with or without immunization with SSS-III; furthermore, priming does not alter the TNP-specific antibody response of mice immunized with TNP_{11}-SS-III. Thus, the phenomenon of low-dose paralysis is highly antigen-specific with respect to both its induction and expression. Although the suppression noted in mice treated with Concanavalin A (Con A) is similar in degree and kinetics for expression to that found after the induction of low-dose paralysis, Con A-induced suppression is not antigen-specific. This suggests that a non-specific product released from activated T cells may be responsible for causing both types of suppressive effects; but, in the case of low-dose paralysis, a mechanism exists for focusing the effects of this product on a selected subpopulation (clone) of antibody-forming cells.

*Work supported in part by ONR Contract N00014-76-C-0053

INTRODUCTION

The phenomenon of low-dose paralysis to Type III pneumococcal polysaccharide (SSS-III) provides an excellent experimental model system for examining the effects of thymus-derived (T) lymphocytes on the magnitude of an antibody response (5, 7, 9). Such unresponsiveness, which is T cell dependent (2, 9), can be induced regularly in all strains of mice upon pre-treatment (priming) with a single injection of a subimmunogenic dose of antigen (3, 4). Previous studies have shown that treatment with a low dose of SSS-III does not influence the magnitude of antibody responses to serologically unrelated antigens (9). Although this suggests that low-dose paralysis is antigen-specific with respect to its *induction*, it provides no information on whether the *production* or *expression* of low-dose paralysis is likewise antigen-specific. In view of the many reports indicating that inhibitory products released by T cells are not always antigen-specific in their mode of action (1), the present study was undertaken to investigate, in detail, whether the expression of low-dose paralysis to SSS-III is antigen-specific, and to compare the pattern for the expression of this form of unresponsiveness, to that produced non-specifically by activated T cells under other circumstances.

MATERIALS AND METHODS

Mice

BALB/c female mice (8-10 weeks of age), obtained from the Cumberland View Farms, Clinton, Tennessee, were used throughout this work.

Antigens

The immunologic properties of the Type III pneumococcal polysaccharide (SSS-III) used, as well as the method by which it was prepared, have been described in detail (2, 6-8, 23). For immunization, mice were given a single intraperitoneal (i.p.) injection of an optimally immunogenic dose (0.5 μg) of SSS-III in 0.5 ml saline.

Dextran B-1355, a branched glucose polymer derived from *Leuconostoc mesenteroides* (NRRL-B-1355) was prepared in our laboratory according to the method of Jeanes et al. (21). For immunization, mice were given a single injection (i.p.) of an optimally immunogenic dose (100 μg) in 0.2 ml saline. It should be noted that the antibody response to this antigen is directed against the α 1,3 determinant of the molecule (3, 4).

Trinitrophenyl (TNP)-SS-III was prepared by first making an amino derivative of SSS-III using a modification of the method of Jones et al. (22). Here, 50 mg of SSS-III (10 mg/ml in borate-saline buffer, pH 8.0) was placed in a beaker kept in an ice bath. Then 0.67 ml (0.1 moles) of a solution of ethylene diamine, and 0.25 ml of 0.1 M sodium metaperiodate were added with constant stirring. After one minute, 1.25 ml of 2.0 M sodium borohydride was added and the mixture was stirred for one hour; at the end of this time period, the solution was dialyzed extensively against several changes of borate-saline buffer. After dialysis, 10 μM of 2, 4, 6-trinitrobenzene sulfonic acid, in a volume of 0.2 ml borate-saline buffer, was added to a 2.0 ml portion of the dialyzed amino derivative (2 mg/ml); the mixture was stirred at room temperature for one hour, after which it was dialyzed against several changes of borate-saline buffer. The number of TNP groups present *per* mole of SSS-III (average molecular size 100,000) was determined spectrophotometrically (34) and found to be 11 TNP groups *per* mole of SSS-III (TNP_{11}-SSS-III). For immunization mice were given a single injection (i.p.) of 0.05 μg TNP_{11}-SSS-III in 0.5 ml saline.

Horse erythrocytes (HRBC), collected in Alsever's solution, were obtained from the Ungulate Unit of the Veterinary Resources Branch of the NIH, Bethesda, MD. Prior to use, the cells were washed several times with saline and adjusted to a 10% (v/v) suspension. For immunization, mice were given a single injection (i.p.) of 0.2 ml of the cell suspension.

Detection of antibody-producing cells

Numbers of antibody-producing plaque-forming cells (PFC), specific for each of the antigens used in this work, provided a measure of the magnitude of the antibody response produced after immunization. In this procedure, each plaque or area of complete lysis is the product of single cells synthesizing and secreting antibody specific for the immunizing antigen. PFC making antibody of the IgM class were detected by a slide version of the technique of localized hemolysis-in-gel (10) using indicator sheep erythrocytes sensitized with SSS-III (10), TNP (34) or dextran B-1355 (25) by conventional methods; unsensitized HRBC were used for the detection of PFC making antibody specific for this antigen. In all cases, only PFC specific for the immunizing antigen are considered; such values were obtained by subtracting background PFC counts for unsensitized sheep erythrocytes. The results obtained, which are log-normally distributed (18), are expressed as the geometric mean of the $\log_{10}$ number of PFC/spleen for groups of similarly treated mice. Student's *t* test was used to assess the significance of the differences observed; differences were considered to be significant when probability (p) values of <0.05 were obtained.

Other materials

Concanavalin-A (Con-A) was purchased from Pharmacia Fine Chemicals, Piscataway, NJ. It was dissolved at a concentration of 1 mg/ml in saline and given i.v. in a volume of 0.1 - 0.2 ml.

RESULTS

Characteristics of the phenomenon of low-dose paralysis

Mice were pretreated (primed) with a single injection (i.p.) of a marginally immunogenic dose of 0.005 μg) of antigen and the magnitude of the PFC response produced was assessed, 5 days after immunization. The results obtained were compared to those for mice, not given a low dose of SSS-III prior to immunization.

The data of Table I, which are typical of those described in earlier studies (7, 9), show that pretreatment with an extremely low dose of SSS-III results in a significant ($p <0.005$) decrease in the capacity of mice to respond to subsequent immunization with an optimally immunogenic dose of antigen. Such unresponsiveness, which persists for several weeks or months after priming with a single injection of SSS-III (30), has been termed low-dose paralysis (7, 9) in contrast to the longer lasting form of unresponsiveness (high-dose paralysis) regularly produced in mice given much larger doses (> 50 μg) of SSS-III (15). Low-dose paralysis to SSS-III has been induced in every strain of mice examined thus far; thisincludes approximately 24 different strains of inbred mice. Therefore, it is a general phenomenon, the expression of which is not dependent upon the major histocompatibility (H-2) type of the strain of mice employed or the capacity to respond to SSS-III (3, 4).

In order to establish the minimal dose of antigen required to induce low-dose paralysis, mice were primed with a single injection (i.p.) of different amounts (0.005-0.05 μg) of SSS-III. Three days later, they were immunized with an optimally immunogenic dose (0.5 μg) of antigen and the magnitude of the PFC response produced was measured, 5 days after immunization; the values obtained were compared to those for immunized (unprimed) controls. A significant ($p <0.005$) reduction in the capacity of mice to response to an optimally immunogenic dose of SSS-III was noted with all priming doses examined (Figure 1). Reductions of 47.2%, 94.5% and 98.8% were obtained for mice primed with 0.005 μg, 0.005 μg of SSS-III, respectively. Since priming with 0.005 μg of SSS-III regularly induces convincing (>80%) unresponsiveness without the formation of detectable serum antibody (2, 4, 7, 9), this dose of antigen was selected for routine use in subsequent studies.

If mice are given 0.005 μg of SSS-III either at the same time or within 2-4 hrs before immunization with 0.5 μg SSS-III, low-dose paralysis is not expressed; thus, some period of time must elapse between priming and subsequent immunization for low-dose paralysis to be induced (7). In order to obtain more precise information on the

TABLE I

Effect of Prior Treatment with a Marginally Immunogenic Dose of SSS-III on the Magnitude of the PFC Response to an Optimal Dose (The Phenomenon of Low-dose Paralysis)

Treatment		
Priming Dose[1]	Immunizing Dose	SSS-III Specific PFC/Spleen
—	0.5 μg SSS-III	4.285 ± 0.083[2] (19,290)
0.005 μg SSS-III	0.5 μg SSS-III	3.051 ± 0.185 (1,124)

1 Mice were given a single injection (i.p.) of 0.005 μg SSS-III, 3 days before immunization (i.p.) with 0.5 μg SSS-III

2 Log_{10} PFC/spleen ± S.E.M. for 10 mice, 5 days after immunization; geometric mean are in parentheses.

length of this inductive period, mice were primed with 0.005 μg of SSS-III at different time intervals before immunization with an optimally immunogenic dose of antigen; values for PFC/spleen were determined, 5 days after immunization and the results obtained were compared to those for unprimed immunized mice (controls) to calculate the percent suppression observed for each time interval considered. The data of Table 2 show that significant low-dose paralysis (about 23%) is demonstrable as early as 12 hrs after priming with a low-dose of antigen; the degree of paralysis expressed increases with the length of the inductive period and is maximally expressed within 48-72 hrs after priming. These findings are in complete agreement with the results of other kinetic studies showing that suppressor T cells are activated within 24 hrs after immunization and reach maximal activity at about 72 hrs (23).

Specificity of low-dose paralysis

Groups of mice were primed with 0.005 μg of SSS-III. Three days later they were immunized with 0.5 μg SSS-III, as well as an optimally immunogenic dose of either dextran B-1355 (100 μg) or horse erthrocytes (HRBC). The magnitude of the PFC response produced in response to each immunizing antigen was assayed, 4-5 days after immunization and compared to that of mice, not given a low dose of SSS-III before immunization. The data of Table 3 show that, although priming with a low dose of SSS-III greatly reduced the capacity of mice to respond

TABLE II

Time Required for the Induction of Low-Dose Paralysis to SSS-III

Time of Priming[1]	% Decrease in the Magnitude of the PFC Response[2]
-12 hrs	22.8 ± 7.2
-18 hrs	55.1 ± 9.4
-24 hrs	67.6 ± 5.7
-48 hrs	85.0 ± 7.2
-72 hrs	84.2 ± 4.4

1 Time relative to immunization with 0.5 μg SSS-III at which mice were primed with 0.005 μg SSS-III.

2 % decrease in SSS-III-specific PFC/spleen ± S.E.M. for groups of 10 mice immunized with 0.5 μg SSS-III. Unprimed mice immunized with 0.5 μg SSS-III served as controls.

TABLE III

Effect of Inducing Low-dose Paralysis on the PFC Response to Both SSS-III and Dextran

Priming[1]	Immunization: SSS-III	Immunization: Dextran	PFC/Spleen vs SSS-III	PFC/Spleen vs Dextran
-	0.5 μg	100 μg	3.889 ± 0.083[2] (7,753)	5,052 ± 0.040 (112,762)
0.005 μg SSS-III	0.5 μg	100 μg	2.525 ± 0.308 (422)	5.038 ± 0.052 (109,032)

1 0.005 μg of SSS-III was given (i.p.), 3 days before immunization (i.p.) with both SSS-III and Dextran.

2 Log_{10} PFC/spleen ± S.E.M. for 10 mice, 5 days after immunization with both SSS-III and dextran.

to an optimally immunogenic dose of SSS-III ($p < 0.005$), it had no significant effect ($p > 0.05$) on the antibody response to dextran, the second immunizing antigen. Similar results were obtained in the case of primed mice immunized with both SSS-III and HRBC (Table 4); only the PFC response to an optimally immunogenic dose of SSS-III was reduced ($p < 0.005$) as a consequence of priming.

In another study, mice primed with 0.005 μg SSS-III were immunized with 0.05 μg of TNP_{11}-SSS-III and the magnitude of the PFC response to both TNP and SSS-III was determined 4 days later; the results obtained were compared to those of unprimed mice immunized with 0.05 μg TNP_{11}-SSS-III. The data of Table 5 show that priming with a lose dose of SSS-III greatly reduced the magnitude of the PFC response to SSS-III ($p < 0.005$); however, it had no effect on the magnitude of the TNP response produced ($p > 0.05$). This was also the case, even in mice given a large dose (50 μg) of SSS-III to induce high-dose paralysis (Table 6). All of the above studies clearly attest to the fact that the expression of low-dose paralysis is highly antigen-specific. Such unresponsiveness cannot be directed to other haptenic groups covalently bound to SSS-III, the immunizing antigen.

TABLE IV

Effect of Inducing Low-Dose Paralysis on the PFC Response to Both SSS-III and HRBC

	Immunization		PFC/spleen vs	
Priming[1]	SSS-III	HRBC	SSS-III	HRBC
–	0.5 μg	0.2 ml 10%	4.101 ± 0.058 (12,627)	4.709 ± 0.063 (51,139)
0.005 μg SSS-III	0.5 μg	0.2 ml 10%	2.958 ± 0.342 (907)	4.908 ± 0.038 (80,898)

1 0.005 μg of SSS-III was given (i.p.), 3 days before immunization (i.p.) with both SSS-III and HRBC.

2 Log_{10} PFC/spleen ± S.E.M. for 10 mice, 4 days after immunization with both SSS-III and HRBC.

Relationship between low-dose paralysis and Con-A induced suppression

The results of a previous study (28) showed that the i.p. injection of a single dose of Con A, at the time of immunization (i.p.) with SSS-III, caused a profound suppression in the magnitude of the PFC response to SSS-III; both the degree of suppression observed and the kinetics for the expression of such suppression resembled that observed following the induction of low-dose paralysis (28). In order to determine whether such suppression may have been due to an interaction between Con A and SSS-III, both of which were given i.p., we decided to examine whether suppression would also be obtained if SSS-III and Con-A were given by different routes. To this end, mice were given a single injection (i.v.) of different amounts of Con A at the time of immunization (i.p.) with an optimally immunogenic dose (0.5 μg) of SSS-III; numbers of PFC/spleen were determined, 5 days later and compared to those of mice, not treated with Con A. The data of Table 7 show that significant ($p < 0.05$) suppression of the PFC response to SSS-III was obtained with all doses of Con A tested; such suppression was dose-dependent and increased with the dose of Con A employed. Thus, the ability of Con A to induce suppression appeared to be independent of the route of injection.

TABLE V

Effect of Inducing Low-Dose Paralysis on the PFC Response to SSS-III and TNP in Mice Immunized with TNP_{11}-SSS-III

Treatment[1]		PRC/Spleen vs	
SSS-III	TNP_{11}-SSS-III	SSS-III	TNP
-	0.05 μg	3.734 ± 0.058[2] (5,423)	3.650 ± 0.120 (4,464)
0.005 μg	0.05 μg	2.105 ± 0.262 (127)	3.727 ± 0.076 (5,329)

1 0.005 μg SSS-III was given (i.p.), 4 days before immunization (i.p) TNP_{11}-SSS-III.

2 Log_{10} PFC/spleen $\pm$ S.E.M. for 10 mice, 4 days after immunization with TNP_{11}-SSS-III; geometric means are in parentheses.

TABLE VI

Effect of Inducing High-Dose Paralysis on the PFC Response to SSS-III and TNP in Mice Immunized with TNP_{11}-SSS-III

Treatment[1]		PFC/Spleen vs	
SSS-III	TNP_{11}-SSS-III	SSS-III	TNP
-	0.05 μg	4.020 ± 0.079[2] (10,479)	3.137 ± 0.163 (1,370)
50 μg	0.05 μg	0.961 ± 0.396 (9.1)	3.282 ± 0.148 (1,913)

1 50 μg of SSS-III was given (i.p.), 8 days before immunization (i.p.) with TNP_{11}-SSS-III.

2 Log_{10} ± S.E.M. for 10 mice, 4 days after immunization with TNP_{11}-SSS-III; geometric means are in parentheses.

In order to compare the kinetics for the expression of both low-dose paralysis and Con A-induced suppression, mice were given a single injection (i.v.) of 150 μg of Con A at the time of immunization with 0.5 μg SSS-III; numbers of PFC/spleen were determined at 2, 3, 4, 5 and 6 days after immunization and the results obtained were compared to those for (a) mice immunized with 0.5 μg SSS-III, 3 days after priming with 0.005 μg of SSS-III (low-dose paralysis), and (b) mice given only 0.5 μg SSS-III (immunized unprimed controls). The data of Figure 2 show that the expression of both Con A-induced suppression and low-dose paralysis followed an identical kinetic pattern; in both cases, suppression was first noted, 3 days after immunization and was most pronounced at about 4-5 days after immunization. Furthermore, the degree of suppression found was similar in both instances. These findings are in agreement with those reported in an earlier study (28), in which Con A was given intraperitoneally and further attest to the fact that the type of suppression induced by Con A is similar in both degree and the kinetics for its expression to the unresponsiveness observed following the induction of low-dose paralysis. The kinetics for the expression of Con-A-induced suppression are also independent of the route of administration of Con A.

DISCUSSION

Thymus-derived (T) lymphocytes are known to exert significant suppressive or inhibitory effects on the expression of a variety of

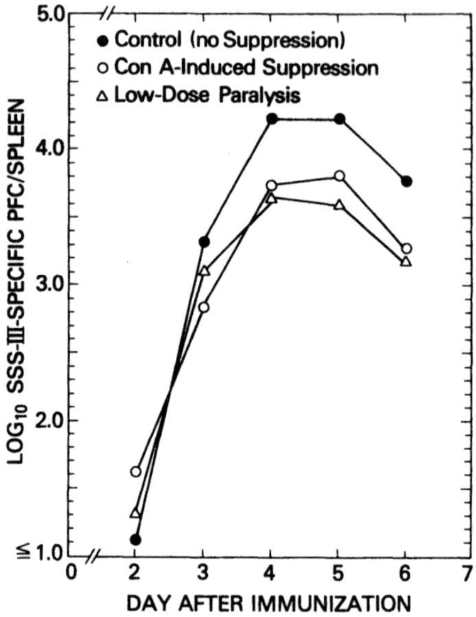

Fig. 1. Effect of priming with different low doses of SSS-III on the magnitude of a 5 day PFC response to an optimally immunogenic dose (0.5 μg) of SSS-III. The data shown represent the mean ± S.E.M. for groups of 10 mice, immunized 3 days after priming. Values in parentheses represent the mean percent suppression observed with reference to control (unprimed) mice.

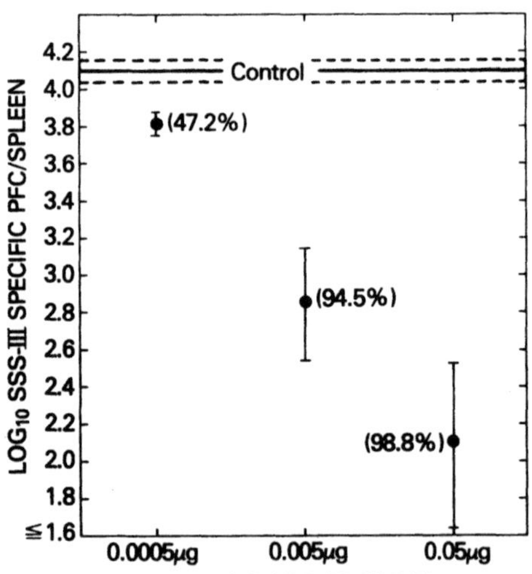

Fig. 2. Kinetics for the expression of Con A-induced suppression and low-dose paralysis. Each data point represents the mean value for groups of 10 similarly treated mice.

immune responses (11); however, such effects are not always antigen-specific. Among these effects might be included the phenomenon of antigenic-competition, in which prior exposure or immunization with one antigen will alter the magnitude and/or the quality of an antibody response to another unrelated antigen (17, 27); carrier-induced suppression, in which pretreatment with a carrier will suppress the magnitude of an antibody response to hapten bound to the same carrier molecule (31, 35, 36); and, the suppression observed after treatment with various T cell stimulants such as allogeneic cells (12,33) or Concanavalin-A (32, 33). To date, neither the T cell product(s) nor the mechanisms involved in the expression of these inhibitory effects have been defined.

Low-dose paralysis to SSS-III (Table 1) represents one of the first examples described of immunological unresponsiveness mediated by suppressor T cells (5, 7, 9). This form of unresponsiveness which is demonstrable for several weeks or months after prior ex-

TABLE VII

Suppression of the PFC Response to SSS-III by Treatment with Concanavalin-A (Con A)

Dose of Con-A[1]	SSS-III-Specific PFC/Spleen[2]	% Suppression[3]
0	4.020 ± 0.053 (10,480)	-
50 μg	3.739 ± 0.071 (5,488)	47.5
100 μg	3.635 ± 0.064 (4,312)	58.9
150 μg	3.413 ± 0.112 (2,589)	75.3

1 Con-A was given (i.v.) at the time of immunization (i.p.) with SSS-III.

2 Log_{10} PFC/spleen ± S.E.M. for 10 mice, 5 days after immunization with 0.5 μg SSS-III.

3 Relative to control group, i.e., mice not given Con-A

posure (priming) to a single sub-immunogenic dose of antigen (30), requires T cells in order to be induced and can be eliminated by treatment with T cell-depleting agents (5, 7, 9). The ability to induce low-dose paralysis in mice unable to make a serum antibody response to SSS-III attests to the fact that it is not due to the formation of circulating antigen-antibody complexes or to antibody-mediated feedback inhibition (29). In the present work, the phenomenon of low-dose paralysis was examined in great detail with respect to antigen-specificity as well as the kinetics for its induction and expression to determine whether similarities exist between this form of unresponsiveness and that induced by Concanavalin-A (Con-A), a non-specific stimulator of T cells.

Previous studies have shown that priming with a subimmunogenic dose of SSS-III, which reduces the capacity of mice to make an antibody response after subsequent immunization with SSS-III, does not influence the antibody response to serologically unrelated antigens (9). This suggests that low-dose paralysis is antigen-specific with respect to its induction. But, the possibility remained that a second injection of SSS-III (subsequent immunization) might lead to the more active synthesis and release of inhibitory products from primed T cells; such products could then suppress the magnitude of antibody responses to other antigens given at the time of immunization with SSS-III. The results of the present work show that this does not occur in the case of primed mice immunized with SSS-III in addition to dextran (Table 3) and HRBC (Table 4). More important, unlike the phenomenon of carrier-induced suppression of the antibody response to a hapten (TNP) bound to SSS-III (Tables 5 and 6). These findings clearly show that low-dose paralysis is antigen-specific with respect to both its induction and expression. Also, the results obtained with TNP_{11}-SSS-III (Tables 5 and 6) negate the possibility that low-dose paralysis is due simply to physical factors such as the sequestration of immunogenic amounts of antigen by primed T cells, or the formation of an "antigen bridge" between antigen-stimulated suppressor T cells and antibody-forming B cells.

Although significant unresponsiveness could be detected in mice primed with as little as 0.0005 μg of SSS-III, profound low-dose paralysis was regularly expressed in mice primed with 0.005 μg of SSS-III (Figure 1); the latter constitutes a marginally immunogenic dose of SSS-III since it is capable of eliciting only an extremely low PFC response - at best - in less than 50% of all primed mice (9). The induction of low-dose paralysis was evident as early as 12 hrs after priming; but, the degree of unresponsiveness attained increased progressively with time after priming and did not reach maximal levels until 48-72 hrs after priming (Table 2). Consequently, in all definitive experiments, mice were immunized with an optimally immunogenic dose of SSS-III, 3 days after priming with 0.005 μg of SSS-III; these appear to be the optimal conditions for demonstrating low-dose paralysis to SSS-III.

The kinetics for the expression of low-dose paralysis parallel those for the expression of Con-A induced suppression (Figure 2); in both instances an inhibitory or suppressive effect is first noted, 3 days after immunization and is maximally expressed at about 5 days after immunization. Although this kinetic pattern suggests that both low-dose paralysis and Con-A induced suppression share a common mechanism by which unresponsiveness is expressed (28), low-dose paralysis is an antigen-specific phenomenon (Tables 3-6), whereas the suppression induced by treatment with Con-A is generally considered to be due to a non-specific stimulatory effect on T cells (14, 29, 32). How might this be explained? One possibility is that the same inhibitory product is synthesized and released by suppressor T cells in both situations; however, in the case of low-dose paralysis, a recognition mechanism exists to permit the activity of the inhibitory product to be focused upon a selected subpopulation (clone) of B cells. Such a recognition mechanism would then permit a low molecular weight non-specific product which is surely made in extremely small quantitities during the induction of low-dose paralysis, to act in a manner that appears to be highly antigen-specific. Since there is evidence to suggest that T cells are capable of recognizing SSS-III directly (11, 13, 16, 19, 20, 24, 26), the most likely possibility is that they recognize the idiotypic determinant of cell-associated antibody present on B cells stimulated by SSS-III; this would provide both an efficient means to focus the activities of suppressor T cells on selected clones of B cells and the high degree of antigen-specificity associated with the phenomenon of low-dose paralysis (4). Evidence is now being sought in support of this hypothesis.

REFERENCES

1. Asherson, G. L., and Zembala, M., 1975, Inhibitory T Cells. Current Topics. Microbiol. Immunol. 72: 55.

2. Baker, P. J., 1975, Homeostatic control of antibody responses: a model based on the recognition of cell-associated antibody by regulatory T cells. Transplant. Rev. 26: 3.

3. Baker, P. J., Amsbaugh, D. F., Prescott, B., and Stashak, P. W., 1976, Genetic control of the antibody response to Type III pneumococcal polysaccharide in mice. III. Analysis of genes governing the expression of regulatory T cell activity. J. Immunogenetics 3: 275.

4. Baker, P. J., Amsbaugh, D. F., Prescott, B., Stashak, P. W., and Rudbach, J. A., 1978, Multigenic control of the antibody response to Type III pneumococcal polysaccharide and other helper T cell independent antigens, p. 67-83. In H. Friedman, T. J. Linna, and P. E. Prier (ed.),"Infection, immunity and genetics". University Park Press, Baltimore, MD.

5. Baker, P. J., Burns, W. H., Prescott, B., Stashak, P. W., and Amsbaugh, D. F., 1974, The role of suppressor T cells in the development of low-dose paralysis to Type III pneumococcal polysaccharide, P. 493-502. In, D. H. Katz and B. Benacerraf (ed.), "Immunological tolerance: mechanisms and potential therapeutic applications. Academic Press, Inc., New York, NY.

6. Baker, P. J., and Stashak, P. W., 1969, Quantitative and qualitative studies on the primary antibody response to pneumococcal polysaccharides at the cellular level. J. Immunol. 103: 1342.

7. Baker, P. J., Stashak, P. W., Amsbaugh, D. F., and Prescott, B., 1971, Characterization of the antibody response to Type III pneumococcal polysaccharide at the cellular level. I. Dose-response studies on the effect of prior immunization on the magnitude of the antibody response. Immunology. 20: 469.

8. Baker, P. J., Stashak, P. W., Amsbaugh, D. F., and Prescott, B., 1971, Characterization of the antibody response to Type III pneumococcal polysaccharide at the cellular level. II. Studies on the relative role of antibody synthesis and release by antibody-producing cells. Immunology. 20: 481.

9. Baker, P. J., Stashak, P. W., Amsbaugh, D. F., and Prescott, B., 1974, Regulation of the antibody response to Type III pneumococcal polysaccharide. IV. Role of suppressor T cells in the development of low-dose paralysis. J. Immunol. 112: 2020.

10. Baker, P. J., Stashak, P. W., and Prescott, B., 1969, Use of erythrocytes sensitized with purified pneumococcal polysaccharides for the assay of antibody and antibody-producing cells. Appl. Microbiol. 17: 422.

11. Braley-Mullen, H., 1974, Regulatory role of T cells in IgG antibody formation and immune memory to Type III pneumococcal polysaccharide. J. Immunol. 113: 1909.

12. Byfield, P., Christie, G. H., Howard, J. G., 1973, Alternating potentiating and inhibitory effects of the GVH reaction on the formation of antibodies against a thymus-independent polysaccharide. (S-III). J. Immunol. 111:72.

13. Davies, A. J. S., Carter, R. L., Leuchars, E., Wallis, V., and Dietrick, F. M., 1970, The morphology of immune reactions in normal, thymectomyzed and reconstituted mice. III. Response to bacterial antigens, Salmonellar flagellar antigen, and pneumococcal polysaccharide. Immunology. 19: 945.

14. Dutton, R. W., 1972, Inhibitory and stimulatory effects of Concanavalin-A on the response of mouse spleen cell suspensions to antigen. I. Characterization of the inhibitory cell activity. J. Exp. Med. 136: 1445.

15. Felton, L. D., Kauffman, G., Prescott, B., and Ottinger, B., 1955, Studies on the mechanism of immunological paralysis induced in mice by pneumococcal polysaccharides. J. Immunol. 74: 17.

16. Gerety, R. J., Ferraresi, R. W., and Raffel, S. J., 1970, Polysaccharide in delayed hypersensitivity. I. Pneumococcal polysaccharide as inducer and elicitor of delayed reactivity in guinea pigs. J. Exp. Med. 131: 189.

17. Gershon, R. K., and Kondo, K., 1971, Antigenic competition between heterologous erythrocytes. I. Thymic dependency. J. Immunol. 106: 1524.

18. Gottlieb, C. F., 1974, Application of transformations to normalize the distribution of plaque-forming cells. J. Immunol. 113: 51.

19. Howard, J. G., Christie, G. H., Courtenay, B. M., Leuchars, E., and Davies, A. J. S., 1971, Studies on immunological paralysis. VI. Thymic-independence of tolerance and immunity to Type III pneumococcal polysaccharide. Cell. Immunol. 2: 614.

20. Humphrey, J. H., Parrott, D. M. V., and East, J., 1964, Studies on globulin and antibody production in mice at birth. Immunology 7: 419.

21. Jeanes, A., Wilham, C. A., and Miers, J. C., 1948, Preparation and characterization of dextran from Leuconostoc mesenteroides. J. Biol. Chem. 176:603.

22. Jones, J. M., Amsbaugh, D. F., and Prescott, B., 1976, Kinetics of the antibody response to Type III pneumococcal polysaccharides (SSS-III). I. Use of ^{125}I-labeled SSS-III to study serum antibody levels, as well as the distribution and excretion of antigen after immunization. J. Immunol. 116: 41.

23. Jones, J. M., Amsbaugh, D. F., Stashak, P. W., Prescott, B., Baker, P. J., and Alling, D. W., 1976, Kinetics of the antibody response to Type III pneumococcal polysaccharide. III. Evidence that suppressor cells function by inhibitory the recruitment and proliferation of antibody producing cells. J. Immunol. 116: 647.

24. Kurger, J., and Gershon, R. K., 1972, DNA synthetic response of thymocytes to a variety of antigens. J. Immunol. 108: 581.

25. Leon, M. A., Young, N. M., and McIntire, K. R., 1970, Immunochemical studies of the reaction between a mouse myeloma macroglobulin and dextrans. Biochem. 9: 1023.

26. Lerman, S. P., Roman, T. J., Mond, J. J., Heidelberger, M., and Thorbecke, G. T., 1975, Induction of primary and inhibition of secondary antibody responses to hapten conjugates of Type III pneumococcal polysaccharides. Cell. Immunol. 15: 321.

27. Liacopoulos, P., and Ben-Efraim, S., 1975, Antigenic competition. Prog. Allergy. 18: 97.

28. Markham, R. B., Stashak, P. W., Prescott, B., Amsbaugh, D. F., and Baker, P. J., 1977, Effect of Concanavalin A on lymphocyte interactions involved in the antibody response to Type III penumococcal polysaccharide. I. Comparison of the suppression induced by Con A and low-dose paralysis. J. Immunol. 118: 952.

29. Markham, R. B., Stashak, P. W., Prescott, B., Amsbaugh, D. F., and Baker, P. J., 1978, Generation of low-dose paralysis in the absence of the ability to secrete antibody. J. Immunol. 120: 986.

30. Morse, H. C., III, Prescott, B., Cross, S. S., Stashak, P. W., and Baker, P. J., 1976, Regulation of the antibody response to Type III pneumococcal polysaccharide. V. Ontogeny of factors influencing the magnitude of the plaque-forming cell response. J. Immunol. 116: 279.

31. Okumura, K., and Tada, T., 1973, Suppression of the hapten-specific antibody response by carrier-specific T cells. Nature (New Biol.) 245: 180.

32. Pierce, C. W., and Kapp, J. A., 1975, Regulation of immune responses by suppressor T cells. Contemp. Top. Immunobiol. 5: 91.

33. Rich, S. S., and Rich, R. R., 1974, Regulatory mechanisms in cell-mediated immune responses. I. Regulation of mixed lymphocyte reactions by allo-antigen-activated thymus-derived lymphocytes. J. Exp. Med. 140: 1588.

34. Rittenberg, M. B., and Pratt, K. L., 1969, Anti-trinitrophenyl (TNP) plaque assay. Primary response of BALB/c mice to soluble and particulate immunogen. Proc. Soc. Exp. Biol. Med. 132: 575.

35. Tada, T., Taniguchi, M., and Takemori, T., 1975, Properties of primed suppressor T cells and their products. Transplant. Rev. 26: 106.

36. Tada, T., and Takemori, T., 1974, Selective roles of thymus-derived lymphocytes in the antibody response. I. Differential suppressive effect of carrier-primed T cells on the hapten-specific IgM and IgG antibody response. J. Exp. Med. 140: 239.

EFFECTS OF STAPHYLOCOCCAL CELL WALL PRODUCTS ON IMMUNITY

Roman Dziarski

Department of Microbiology, Immunology and Pathology
Pennsylvania College of Podiatric Medicine
Philadelphia, PA 19107

INTRODUCTION

A number of bacterial products from a variety of bacteria can affect a host's immunity by modulating its specific immune response and/or nonspecific resistance mechanisms. Staphylococcus aureus is a particularly good model for such studies, as it is a very ubiquitous microorganism present as normal flora on the mucous membranes and skin of man and animals, yet it is capable of causing serious infections in almost every part of the body. Staphylococcal cell wall is one of the important virulence factors of this microorganism, facilitating establishment and persistence of an infection (26, 36, 41-44, 70, 77, 78, 120, 121, 123, 167, 174, 176). Furthermore, even if the host's bactericidal mechanisms are efficient, staphylococcal cells or cell wall fragments can persist undegraded in the host's tissues for a long period of time (36, 48). It is conceivable that at both of these stages staphylococcal cell wall products can modulate the immunity of the host.

The major constituents of the S. aureus cell wall are: capsule, clumping factor, protein A, protein B, teichoic acid, and peptidoglycan. Their biological properties are summarized in Tables 1, 2, and 3.

CAPSULE

Capsule is found in 5 to 45% of S. aureus strains (174, 180). It is usually composed of acidic polysaccharides containing uronic acid, galactose, aminosugars, and some amino acids (39, 94, 147). Unusual aminosugars, e.g. D-aminogalacturonic acid, D-fucosamine, D-aminoglucuronic acid and D-aminomannuronic acid, are found in the

TABLE I

Biological properties of S. aureus cell wall constituents

Product	Properties	References
Capsule	Inhibition of phagocytosis	77,78,120,123,174,176
Clumping Factor	Paracoagulation	5,14,27,28,96,162
Protein A	Reaction with Fc fragment of immunoglobulins	45,49,72,89,91,98,119
	Complement activation	90,126,151,157-159
	Generation of chemotaxis	60,61
	Coagulation	181
	Platelet injury	61,62
	Inhibition of phagocytosis	26,43,44,121
	Hypersensitivity	54,55,63,64
	Histamine release from leukocytes	124
	Mitogenicity	7,46,128,136
	Polyclonal activation	105
	Induction of lymphocyte colonies	149
Teichoic acid	Hypersensitivity	101,102,179
	Immunosuppression	39
	Cytotoxicity	30, this paper
Peptidoglycan	See Tables 2 and 3	

capsular material, and capsules from different staphylococcal strains differ in their chemical composition (59,94,95,178). Capsule was shown to inhibit phagocytosis of staphylococci by interfering with effective opsonization (77, 78, 120,123,174,176).

CLUMPING FACTOR

Clumping factor is a protein with a molecular weight of 20,000 present on the surface of all S. aureus strains (162). It causes paracoagulation of human and animal plasma. The substrate for this reaction is fibrinogen or the soluble fibrin monomer complexes and the reaction results in clumping of staphylococci in the presence

TABLE II

In vivo biological properties of peptidoglycan (PG)

Property	Hosts	Microbial sources of PG	References
Adjuvanticity	Mouse, guinea pig, rat, rabbit	*Staphylococcus aureus*, *Staphylococcus epidermidis*, *Streptococcus pyogenes*, *Streptococcus mutans*, *Micrococcus roseus*, *Neisseria*, *Escherichia coli*, *Proteus*, *Moraxella*, *Bacillus megaterium*, *Bacillus cereus*, *Lactobacillus plantarum*, *Clostridium*, *Corynebacterium parvum*, *Mycobacterium smegmatos*. *Nocardia*. *Streptomyces*, *Brevibacterium divaricatum*	2-4, 34, 71 73, 75, 87, 108, 117, 118 126
Arthritogenicity	Rat, rabbit	*S. aureus*, *S. epidermidis*, *S. pyogenes*, *S. mutans*, *Streptococcus faecalis*, *Streptococcus salivarius*, *Streptococcus* gr. N, *L. plantarum*, *B. megaterium*, *Clostridium botulinum*, *Mycobacterium tuberculosis*, *M. smegmatis*, *Streptomyces*	20, 79-85, 146
Skin lesions: dermonecrosis, nodular aseptic abscesses	Rabbit, rat, guinea pig, humans	*S. aureus*, *S. epidermidis*, *S. pyogenes*, *Streptococcus* gr. B, C, D, E, *Gaffkya tetragena*, *B. cereus*, *Lactobacillus casei*, *Actinomyces*	1, 66-68, 99, 114, 141, 142, 145

Table II (continued)

Property	Hosts	Microbial sources of PG	References
		israeli, *Odontomyces viscosus*, *Chromobacterium violaceum*	
Chronic inflammatory lesions in heart	Mouse, rabbit	*S. pyogenes*, *S. aureus*	19, 36, 107, 115, 131
Chronic inflammatory lesions in liver	Mouse, rat	*S. aureus*, *S. pyogenes*, *Streptococcus* gr. D	19, 36, 69
Pyrogenicity	Rabbit	*S. aureus*, *S. epidermidis*, *S. pyogenes*, *Streptococcus* gr. B and L, *Streptococcus pneumoniae*, *E. coli*, *Spirillum serpens*	6, 37, 58, 68, 130-133
Virulence factor	Mouse, humans	*S. aureus*	36, 41, 42, 70, 167
Immediate hypersensitivity	Mouse guinea pig	*S. aureus*	31, 36, 56, 88, 126
Delayed hypersensitivity	Guinea pig, mouse	*S. aureus*, *S. pyogenes*, *Mycobacterium*	31, 36, 38, 56, 82, 126, 144, 164-166
Local Shwartzman reaction	Rabbit	*S. aureus*, *S. epidermidis*, *S. pyogenes*	129, 131

Table II (continued)

Property	Hosts	Microbial sources of PG	References
Leukopenia followed by leukocytosis	Rabbit	*S. pyogenes*	58
Increase in serum lysozyme level	Rabbit	*S. aureus*	37
Nonspecific resistance to bacterial infection	Mouse	*S. pyogenes*	132
Reticuloendothelial system stimulation	Mouse	*S. aureus*	30
Induction of colony stimulating factor	Mouse	*E. coli*	156
Generation of chemotaxis	Rabbit	*S. aureus*	53
Induction of interferon	Mouse	*Nocardia*	8
Immunosuppression	Mouse	*S. aureus*	32-34
Antitumor activity	Rat	*B. megaterium*	109

Table II (continued)

Property	Hosts	Microbial sources of PG	References
Increased capillary permeability	Guinea pig, rat	*S. pyogenes*	116
Sleep disturbance	Rat	*S. pyogenes*	103

TABLE III

In vitro biological properties of peptidoglycan

Property	Hosts	Microbial sources of PG	References
Mitogenicity	Mouse, rabbit, humans, rat	*S. aureus*, *B. megaterium*, *E. coli*, *Nocardia*	12, 13, 17, 22 34, 35, this paper
Polyclonal activation	Mouse, humans	*S. aureus*, *Nocardia*	10, 11, 93, this paper
Adjuvanticity	Mouse	*S. aureus*	34
Complement activation	Humans, guinea pig, mouse	*S. aureus*, *S. epidermidis*, *S. pyogenes*, *Micrococcus lysodeikticus*, *Micropolyspora faeni*	9, 50, 126, 154, 175

Table III (continued)

Property	Hosts	Microbial sources of PG	References
Generation of chemotaxis	Rabbit, humans	*S. aureus*, *S. pyogenes*, *Bordetella pertussis*	53, 68, 139
Macrophage activation	Mouse, rat	*S. pyogenes*	25, 152
Promotion of opsonization	Humans	*S. aureus*, *M. lysodeikticus*	74, 122, 148, 176
Macrophage and leukocyte migration Inhibition	Rat, guinea pig, mouse, humans	*S. aureus*, *S. epidermidis*, *S. pyogenes*, *Streptococcus* gr. B	15, 52, 65-67, 165, 169
Inhibition of phagocytosis	Rabbit, rat	*S. pyogenes*	76, 153
Toxicity for phagocytes and kidney cells	Mouse, rabbit	*S. aureus*, *S. pyogenes*	30, 76
Immunosuppression	Mouse	*S. aureus*	33
Thrombocytolysis	Rabbit, rat	*S. aureus*, *S. pyogenes*, *S. pneumoniae*	127, 134, 135
Release of endogenous viruses	Mouse	*Nocardia*	125

Table III (continued)

Property	Hosts	Microbial sources of PG	References
Gelation of Limulus lysate	Horseshoe crab	*S. aureus*, *S. epidermidis*, *S. pyogenes*, *M. lysodeikticus*	173

of plasma (5, 14, 27, 28, 96, 162). The biological significance of this phenomenon has not been fully explained and is discussed elsewhere (162). It is conceivable, however, that clumping of staphylococci may interfere with phagocytosis.

PROTEIN A

Protein A is a major protein component of *S. aureus* cell walls (112, 150). Its molecular weight is about 42,000. It is not present in *Staphylococcus epidermidis* and *Micrococcus* strains. In *S. aureus* it is found in 90% of human strains, but it is not usually present in strains isolated from animals (with the exception of cows) (57).

Protein A (Table 1) can react nonspecifically with the Fc fragment of immunoglobulins, primarily of the IgG class, but also IgA and IgM (45, 49, 72, 89, 91, 98, 119), and most of its biological activities are in vivo or in vitro consequences of this reaction. Protein A - immunoglobulin complexes can activate complement (90, 126, 151, 157-159), which in turn can lead to a generation of chemotactic factors (60, 161), blood coagulation (181), platelet injury (61, 62), or release of histamine from leukocytes (124). Reaction of protein A with immunoglobulins is also responsible for the inhibition of phagocytosis of staphylococci (26, 43, 44, 121) and symptoms of immediate hypersensitivity (54, 55, 63). Protein A can also induce and elicit delayed hypersensitivity (63, 64).

Protein A is mitogenic for human T and B lymphocytes (7, 46, 128, 136) and is a polyclonal B cell activator in mice (105). These properties are probably not related to its ability to interact with the Fc fragment of immunoglobulins (105). Protein A can also induce the formation of lymphocyte colonies from human cord and peripheral blood (149). It is not known, however, whether this activity is related to the Fc-binding property of protein A.

S. aureus cell wall also contains a small amount of protein B (113). Its physicochemical properties are similar to the properties of protein A but it does not react with the Fc fragment of immunoglobulins. At present, its biological activities and significance are not known.

TEICHOIC ACID AND PEPTIDOGLYCAN

Teichoic Acid

The majority of *S. aureus* strains possess ribitol teichoic acid (TA), composed of 7 to 36 phosphoribitol units, with L-alanine and α- or β-N-acetylglucosamine as substituents (29, 137). It is bound to the muramic acid of peptidoglycan via three phosphoglycerol units (18). Sugar substituents of TA are the major antigenic determinants of staphylococcal cell walls. Anti-TA antibodies are found in normal human sera (24) and in patients with staphylococcal infections (21, 39, 100, 102, 106). This accounts for an immediate hypersensitivity to staphylococcal TA which is frequently observed in humans (101, 102, 179). Soluble complexes of TA with peptidoglycan fragments, that have a molecular weight of about 8,000, were often isolated from staphylococcal cells. They are usually referred to as polysaccharides. Depending on the type of teichoic acid and sugar substituents, they are known as polysaccharide A, B, C (H), P, V, and 187 (110, 111, 113). Their serological properties are similar to that of purified TA.

Purified TA's have very few biologic activities. Except for the above-mentioned hypersensitivity, staphylococcal TA was shown to suppress antibody response in mice (39) and to possess cytotoxic properties in vitro (30). However, high doses of TA were required to produce these effects. Our recent studies on other biological activities of TA will be discussed in the following sections of this monograph.

Lipoteichoic acids, which are membrane TA's combined with glycolipids or phospholipids of the cell membrane, have more biological activities than purified cell wall TA (171, 172), but since they are not cell wall components, a discussion of them is beyond the scope of this presentation.

Peptidoglycan

Peptidoglycan (PG) is a heteropolymer present in cell walls of bacteria, actinomycetes and blue-green algae (cyanobacteria) (138). It is composed of polysaccharide chains made up of N-acetylglucosamine and N-acetylmuramic acid residues, linked by β-1, 4 glycosidic bonds and cross-linked through short peptides. The peptide moiety of *S. aureus* PG is composed of L-alanine, D-glutamine, L-tyrosine, D-alanine and a pentaglycine bridge bound to an identical peptide of the adjacent PG chain. PG from different bacteria differ in the composition of the peptide part of the molecule and the extent of cross-linking between the adjacent chains (138).

Peptidoglycans possess numerous biological activities which in the last decade were the subject of intensive research, and detailed reviews of the biology of PG have been published (65, 68, 129). For this reason, I will only present a brief review of all the activities of PG and then concentrate on our own recent studies on the effects of staphylococcal PG on immunity. Various in vivo and in vitro biological properties of PG are summarized in Tables 2 and 3. It is apparent that PG can modulate both specific immune responses and nonspecific resistance mechanisms in a variety of in vivo and in vitro systems. The arrangement of different activities of PG in these tables is quite arbitrary and has been designed to illustrate the research efforts devoted to each property and their related biological significance (as judged by the author).

Relation of Peptidoglycan Structure to Activity

Because of the similar structure, PG from different bacteria possess similar biological properties. Most of the activities listed in Tables 2 and 3 are also associated with staphyloccal PG. It should be noted also that various PG preparations, differing in molecular size, homogeneity, solubility, and purity, were used in the above studies. For a number of biological activities, e.g. complement activation, mitogenicity, or arthritogenicity, the molecular size of the PG preparation was of crucial importance. Until now it was possible to define the exact chemical structure and molecular weight of PG fragments responsible for a given biological activity in only a few cases. The best examples are the studies on the adjuvant properties of PG that associated this activity with the soluble monomeric subunits composed of sugar-peptide complexes (3, 108). Subsequent experiments on the synthetic analogues of naturally occurring PG defined N-acetyl-muramyl-L-alanyl-D-isoglutamine (MDP, for muramyl dipeptide) as the smallest adjuvant-active molecule (4, 87, 104). This discovery provoked an extensive research effort aimed at characterization of other biological properties of MDP and synthesis of other biologically active MDP analogues (reviewed in 16). The properties and application of these synthetic compounds are discussed by Chedid (this volume).

Studies on the relationships between the structure and other activities of PG are less advanced. It appears, however, that different PG fragments, or at least fragments of different molecular weight, are responsible for different activities of PG. The minimal structure required for the induction of an adjuvant arthritis in rats is composed of at least two or more disaccharide units; however, more severe symptoms required larger molecules. Disaccharide-peptide fragments were not active (79, 80, 85).

The minimal structure of staphylococcal PG active in migration inhibition of peritoneal macrophages from unsensitized guinea pigs was a complex of N-acetylamino-sugars and peptide with a molecular weight of approximately 1,000. Smaller molecules (trisaccharides, tetrasaccharides, monomeric pentpeptides, two tetrapeptides linked by a pentaglycine bridge, and N-aceylmuramic acid-peptide) had no activity (52).

The generation of chemotaxis by PG occurs via activation of complement and the release of complement split products with chemotactic properties. For this activity a molecular weight of about 2,000 was a critical lower limit for the PG molecule (53).

Association of the other activities of PG with chemically defined structures and molecular weight is much less certain. Pyrogenic activity appears to be associated with the MDP molecule (86) but this needs to be confirmed. The structure responsible for the mitogenic activity appears to depend on the bacterial source of PG, animal species studied, and the culture conditions. MDP was distinctly mitogenic for guinea pig lymphocytes (163), while it had a very weak, if any, blastogenic activity for mouse lymphocytes (155, 163). However, 4 or 5 day cultures in a serum-free medium supplemented with 2-mercaptoethanol rendered MDP mitogenic for mouse lymphocytes (23). This may indicate potentiation of mitogenic properties of 2-mercaptoethanol by MDP. Fragments of Nocardia PG solubilized by lysostaphin treatment were mitogenic for both mouse and rabbit lymphocytes (17), indicating that intact glycan strands substituted by tetra- or tripeptides are required for the mitogenic activity. Soluble fragments of staphylococcal PG, obtained by extensive disintegration of PG with ultrasonics, were not mitogenic for murine or human lymphocytes (34, Dziarski, Dziarski, and Levinson, unpublished). The minimal structure required for the mitogenic activity of staphylococcal PG remains, therefore, to be determined, especially as the peptide part of PG from Gram-positive cocci is different from that of Gram-negative and Gram-positive rods (138).

Immunomodulating Activity

The majority of adjuvants act as immunomodulators and can either enhance or suppress the immune response, depending on the timing in relation to the antigenic stimulation and the dosage of both the antigen and immunomodulator (143, 170).

Staphylococcal PG (particulate preparation, used in most of our studies) was shown to suppress the primary IgM antibody response to sheep erythrocytes (SRBC) in mice when injected in a large dose (400 μg) before antigenic stimulation (Table 4) (32, 34). Both the delay in the antibody response and the overall decreased response were responsible for the suppression. PG did not suppress the antibody response to thymus-independent antigens. A small dose of PG (10 μg) was immunostimulatory in BALB/c mice (34) but was still immunosuppressive in Swiss mice (32). When PG was solubilized by extensive treatment with ultrasonics, it lost its immunosuppressive activity and both high and low doses were adjuvant-active when given either before or simultaneously with the antigenic stimulus (34).

Both particulate and soluble PG preparations were adjuvant-active for mouse splenocytes in vitro immunized with SRBC (34). A dose-dependent effect was observed and optimal adjuvant concentration of particulate PG was 25 μg/ml and of soluble PG - 200 μg/ml. Particulate PG was more active than the soluble PG and caused both an acceleration of the immune response and an overall increase in

TABLE IV

Effect of PG on in vivo anti-SRBC PFC response in mice

	% of control PFC	
Treatment[a]	Swiss	BALB/c
Particulate PG, 400 μg		
Day 0	73	66[b]
Day -1	16[b]	27[b]
Day -2	21[b]	28[b]
Day -3	7[b]	74[b]
Day -5	79	n.t.[c]
Particulate PG, 10 μg		
Day 0	127	133[b]
Day -1	109	125[b]
Day -2	24[b]	103
Day -3	77	n.t.
Soluble PG, 400 μg		
Day 0	n.t.	184[b]
Day -1	n.t.	137[b]
Day -2	n.t.	156[b]
Day -3	n.t.	187[b]
Soluble PG, 10 μg		
Day 0	n.t.	165[b]
Day -1	n.t.	150[b]
Day -2	n.t.	105

[a] Mice received intravenous injection of SRBC on day 0 and of PG on day 0 or on one of the indicated days prior to SRBC injection; PFC's were assayed on day 4; from (32) and (34).

[b] Significantly different from control ($p < 0.05$).

[c] n.t., not tested.

the response during the 7 day culture period. The acceleration was not so apparent with soluble PG and an increase in the magnitude of the immune response was observed during the first 4 days of culture. Doses of PG up to 500 μg/ml were not directly suppressive for the in vitro immune response.

These results differ from the data recently reported for PG from Brevibacterium divaricatum (73). This soluble PG monomer was immunostimulatory in vivo but was not active in vitro. This discrepancy can be explained by the differences in the in vitro culture system used by these authors. This is consistent with the fact that in the culture systems similar to that used by us, MDP was shown to be active as an adjuvant (40, 97, 155). The exact mechanism of the adjuvant activity of PG is still not known. Recent studies on MDP identified T lymphocytes and macrophages as the mediators of its adjuvant activity (40, 97, 160). However, additional studies are required since there are also data suggesting a direct effect of MDP on B cells (92, 168). It remains to be elucidated which mechanism is responsible for the adjuvant activity of PG.

Studies on the mechanism of PG-induced immunosuppression (33) revealed that the suppression could be transferred into normal recipients by syngeneic spleen cells from PG-treated mice, while the transfer of spleen cell sonicates was not effective. Anti-SRBC plaque forming cell (PFC) response of in vitro immunized spleen cells from PG-treated mice was about 20% of the antibody response of splenocytes from untreated animals. Spleen cells from PG-injected mice suppressed the in vitro PFC response of normal splenocytes when added at the initiation of the cultures (Table 5). Living cells were required for the suppression and the early stage of the immune response was affected. Cell fractionation revealed that the adherent cells from PG-injected animals were immunosuppressive. These cells comprised 90% macrophages and could also be made immunosuppressive by in vitro treatment with PG. The exact mechanism of this suppression remains to be elucidated. Macrophages are known to regulate the immune responses by both secretion of immunoregulatory products and by direct contact with the responding lymphocytes (47, 177).

In Vivo Effect on Blastogenic Responsiveness

As indicated in the preceding section, in vivo PG treatment modulated the subsequent in vivo and in vitro antibody response. It was of interest to determine whether similar in vivo PG treatment would change the subsequent blastogenic responsiveness to a number of mitogens (Dziarski, manuscript in preparation). Mice were injected with different doses of PG (50-1,000 μg), and 2 days later the in vitro response to phytohemagglutinin (PHA), concanavalin A (Con A), lipopolysaccharide (LPS), and pokeweed mitogen (PWM) was studied. Such treatment caused a significant increase in the responsiveness to PHA and PWM, with a dose of 400 μg of PG being the most effective (two-fold increase). Responsiveness to Con A was also somewhat increased while the responsiveness to LPS in mice treated with 1,000 μg of PG was decreased. These changes were apparent both in terms of the stimulation indexes and the actual thymidine incorporation.

Response to PHA and LPS was chosen for further studies. It was shown that the increased PHA or decreased LPS responses were not due to a change in the kinetics of the response, but were observed over the entire culture period. Time kinetics studies also showed that the increased responsiveness to PHA in mice injected with 400 μg of PG lasted for several days, while the variations in the responsiveness to LPS were much smaller and less persistent (Fig. 1). Simultaneous monitoring of the background thymidine incorporation in the cultures of cells from PG injected mice revealed a 40% increase be tween days 5 and 14 after the PG treatment, which accounts for some decrease of the stimulation indexes at that time.

The mechanism of this increased responsiveness to mitogens in terms of the involvement of different cell types is not clear and is currently under investigation.

<u>Mitogenic Activity</u>

Staphylococcal PG is mitogenic for mouse splenocytes and human peripheral blood lymphocytes, and B lymphocytes are the PG-responding cells in mouse splenocyte cultures (Table 6) (35). Soluble PG is not mitogenic for either mouse splenocytes (34) or human peripheral blood lymphocytes (Dziarski, Dziarski and Levinson, unpublished). This indicated that the mitogenic activity of PG can be dissociated from its adjuvant activity, possibly suggesting different mechanisms responsible for these two phenomena (34).

The mitogenic effect of <u>S. aureus</u> purified cell wall (CW), which is a PG-TA complex, and TA alone on mouse, human and rat lymphocytes was also studied (Dziarski, Dziarski and Levinson, manuscript in preparation). CW was less mitogenic for mouse splenocytes than PG and at higher concentrations (50-400 μg/ml) it was actually cytotoxic, as indicated by a drop in the viability and an inhibition of the background thymidine incorporation (Table 7). TA was not mitogenic for mouse splenocytes and at higher concentrations it also caused a decrease in the viability and background DNA synthesis (Table 7).

Similar results were obtained with human peripheral blood lymphocytes (Table 8). CW was mitogenic at lower concentrations and it was toxic at a high concentration, while TA had no mitogenic activity, exhibiting toxic effects only.

TABLE V

Effect of spleen cells from PG-treated mice and macrophages cultured with PG on in vitro anti-SRBC PFC response[a]

Cells added to normal spleen cell cultures[b]	% of control response[c]
Normal spleen cells	112
Normal adherent cells	98
Cells from PG-injected mice	
spleen cells, day 0	66[d]
spleen cells, day +1	112
spleen cells, day +2	98
spleen cells, day +3	103
spleen cells, 56°, 30'	118
nonadherent cells	126
adherent cells	65[d]
Normal adherent cells cultured in vitro	106
Adherent cells cultured in vitro with PG	70[d]

[a] 10^7 spleen cells immunized with SRBC.

[b] 20% of spleen cells or nonadherent cells or 2% of adherent cells added.

[c] Mean of 8 to 28 cultures from 2 to 7 experiments.

[d] Significantly lower than control ($p < 0.05$).
From (33).

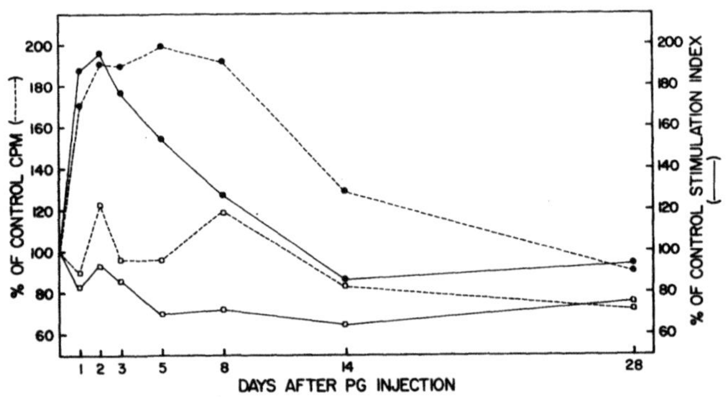

Fig. 1. Effect of in vivo PG treatment on in vitro blastogenic responsiveness. Groups of 3 mice were injected with 400 µg of PG and their mitogenic responses to PHA (●) and LPS (□), evaluated in quadruplicate cultures on the indicated days, were compared to the responses of uninjected controls. The values are means of two experiments. From: Dzarski (manuscript in preparation).

TABLE VI

Mitogenic effect of PG on mouse spleen lymphocytes

Stimulant added	Concen μg/ml	Stimulation index with the following cells		
		T + B	B[a]	T[b]
PG	1	1.8	4.0	1.0
	10	4.0	6.5	1.2
	50	9.7	13.0	1.5
	100	12.4	17.0	1.5
	400	25.7	27.4	1.4
	1,000	21.5	29.1	1.1
PHA	38	15.9	0.8	94.1
LPS	100	56.6	49.4	3.7

[a] Spleen cells from athymic nude mice.

[b] Spleen lymphocytes purified on glass wool and nylon wool columns. From (35).

PG was also mitogenic for rat splenic lymphocytes, while CW and TA were not mitogenic, showing toxic effects at high concentrations. The response of rat lymph node cells to PG was much lower than that of splenic lymphocytes, while CW and TA were again not mitogenic but had some cytotoxic activity. PG was not cytotoxic for mouse, human and rat lymphocytes.

From these studies it appears that TA when bound to PG can somehow mask the mitogenic activity of PG and render CW cytotoxic.

In Vitro Effect on Blastogenic Responsiveness

PG can modulate both the in vivo and in vitro immune response and is a potent mitogen. It was of interest to determine how it affects the blastogenic response to other mitogens. The effect of CW and TA on blastogenic responsiveness was also studied to determine whether the cytotoxic effect of these substances was strong enough to inhibit the blastogenic response of lymphocytes (Dziarski, Dziarski and Levinson manuscript in preparation).

Mouse lymphocyte cultures containing PHA or LPS and either PG, CW or TA were established, and the stimulation of these cultures was compared to the stimulation obtained in cultures treated with one mitogen only. To assess stimulation or suppression of the blastogenic response, an index used for the studies on synergistic

TABLE VII

Mitogenic effect of CW and TA on mouse spleen lymphocytes[a]

Stimulant added	Concen μg/ml	cpm	Viability % of control
None		3,446	
CW	1	8,929	95
	10	12,993	35
	50	646	19
	100	185	17
	400	128	8
None		1,392	
TA	1	2,295	117
	10	2,711	96
	50	1,721	75
	100	727	40
	400	176	33
PG	400	34,581	98
PHA	38	25,036	53
LPS	100	48,244	113

[a] Mean values determined from 8 cultures in 2 experiments.
From: Dziarski, Dziarski and Levinson (manuscript in preparation.

effects of two mitogens (140) was adapted (Table 9). If two mitogens were responding independently of each other the % of expected cpm for the cultures stimulated with these two mitogens would be 100%. If there is a synergistic effect, the value is more than 100%; if interference occurs, the value is less than 100%. Co-stimulation with PHA and PG (both at optimal mitogenic concentrations) resulted in inhibition of stimulation by one of the mitogens, even though PHA acts primarily on T cells, whereas PG is a B cell mitogen. Similar results were obtained with a low (mitogenic) concentration of CW, while higher concentrations of CW and TA significantly inhibited lymphocyte stimulation by PHA. Similar data were obtained with co-stimulation with LPS and staphylococcal fractions (Table 9).

The results of analogous co-stimulation experiments performed on human peripheral blood lymphocytes with PHA, Con A or PWM and PG or CW were essentially similar to the studies on mice (Table 10). The important difference was the effect of TA on the PHA and Con A responses. Co-stimulation of human lymphocytes with 50 μg/ml

TABLE VIII

Mitogenic effect of CW, TA and PG on human peripheral blood lymphocytes[a]

Stimulant added	Concen µg/ml	cpm	Viability % of control
None		1,394	
CW	1	2,905	93
	10	13,861	99
	50	11,160	73
	100	4,044	24
	400	128	0
TA	1	1,201	101
	10	1,069	86
	50	419	45
	100	172	28
	400	70	0.4
PG	400	18,757	105
PHA	0.12	27,974	218
Con A	1.5	24,815	142

[a] Mean values determined from 12 cultures in 3 experiments with lymphocytes from 3 different donors.

From: Dziarski, Dziarski and Levinson (manuscript in preparation).

of TA and PHA or Con A resulted in an increase (up to two-fold) in the blastogenic response. The significance of this phenomenon is presently not known and its mechanism is under investigation. An increase in the responsiveness of human lymphocytes to PHA and Con A by a non-mitogenic preparation of bacterial LPS was previously described (140).

Polyclonal Activation

The majority of B cell mitogens are also able to induce differentiation of lymphocytes resulting in the synthesis and secretion of polyclonal antibodies (polyclonal activation). The ability of staphylococcal PG to induce polyclonal activation was studied in mice and humans. An increase in the number of immunoglobulin-secreting cells was studied with an application of the reverse

TABLE IX

In vitro effect of PG, CW and TA on blastogenic response of mouse spleen cells to PHA and LPS

Mitogens (μg/ml)	% of expected cpm[a]
PHA + PG	53
PHA + CW (10)	62
PHA + CW (50)	5
PHA + CW (400)	0.6
PHA + TA (50)	5
PHA + TA (400)	0.7
LPS + PG	64
LPS + CW (10)	27
LPS + CW (50)	0.4
LPS + CW (400)	0.2
LPS + TA (50)	23
LPS + TA (400)	0.2

a

$$\% \text{ of expected cpm} = \frac{\text{net cpm (M1 + M2)}}{\text{net cpm M1 + Net cpm M2}} \times 100\%;$$ determined from 8 cultures in 2 experiments.

From: Dziarski, Dziarski, Levinson (manuscript in preparation).

hemolytic PFC assay (51) with protein A-coated SRBC as target cells and anti-immunoglobulin sera as developing reagents.

Four day cultures of mouse splenic lymphocytes with optimal concentrations of LPS (50 μg/ml) or PG (400 μg/ml) resulted in a substantial increase in the numbers of immunoglobulin secreting cells, as assayed by the reverse PFC assay (Table 11). PFC's were developed with an application of a polyvalent anti-immunoglobulin serum. Polyclonal activation of lymphocytes from both BALB/c and athymic nude (nu/nu) mice was observed, indicating that the effect was T cell independent. Pg was more effective than LPS. Application of specific anti-IgM, anti-IgG (IgG1 and IgG2a), and anti-IgA sera revealed the production of these three major immunoglobulin classes in PG and LPS stimulated cultures (Dziarski, unpublished).

PG was also a very effective polyclonal activator of human peripheral blood lymphocytes with the activity comparable to that of PWM (Table 12) (Levinson, Dziarski and Dziarski, unpublished). These data indicate that PG is a polyclonal B cell activator in humans.

TABLE X

In vitro effect of Pg, CW and TA on blastogenic responses of human peripheral blood lymphocytes to PHA, Con A and PWM

Mitogens (μg/ml)	% of expected cpm[a]
PHA + PG	80
PHA + CW (10)	68
PHA + CW (400)	1
PHA + TA (50)	197
PHA + TA (400)	57
Con A + PG	65
Con A + CW (10)	77
Con A + CW (400)	1
Con A + TA (50)	139
Con A + TA (400)	0.2
PWM + PG	25
PWM + CW (10)	47
PWM + CW (400)	0.3
PWM + TA (50)	55
PWM + TA (400)	0.2

a Determined from 8 cultures in 2 experiments with lymphocytes from 2 different donors; % of expected cpm was calculated as in Table 9.

From: Dziarski, Dziarski and Levinson (manuscript in preparation.

CONCLUSIONS AND PERSPECTIVES

From this brief review it is apparent that PG is biologically the most active part of the staphylococcal cell wall (Tables 2 and 3). Its properties include adjuvanticity, arthritogenicity, mitogenicity, polyclonal B cell activation, in vivo and in vitro toxicity, pyrogenicity, complement activation, enhancement of virulence, and activation of the reticuloendothelial system. Complexes of TA and PG, naturally occurring in staphylococcal cell wall, have somewhat different properties than purified PG. They are more toxic and can persist longer in tissues causing more chronic inflammatory changes. They are also less mitogenic and less stimulatory for the reticuloendothelial system.

Peptidoglycan can affect nonspecific resistance mechanisms and modulate activities of various compartments of the specific immune response. However, the exact mechanism(s) of its action is

TABLE XI

Polyclonal activation of mouse spleen lymphocytes by PG and LPS[a]

Lymphocyte donor	Stimulant	Igs PFC/10^4 ± SEM[b]
BALB/c	None	98 ± 10
	LPS	505 ± 46
	PG	719 ± 23
nu/nu	None	152 ± 7
	LPS	542 ± 27
	PG	818 ± 31

[a] Cultures of 5×10^5 spleen cells were incubated for 4 days with the indicated material (LPS, 50 μg/ml; PG, 400 μg/ml) and assayed for immunoglobulin-secreting cells (Igs PFC) with protein A-coated SRBC and polyvalent anti-immunoglobulin serum (51).

[b] Means of 4 cultures.

From: Dziarski (unpublished).

TABLE XII

Polyclonal activation of human peripheral blood lymphocytes by PG and PWM[a]

Stimulant added	Igs PFC/10^4 with the following donors		
	N.M.	D.A.	M.A.
None	1	21	12
PG	164	132	240
PWM	291	134	206

[a] Cultures of 10^6 lymphocytes were incubated for 5 days with the indicated material PG, 400 μg/ml; PWM, 1:1000) and assayed as described in footnote "a" to Table XI; 4 cultures of cells from each donor were pooled before the assay.

From: Levinson, Dziarski, and Dziarski (unpublished).

(are) not known. Future studies should concentrate on defining its active structures and the mechanisms of action in terms of the cell types involved, the cell receptors interacting with the defined PG structures, and an induction of mediators of its activities. The differences between the activities of PG and CW (PG-TA complex) should also be studied, since under natural conditions of staphylococcal infection the host is usually exposed to CW rather than purified PG.

Protein A also possesses a number of interesting biological activities (Table 1), most of them affecting nonspecific resistance mechanisms. Its effects on the specific immune response, as well as the mechanisms of action, are certainly worth investigating. Due to its interaction with the Fc fragment of immunoglobulins, protein A is also an extremely useful immunological reagent.

Precise characterization of the interactions between the immune system and the above mentioned bacterial products will provide a valuable tool for studying immunoregulatory mechanisms or the function of lymphocytes in different immunologic disorders.

ACKNOWLEDGEMENTS

I am grateful to my wife, Agnes, and Arnol Levinson for stimulating collaboration and performing the experiments on human lymphocytes, to David Axler for his critical comments and reviewing the manuscript, and to Ann Rulinski for her skillful secretarial assistance.

This work was supported by grants from the National Foundation for Infectious Diseases and the Pennsylvania College of Podiatric Medicine.

REFERENCES

1. Abdulla, E. M., and Schwab, J. H., 1966, Biological properties of streptococcal cell wall particles. III. Dermonecrotic reaction to cell wall mucopeptides. J. Bacteriol. 91: 374.

2. Adam, A., Ciorbaru, R., Petit, J. F., Lederer, E., Chedid, L., Lamensans, A., Parant, F., Parant, M., Rosselet, J. P., and Berger, F. M., 1973, Preparation and biological properties of water-soluble adjuvant fractions from delipidated cells of Mycobacterium smegmatis and Nocardia opaca. Infect. Immun. 7: 855.

3. Adam, A., Ciorbaru,R., Elluoz, F., Petit, J. F., and Lederer, E., 1974, Adjuvant activity of monomeric bacterial cell wall peptidoglycans. Biochem. Biophys. Res. Commun. 56: 561.

4. Adamm A., Elluoz, F., Ciorbaru, R., Petit, J. F., and Lederer, E., 1975, Peptidoglycan adjuvants: minimal structure required for activity. *Z. Immunitaetsforsch. Exp. Klin. Immunol*. 149: 341.

5. Allington, J. M., 1967, Fibrinogen and fibrin degradation products and the clumping of staphylococci in serum. *Brit. J. Haematol.* 13: 550.

6. Atkins, E., and Morse, S. I., 1967, Studies in staphylococcal fever. VI. Responses induced by cell walls and various fractions of Staphylococci and their products. *Yale J. Biol. Med*. 39: 297.

7. Atuio, K., Turunen, O., Lundqvist, C., and Schroder, J., 1978, Activation of lymphocytes in CLL by protein A from *Staphylococcus aureus*. *Clin. Exp. Immunol.* 34: 188.

8. Barot-Ciorbaru, R., Wietzerbin, J., Petit, J. F., Chedid, L., Falcoff, E., and Lederer, E., 1978, Induction of interferon synthesis in mice by fractions from *Nocardia*. *Infect. Immun.* 19: 353.

9. Bokisch, V. A., 1975, Interactions of peptidoglycans with anti-IgGs and with complement. *Z. Immunitaetsforsch. Exp. Klin. Immunol*. 149: 320.

10. Bona, C., 1979, Modulation of immune responses by *Nocardia* immunostimulants. *Prog. Allergy* 26: 97.

11. Bona, C., Broder, S., Dimitru, A., and Waldman, T. A., 1979, Polyclonal activation of human B lymphocytes by *Nocardia* water-soluble mitogen (NWSM). *Immunol. Rev.* 45: 69.

12. Bona, C., Chedid, L., Damais, C., Ciorbaru, R., Shek, P.N., Dubiski, S., and Cinader, B., 1975, Blast transformation of rabbit B-derived lymphocytes by a mitogen extracted from *Nocardia*. *J. Immunol*. 114: 348.

13. Brochier, J., Bona, C., Ciorbaru, R., Revillard, J. P., and Chedid, L., 1976, A human T-independent B lymphocyte mitogen extracted from *Nocardia opaca*. *J. Immunol*. 117: 1434.

14. Brown, A. E., and Faruque, A. A., 1963, The clumping of *Staphylococcus pyogenes* in serum and fibrinogen-free plasmas. *J. Clin. Pathol*. 16: 457.

15. Bultmann, B., Heymer, B., Schleifer, K. H., Seidl, H. P., and Haferkamp, O., 1975, Migration inhibition of peritoneal macrophages by peptidoglycan. *Z. Immunitaetsforsch. Exp. Klin. Immunol*. 149: 289.

16. Chedid, L., and Audibert, F., 1977, Recent advances in the use of synthetic immunoadjuvants, muramyl dipeptide and analogues, p. 388-394. In D. Schlessinger (ed.), Microbiology, 1977. American Society for Microbiology, Washington, DC.

17. Ciorbaru, R., Petit, J. F., Lederer, E., Zissman, E., Bona, C., and Chedid, L., 1976, Presence and subcellular localization of two distinct mitogenic fractions in the cells of Nocardia rubra and Nocardia opaca: preparation of soluble mitogenic peptidoglycan fragments. Infect. Immun. 13: 1084.

18. Coley, J., Archibald, A. R., and Baddiley, J., 1976, A linkage unit joining peptidoglycan to teichoic acid in Staphylococcus aureus H. FEBS Letters 61: 240.

19. Cromartie, W. J., and Craddock, J. G., 1966, Rheumatic-like cardiac lesions in mice. Science 154: 285.

20. Cromartie, W. J., Craddock, J. G., Schwab, J. H., Anderle, S. K., and Yang, C. H, 1977, Arthritis in rats after systemic injection of streptococcal cells or cell walls. J. Exp. Med. 146: 1585.

21. Crowder, J. G., and White, A., 1972, Teichoic acid antibodies in staphylococcal and nonstaphylococcal endocarditis. Ann. Int. Med. 77: 87.

22. Damais, C., Bona, C., Chedid, L., Fleck, J., Nauciel, C., and Martin, M. P., 1975, Mitogenic effect of bacterial peptidoglycans possessing adjuvant activity. J. Immunol. 115: 268.

23. Damais, C., Parant, M., and Chedid, L., 1977, Nonspecific activation of murine spleen cells in vitro by a synthetic immunoadjuvant (N-acetyl-muramyl-L-alanyl-D-isoglutamine). Cell. Immunol. 34: 49.

24. Daugharty, H., Martin, R. R., and White, A., 1967, Antibodies against staphylococcal teichoic acids and type-specific antigens in man. J. Immunol. 98: 1123.

25. Davis, P., Page, R. C., and Allison, A. C., 1974, Changes in cellular enzyme levels and extracellular release of lysosomal acid hydrolases in macrophages exposed to group A streptococcal cell wall substances. J. Exp. Med. 139: 1262.

26. Dossett, J. H., Kronvall, G., Williams, R. C.,and Quie, P. G., 1969, Antiphagocytic effect of staphylococcal protein A. J. Immunol. 103: 1405.

27. Dutie, E. S., 1954, Evidence of two forms of staphylococcal coagulase. J. Gen. Microbiol. 10: 427.

28. Duthie, E. S., 1955, The action of fibrinogen on certain pathogenic cocci. J. Gen. Microbiol. 13: 383.

29. Dziarski, R., 1976, Teichoic acids. Curr. Topics Microbiol. Immunol. 74: 113.

30. Dziarski, R., 1977, Stimulation of reticuloendothelial system and toxicity to macrophages of Staphylococcus aureus cell wall, peptidoglycan and teichoic acid. Zentralbl. Bakteriol. Parasitendk. Infektionskr. Hyg. Abt. 1 A238: 320.

31. Dziarski, R., 1978, Delayed type hypersensitivity to Staphylococcus aureus peptidoglycan in guinea pigs. Zentralbl. Backteriol. Parasitenkd. Infektionskr. Hyg. Abt. 1 A240: 165.

32. Dziarski, R., 1978. Immunosuppressive effect of Staphylococcus aureus peptidoglycan on antibody response in mice. Int. Arch. Allergy Appl. Immunol. 57: 304.

33. Dziarski, R., 1979, Splenic macrophages: mediators of immunosuppressive activity of staphylococcal peptidoglycan. RES. J. Reticuloendothel. Soc. 26: 239.

34. Dziarski, R., 1979, Relationships between adjuvant, immunosuppressive, and mitogenic activities of staphylococcal peptidoglycan. Infect. Immun. 26: 508.

35. Dziarski, R., and Dziarski, A., 1979, Mitogenic activity of staphylococcal peptidoglycan. Infect. Immun. 23: 706.

36. Dziarski, R., and Kwarecki, K., 1976, Biological effects of staphylococcal cell wall and its components in mice. Zentralbl. Baketiol. Parasitenkd. Infektionskr. Hyg. Abt. 1 Suppl. 5: 393.

37. Dziarski, R., Kwarecki, K., Kowalski, W., and Mezykowski, T., 1976, Pyrogenicity of staphylococcal peptidoglycan. Zentralbl. Bakteriol. Parasitenkd. Infektionskr. Hyg. Abt. 1 Suppl. 5: 407.

38. Easmon, C. S. F., and Glynn, A. A., 1978, Role of Staphylococcus aureus cell wall antigens in the stimulation of delayed hypersensitivity after staphylococcal infection. Infect. Immun. 19: 341.

39. Ekstedt, R. D., 1974, Immune response to surface antigens of Staphylococcus aureus and their role in resistance to staphylococcal disease. Ann. N.Y. Acad. Sci. 236: 203.

40. Febrier, M., Birrien, J. L., Leclerec, C., Chedid, L., and Liacopoulos, P., 1978, The macrophage, target cell for the synthetic adjuvant muramyl dipeptide. Eur. J. Immunol. 8: 558.

41. Fisher, S., 1965, Experimental staphylococcal infection of the subcutaneous tissue of the mouse. II. Promotion of the infection with staphylococcal cells and products. J. Infect. Dis. 113: 213.

42. Fisher, S., 1965, Experimental staphylococcal infection of the subcutaneous tissue of the mouse. III. Further observations on the cellular aggressin of coagulase-producing staphylococci. J. Infect. Dis. 115: 285.

43. Forsgren, A., and Quie, P. G., 1974, Effects of staphylococcal protein A on heat labile opsonins. J. Immunol. 112: 117.

44. Forsgren, A., and Nordstrom, K., 1974, Protein A from Staphylococcis aureus. The biological significance of its reaction with IgG. Ann. N.Y. Acad. Sci. 236: 252.

45. Forsgren, A., and Sjoquist, J., 1966, Protein A from Staphylococcus aureus. I. Pseudoimmune reaction with human γ-globulin. J. Immunol. 99: 822.

46. Forsgren, A., Svedjelund, A., and Wigzell, H., 1976, Lymphocyte stimulation by protein A of Staphylococcus aureus. Eur. J. Immunol. 6: 207.

47. Gery, I., and Davies, P., 1979, Immunoregulatory products of macrophages, p. 347-367. In Biology of the lymphokines. Academic Press, Inc., London.

48. Ginsburg, I., and Sela, M. N., 1976, The role of leukocytes and their hydrolases in the persistence, degradation, and transport of bacterial constituents in tissues: relation to chronic inflammatory processes in staphylococcal, streptococcal, and mycobacterial infections and in chronic periodontal disease. CRC Critical Rev. Microbiol. 4: 249.

49. Goudswaard, J., van der Donk, J. A., Noordzij, A., van Dam, R. H., and Vaerman, J. P., 1978, Protein A reactivity of various mammalian immunoglobulins. Scand. J. Immunol. 8: 21.

50. Greenblatt, J., Boackle, R. J., and Schwab, J. H., 1978, Activation of the alternate complement pathway by peptidoglycan from streptococcal cell wall. Infect. Immun. 19: 296.

51. Gronowicz, E., Coutinho, A., and Melchers, F., 1976, A plaque assay for all cells secreting Ig of a given type or class. Eur. J. Immunol. 6: 588.

52. Grov, A., Helgeland, S., and Endersen, C., 1976, Inhibition of leukocyte migration by peptidoglycan fragments. Zentralbl. Bakteriol. Parasitenkd. Infektionskr. Hyg. Abt. 1 Supple. 5: 389.

53. Grov., A., and Sveen, K., 1978, Induction of leukochemotaxis by peptidoglycan of Staphylococcus aureus. Acta Path. Microbiol. Scand. B86: 375.

54. Gustafson, G. R., Sjoquist, J., and Stalenheim, G., 1976., "Protein A" from Staphylococcus aureus. II. Arthus-like reaction produced in rabbits by interaction of protein A and human γ-globulin. J. Immunol. 96: 1178.

55. Gustafson, G. R., Stalenheim, G., Forsgren, A., and Sjoquist, J., 1968, "Protein A" from Staphylococcus aureus. IV. Production of anaphylaxis-like cutaneous and systemic reactions in non-immunized guinea pigs. J. Immunol. 100: 530.

56. Gutkowski, P., Pryjma, J., and Heczko, P. G., 1973, Delayed hypersensitivity and experimental staphylococcal infection, p. 255-257. In J. Jeljaszewicz (ed.), Staphylococci and staphylococcal infections. S. Karger, Basel.

57. Hajek, V., and Marsalek, E., 1976, Evaluation of classificatory criteria for staphylococci. Zentralbl. Bakteriol. Parasitenkd. Infektionskr. Hyg. Abt. 1 Suppl. 5: 11.

58. Hamada, S., Narita, T., Kotani, S., and Kato, K., 1971, Studies on cell walls of group A Streptococcus pyogenes , type 12.II. Pyrogenic and related biological activities of the higher molecular weight fraction of an enzymatic digest of the cell walls. Bikien J. 14: 217.

59. Hanessian, S., and Haskell, T. H., 1964, Structural studies on staphylococcal polysaccharide antigen. J. Biol. Chem. 239: 2758.

60. Harvey, R. L., Kronvall, G., Troup, G. M., Anderson, R. F., and Williams, R. C., 1970, Chemotaxis of polymorphonuclear leukocytes by protein A of the staphylococcus. Proc. Soc. Exp. Biol. 135: 453.

61. Hawiger, J., Marney, S. R., Calley, D. G., and Des Prez, R. M., 1972, Complement dependent injury of staphylococcal protein A. J. Exp. Med. 136: 68.

62. Hawiger, J., Steckley, S., Hammond, D., Cheng, C., Timmons, S., Glock, A. D., and Des Prez, R. M., 1979, Staphylococci-induced human platelet injury mediated by protein-A and immunoglobulin G Fc-fragment receptor. J. Clin. Invest. 64: 931.

63. Heczko, P. B., Grov, A., and Oeding, P., 1973, In vivo reactions of staphylococcal antigens. I. Hypersensitivity to protein A. Acta Pathol. Microbiol. Scand. B 81: 731.

64. Helgeland, S. M., Naess, R. R., and Grov, A., 1975, Delayed hypersensitivity to staphylococcal protein A detected by leukocyte migration inhibition. Acta Pathol. Microbiol. Scand. C 83: 15.

65. Heymer, B., 1975, Biological properties of the peptidoglycan. Z. Immunitaets-forsch. Exp. Klin. Immunol. 149: 245.

66. Heymer, B., Bultmann, B., and Haferkamp, O., 1971, Toxicity of streptococcal mucopeptides in vivo and in vitro. J. Immunol. 106: 858.

67. Heymer, B., Bultmann, B., Schachenmayr, W., Spancel, R., Hafterkamp, O., and Schmidt, W. C., 1973, Migration inhibition of rat peritoneal cells induced by streptococcal mucopeptide. J. Immunol. 111: 1743.

68. Heymer, B., and rietschel, E. T., 1977, Biological properties of peptidoglycans, p. 344-349. In D. Schlessinger (ed.), Microbiology - 1977. American Society for Microbiology, Washington, D. C.

69. Heymer, B., Schafer, H., Schachenmayr, W., Haferkamp, O., and Schmidt, W. C., 1971, Streptococcal cell wall structure inducing hepatic granuloma. Arch. Pathol. 92: 84.

70. Hill, M. J., 1968, A staphylococcal aggressin. J. Med. Microbiol. 1: 33.

71. Holton, J. B., and Schwab, J. H., 1966, Adjuvant properties of bacterial cell wall mucopeptides. J. Immunol. 96: 134.

72. Howell-Saxton, E., and Wettstein, F. O., 1978, Immunoglobulin M synthesized by human lymphoblastoid cells: interaction with Staphylococcus aureus and protein A. J. Immunol. 121: 1334.

73. Hrsak, I., Tomasic, J., Pavelic, K., and Valinger, Z., 1979, Stimulation of humoral immunity by peptidoglycan monomer from

Brevibacterium divaricatum. Z. Immunitaetsforsch. Exp. Klin. Immunol. 149: 331.

74. Humphreys, D. W., Wheat, L. J., and White, A., 1974, Staphylococcal heat-stable opsonins. J. Lab. Clin. Med. 84: 122.

75. Jolles, P., Migliore-Samour, D., Maral, L., Floc'h, F., and Werner, G. H., 1975, Low molecular weight water-soluble peptidoglycans and immunostimulants. Z. Immunitaetsforsch. Exp. Klin. Immunol. 149: 331.

76. Jones, J. M., and Schwab, J. H., 1970, Effects of streptococcal cell wall fragments on phagocytosis and tissue culture cells. Infect. Immun. 1: 232.

77. Karakawa, W. W., and Young, D. A., 1979, Immunological specificity of heat-stable opsonins in immune and nonimmune sera and their interaction with nonencapsulated strains of Staphylococcus aureus. Infect. Immun. 25: 175.

78. Karakawa, W. W., Young, D. A., and Kane, J. A., 1978, Structural analysis of the cellular constituents of a fresh clinical isolate of Staphylococcus aureus, and their role in the interaction between the organisms and polymorphonuclear leukocytes in the presence of serum factors. Infect. Immun. 21: 496.

79. Koga, T., Kotani, S., Narita, T., and Pearson, C. M., 1976, Induction of adjuvant arthritis in the rat by various bacterial cell walls and their water-soluble components. Int. Arch. Allergy Appl. Immunol. 51: 206.

80. Koga, T., Maeda, T., Onoue, K., Kato, K., and Kotani, S., 1979, Chemical structure required for immunoadjuvant and arthritogenic activities of cell wall peptidoglycans. Molecular Immunol. 16: 153.

81. Koga, T., Pearson, C. M., Narita, T., and Kotani, S., 1973, Polyarthritis induced in the rat with cell walls from several bacteria and two streptomyces species. Proc. Soc. Exp. Biol. Med. 143: 824.

82. Kohashi, O., Pearson, C. M., Beck, F. J. W., and Alexander, M., 1977, Effect of oil composition on both adjuvant-induced arthritis and delayed hypersensitivity to purified protein derivative and peptidoglycans in various rat strains. Infect. Immun. 17: 244.

83. Kohashi, O., Pearson, C. M., Beck, F.J.W., Narita, T., and Kotani, S., 1976, Arthritogenicity in rats of cell walls from

several streptococci, staphylococci and two other bacteria. Proc. Soc. Exp. Biol. Med. 152: 199.

84. Kohashi, O., Pearson, C. M., Watanabe, Y., and Kotani, S., 1977, Preparation of arthritogenic hydrosoluble peptidoglycans from both arthritogenic and non-arthritogenic bacterial cell walls. Infect. Immun. 16: 861.

85. Kohashi, O., Pearson, C. M., Watanabe, Y., Kotani, S., and Koga, T., 1976, Structural requirements for arthritogenicity of peptidoglycans from Staphylococcus aureus and Lactobacillus plantarum and analogous synthetic compounds. J. Immunol. 116: 1634.

86. Kotani, S., Watanabe, Y., Shimono, T., Harada, K., Shiba, T., Kusumoto, S., Yokogawa, K., and Toniguchi, M., 1976, Correlation between the immunoadjuvant activities and pyrogenicities of synthetic N-acetylmuramyl-peptides or -amino acid. Biken J. 19: 9.

87. Kotani, S., Watanabe, Y, Shimono, T., Narita, T., Kato, K., Stuart-Tull, D.E.S., Kinoshita, F., Yokogawa, K., Kawata, S., Shiba, T., Kusumoto, S., and Tarumi, Y., 1975, Immunoadjuvant activities of cell walls, their water-soluble fractions and peptidoglycan subunits, prepared from various Gram-positive bacteria, and synthetic N-acetylmuramyl peptides. Z. Immunitaetsforsch. Exp. Klin. Immunol. 149: 302.

88. Kowalski, J. J., and Berman, D. T., 1971, Immunological activity of cell wall antigens of Staphylococcus aureus. Infect. Immun. 4: 205.

89. Kronvall, G., and Frommel, D., 1970, Definition of staphylococcal protein A reactivity for human immunoglobulin G fragments. Immunochemistry 7: 124.

90. Kronvall, G., and Gewurz, H., 1970, Activation and inhibition of IgG mediated complement fixation by staphylococcal protein A. Clin. Exp. Immunol. 7: 213.

91. Kronvall, G., and Williams, R. C., 1969, Differences in anti-protein A activity among IgG sub-groups. J. Immunol. 103: 828.

92. Leclerc, C., Bourgeois, E., and Chedid, L., 1979, Enhancement by muramyl dipeptide of in vitro nude mice responses to a T-dependent antigen. Immunol. Commun. 8: 55.

93. Lethibichthuy, Ciorbaru, R., and J. Brochier, 1978, Human B cell differentiation. I. Immunoglobulin synthesis induced by Nocardia mitogen. Eur. J. Immunol. 8: 119.

94. Liau, D. F., and Hash, J. H., 1977, Structural analysis of the surface polysaccharide of Staphylococcus aureus M. Infect. Immun. 131: 194.

95. Liau, D. F., Melly, M. A., and Hash, J. H., 1974, Surface polysaccharide from Staphylococcus aureus M that contains taurine, D-aminogalacturonic acid, and D-fucosamine. J. Bacteriol. 119:913.

96. Lipinski, B., Hawiger, J., and Jeljaszewicz, J., 1967, Staphylococcal clumping with stable fibrin monomer complexes. J. Exp. Biol. 126: 979.

97. Lowy, I., Bona, C., and Chedid, L., 1977, Target cells for the activity of synthetic adjuvant: muramyl dipeptide. Cell. Immunol. 29: 195

98. Mackenzie, M. R., Gutman, G. A., and Warner, N. L., 1978, The binding of murine IgM to staphylococcal protein A. Scand. J. Immunol. 7: 367.

99. Mageau, R. P., and Roberson, B. S., 1969, Association of toxic capsule and cell wall mucopeptide with virulence in Gaffkya tetragena. J. Bacteriol. 97: 16.

100. Martin, R. R., 1972, Staphylococcus and teichoic acid. Ann. Int. Med. 77:813.

101. Martin, R. R., Crowder, J. G., and White, A., 1967, Human reaction to staphylococcal antigens. A possible role of leukocyte lysosomal enzymes. J. Immunol. 99: 269.

102. Martin, R. R., Daugharty, H., and White, A., 1965, Staphylococcal antibodies and hypersensitivity to teichoic acids in man. Antimicrob. Ag. Chemother., p 91.

103. Masek, K., Kadlecova, O., and Petrovicky, P., 1975, The effect of some bacterial products on temperature and sleep in rat. Z. Immunitaetsforsch. Exp. Klin. Immunol. 149: 273.

104. Meser, C., Sinay, P., and Adam, A., 1975, Total synthesis and adjuvant activity of bacterial peptidoglycan derivatives. Biochem. Biophys. Res. Commun. 66: 1316.

105. Moller, G., and Landwall, P., 1977, The polyclonal B-cell-activating property of protein A is not due to its interaction with Fc part of immunoglobulin receptors. Scand. J. Immunol. 6:357.

106. Nagel, J. G., Tuazon, C. U., Cardella, T. A., and Sheagren,

J. N., 1975, Teichoic acid serologic diagnosis of staphylococcal endocarditis. Ann. Intern. Med. 82: 13.

107. Narita, T., Hamada, S., Kotani, S., Hasegawa, and Ishida, T., 1971, Studies on cell walls of Group A Streptococcus pyogens, type 12. III. Induction of cardiac lesions in mice by a higher molecular weight fraction from a digest of cell walls with the L-11 enzyme. Biken J. 14: 233.

108. Nauciel, C., and Fleck, J., 1975, Adjuvant activity of bacterial peptidoglycans. Z. Immunitaetsforsch. Exp. Klin. Immunol. 149: 349.

109. Nauciel, C., and Goguel, A. F., 1977, Inhibition of tumor growth by the peptidoglycan from Bacillus megaterium. J. Natl. Cancer Inst. 59: 1723.

110. Oeding, P., 1974, Cellular antigens of staphylococci. Ann. N.Y. Acad. Sci. 236: 15.

111. Oeding, P., and Digranes, A., 1976, Staphylococcus saprophyticus: classification and infections. Zentralbl. Bakteriol. Parasitenkd. Infektionskr. Hyg. Abt. 1 Suppl. 5:113.

112. Oeding, P., and Grov, A., 1972, Cellular antigens, p. 333-356. In J. O. Cohen (ed.), Staphylococci and staphylococcal infections, S. Karger, Basel.

114. Ohanian, S. H., and Schwab, J. H., 1967, Persistence of group A streptococcal cell walls related to chronic inflammation of rabbit dermal connective tissue. J. Exp. Med. 125:1137.

115. Ohanian, S. H., Schwab, J. H., and Cromartie, W. J., 1969, Relation of rheumatic-like cardiac lesions of the mouse to localization of group A streptococcal cell walls. J. Exp. Med. 129: 27.

116. Ohkuni, H., and Kimura, Y, 1976, Increased capillary permeability in guinea pigs and rats by peptidoglycan fraction extracted from group A streptococcal cell walls. Exp. Cell Biol. 44: 83.

117. Ohkuni, H., Norose, Y., Hayama, M., Kimura, Y., Kotani, S., Shiba, T., Kusumoto, S., Yokogawa, K., and Kawata, S., 1977, Adjuvant activities in production of reaginic antibody in mice of bacterial cell wall peptidoglycans or peptidoglycan subunits and of synthetic N-acetylmuramyl dipeptides. Biken J. 20: 131.

118. Ohkuni, H., Norose, Y., Ohta, M., Hayama, M., Kimura, Y., Tsujimoto, M., Kotani, S., Shiba, T., Kusumoto, S., Yokogawa, K., and Kawata, S., 1979, Adjuvant activities in production of reaginic antibody by bacterial cell wall peptidoglycan or synthetic N-acetylmuramyl dipeptides in mice. Infect. Immun. 24: 313.

119. Patrick, C. C., Virella, G., Koistinen, J., and Fudenberg, H. H., 1977, Differential binding of IgA proteins of different subclasses and allotypes to staphylococcal protein A. Z. Immunitaetsforsch. Exp. Klin. Immunol. 153: 466.

120. Peterson, P. K., Kim, Y., Wilkinson, B. J., Schmeling, D., Michael, A. F., and Quie, P. G., 1978, Dichotomy between opsonization and serum complement activation by encapsulated staphylococci. Infect. Immun. 20: 770.

121. Peterson, P. K., Verhoef, J., Sabath, L. D., and Quie, P. G., 1977, The effect of protein A on staphylococcal opsonization. Infect. Immun. 15:750.

122. Peterson, P. K., Wilkinson, B. J., Kim, Y., Schmeling, D., Douglas, S. D., Quie, P. G., and Verhoef, J., 1978, The key role of peptidoglycan in the opsonization of Staphylococcus aureus. J. Clin. Invest. 61: 597.

123. Peterson, P. K., Wilkinson, B. J., Kim, Y., Schmeling, D., and Quie, P. G., 1978, Influence of encapsulation on staphylococcal opsonization and phagocytosis by human polymorphonuclear leukocytes. Infect. Immun. 19: 943.

124. Petersson, B. A., 1975, Induction of histamine release and desensitization in human leukocytes. IgG-mediated histamine release. Scand. J. Immunol. 4: 777.

125. Phillips, S. M., Stephenson, J. R., and Aaronson, S. A., 1977 Genetic factors influencing mouse type C RNA virus induction by naturally occurring B cell mitogens. J. Immunol. 118: 662.

126. Pryjma, J., Pryjma, K., Grov, A., and Heczko, P. B., 1976, Immunological activity of staphylococcal cell wall antigens. Zentralbl. Bakteriol. Parasitenkd. Infectionskr. Hyg. Abt. 1 Suppl. 5: 873.

127. Raskova, H., Ryc, M., Rotta, J., and Masek, K., 1971, Release of 5-hydroxytryptamine and morphological changes in blood platelets induced by mucopeptide of streptococcal cell walls.

J. Infect. Dis. 123: 587.

128. Rodey, G. E., Davis, T., and Quie, P. G., 1972, Response of peripheral blood lymphocytes from noraml, hypogammaglobulinemic and chronic lymphocytic leukemic patients. J. Immunol. 108: 178.

129. Rotta, J., 1975, Endotoxin-like properties of the peptidoglycan. Z. Immunitaetsforsch. Exp. Klin. Immunol. 149: 230.

130. Rotta, J., and Bednar, B., 1969, Biological properties of cell wall mucopeptide of hemolytic streptococci. J. Exp. Med. 130: 31.

131. Rotta, J., Bednar, B., and Ryc, M., 1977, Biological characteristics of peptidoglycans of group A streptococcus and some other bacterial species. I. Tolerance and effect of antibody in fever response, and heart damaging effect in rabbits. J. Hyg. Epidemiol. Microbiol. Immunol. 21: 433.

132. Rotta, J., Prendergast, T. J., Karakawa, W. W., Harmon, C. K., and Krause, R. M., 1965, Enhanced resistance to streptococcal infection induced in mice by cell wall mucopeptide. J. Exp. Med. 122: 877.

133. Rotta, J., and Schleifer, K. H., 1974, Pyrogenic activity of bacterial mucopeptide. J. Hyg. Epidemiol. Microbiol. Immunol. 18: 50.

134. Ryc, M., and Rotta, J., 1975, The thrombocytolytic activity of bacterial peptidoglycans. Z. Immunitaetsforsch. Exp. Klin. Immunol. 149: 265.

135. Ryc, M., and Rotta, J., 1978, Biological characteristics of peptidoglycans of group A streptococcus and some other bacterial species. II. Immunological mechanisms involved in thrombocytolysis. J. Hyg. Epidemiol. Microbiol. Immunol. 22: 435.

136. Sakane, T., and Green, I., 1978, Protein A from Staphylococcus aureus - a mitogen for human T and B lymphocytes but not for L. lymphocytes. J. Immunol. 120: 302.

137. Schleifer, K. H., 1973, Chemical composition of staphylococcal cell walls, p. 13-23. In J. Jeljaszewicz (ed.), Staphylococci and staphylococcal infections. S. Karger, Basel.

138. Schleifer, K. H., and Kandler, O., 1972, Peptidoglycan types of bacterial cell walls and their taxonomic implications. Bacteriol. Rev. 36: 407.

139. Schmeling, D. J., Peterson, P. K., Hammerschmidt, D. E., Kim, Y., Verhoef, J., Wilkinson, B. J., and Quie, P. G., 1979, Chemotaxigenesis by cell surface components of Staphylococcus aureus. Infect. Immun. 26: 47.

140. Schmidtke, J. R., and Najarian, J. S., 1975, Synergistic effects on DNA synthesis of phytohemagglutinin or concanavalin A and lipopolysaccharide in human peripheral blood lymphocytes. J. Immunol. 114: 742.

141. Schuster, G. S., Hayski, J. A., and Bahn, A. M., 1967, Toxic properties of the cell wall of Gram-positive bacteria. J. Bacteriol. 93: 47.

142. Schwab, J. H., 1965, Biological properties of streptococcal cell wall particles. I. Determinants of chronic nodular lesions of connective tissue. J. Bacteriol. 90: 1405.

143. Schwab, J. H., 1975, Suppression of the immune response by microorganisms. Bact. Rev. 39: 121.

144. Schwab, J. H., 1979, Acute and chronic inflammation induced by bacterial cell wall structures, p. 209-214. In D. Schlessinger (ed.), Microbiology 1979. American Society for Microbiology, Washington, DC.

145. Schwab, J. H., and Cromartie, W. J., 1957, Studies on a toxic cellular component of group A streptococci. J. Bacteriol. 74: 673.

146. Schwab, J. H., Cromartie, W. J., Ohanian, S. H., and Craddock, J. G., 1967, Association of experimental chronic arthritis with the persistence of group A streptococcal cell walls in the articular tissue. J. Bacteriol. 94: 1728.

147. Seltmann, G., and Beer, W., 1976, Chemical studies on the capsule material of Staphylococcus aureus strain 1193/74. Zentralbl. Bakteriol. Parasitenkd. Infectionskr. Hyg. Abt. 1 Suppl. 5: 377.

148. Shayegani, M., Hisatsune, and Mudd, S., 1970, Cell wall component which affects the ability of serum to promote phagocytosis and killing of Staphylococcus aureus. Infect. Immun. 2:750.

149. Shibasaki, M., Nemoto, H., Suzuki, S., and Kuroume, T., 1978, Induction of lymphocyte colony formation in vitro by protein A. J. Immunol. 121: 2278.

150. Sjoquist, J., 1973, Structure and immunology of protein A, p. 83-92. In J. Jeljaszewicz (ed.), Staphylococci and staphylococcal infections. S. Karger, Basel.

151. Sjoquist, J., and Stalenheim, G., 1969, Protein A from Staphylococcus aureus. IX. Complement fixing activity of protein A-IgG complexes. J. Immunol. 103: 467.

152. Smialowicz, R. J., and Schwab, J. H., 1977, Cytotoxicity of rat macrophages activated by persistent or biodegradable bacterial cell walls. Infect. Immun. 17: 599.

153. Smialowicz, R. J., and Schwab, J. H., 1978, Inhibition of macrophage phagocytic activity by group A streptococcal cell walls. Infect. Immun. 20: 258.

154. Smith, S. M., Burrell, R., and Synder, I. S., 1978, Complement activation by cell wall fractions of Micropolyspora faeni. Infect. Immun. 22: 568.

155. Specter, S., Cimprich, R., Friedman, H., and Chedid, L., 1978, Stimulation of an enhanced in vitro immune response by a synthetic adjuvant, muramyl dipeptide. J. Immunol. 120: 487.

156. Staber, F. G., Tarcsay, L., and Duktor, P., 1978, Modulation of myelopoiesis in vivo by chemically pure preparations of cell wall components from gram-negative bacteria: effects at different stages. Infect. Immun. 20: 40

157. Stalenheim, G., and Castensson, S., 1971, Protein A from Staphylococcus aureus. XII. Conversion of complement factor C3 by aggregates between IgG and protein A. FEBS Letters. 14: 79.

158. Stalenheim, G., and Malmheden-Ericksson, I., 1971, Protein A from Staphylococcus aureus. XIII. Complement fixation by aggregates between protein and IgG1 or IgG2 from guinea pig. FEBS Letters 14: 82.

159. Stalenheim, G., and Sjoquist, J., 1970. Protein A from Staphylococcus aureus X. Complement fixing activity of complexes between protein A and myeloma IgG or papain fragments of IgG. J. Immunol. 105: 944.

160. Sugimoto, M., Germain, R. N., Chedid, L., and Benacerraf, B., 1978, Enhancement of carrier-specific helper T cell function by the synthetic adjuvant, N-acetylmuramyl-L-alanyl-D-isoglutamine (MDP). J. Immunol. 120: 980.

161. Sveen, K., and Grov., A., 1978, Induction of leukochemotaxis by protein A of Staphylococcus aureus . Acta Path. Microbiol. Scand. B86: 369.

162. Switalski, L. M., 1976, Isolation and characterization of staphylococcal clumping factor. Zentralbl. Bakteriol. Parasitenkd. Infektionskr. Hyg. Abt. 1 Suppl. 5: 413.

163. Takeda, H., Kotani, S., Kusumoto, S., Tarumi, Y, Ikenaka, K., and Shiba, T., 1977, Mitogenic activity of adjuvant-active N-acetylmuramyl-L-alanyl-D-isoglutamine and its analogues. Biken. J. 20: 81.

164. Targowski, S. P., and Berman, D. T., 1974, Passive transfer of delayed-type hypersensitivity to cell walls of Staphylococcus aureus. Infect. Immun. 9: 41.

165. Targowski, S. P., and Berman, D. T., 1975, Cell-mediated immune reactions in vitro to cell walls and peptidoglycan from Staphylococcus aureus. Z. Immunitaetsforsch. Exp. Klin. Immunol. 149: 295.

166. Targowski, S. P., and Berman, D. T., 1975, Cell-mediated immunity to cell wall antigens of Staphylococcus aureus in vitro. II. The production of chemotactic factor by guinea pig peritoneal exudate cells. Z. Immunitaetsforsch. Exp. Klin. Immunol. 149: 417.

167. Van der Vijver, J. C. M., van es-Boon, M. M., and Michel, M. F., 1974, The enhancing effect of cell-wall aggressin on the virulence of Staphylococcus aureus in normal and irradiated mice and in man. Antonie von Leeuwenhoek J. Microbiol. Serol. 40: 49.

168. Watson, J., and Whitlock, C., 1978, Effect of a synthetic adjuvant on the induction of primary immune responses in T cell-depleted spleen cultures. J. Immunol. 121: 383.

169. Weksler, B. B., and Hill, M. J., 1969, Inhibition of leukocyte migration by a staphylococcal factor. J. Bacteriol. 98: 1030.

170. White, R. G., 1976, The adjuvant effect of microbial products on the immune response. Ann. Rev. Microbiol. 30: 579.

171. Wicken, A. J., and Knox, K. W., 1975, Lipoteichoic acids: a new class of bacterial antigen. Science 187: 1161.

172. Wicken, A. J., and Knox, K. W., 1977, Biological properties of lipoteichoic acids, p. 360-365. In D. Schlessinger (ed.), Microbiology - 1977. American Society for Microbiology, Washington, D. C.

173. Wildfeuer, A., Heymer, B., Spilker, D., Schleifer, K. H., Vanek, E., and Haferkamp, O., 1975, Use of Limulus assay to compare the biological activity of peptidoglycan and endotoxin. Z. Immunitaetsforsch. Exp. Klin. Immunol. 149: 258.

174. Wiley, B. B., and Maverakis, N. H., 1974, Capsule production and virulence among strains of Staphylococcus aureus. Ann. N. Y. Acad. Sci. 236: 221.

175. Wilkinson, B. J., Kim, Y., Peterson, P. K., Quie, P. G., and Michael, A. F., 1978, Activation of complement by cell surface components of Staphylococcus aureus. Infect. Immun. 20: 388.

176. Wilkinson, B. J., Peterson, P. K., and Que, P. G., 1979, Cryptic peptidoglycan and the antiphagocytic effect of the Staphylococcus aureus capsule: model for the antiphagocytic effect of bacterial cell surface polymers. Infect. Immun. 23: 502.

177. Wood, D. D., 1977, Role of adherent cell products in the immune response, p. 117-136. In D. O. Lucas (ed.), Regulatory mechanisms in lymphocyte activation. Academic Press, Inc., New York, NY.

178. Wu, T. C. M., and Park, J. T., 1971, Chemical characterization of a new surface antigenic polysaccharide from a mutant of Staphylococcus aureus. J. Bacteriol. 108: 874.

179. Wyszomirska, Z., Stachow, A., and Rudzki, A., 1963, Activity of teichoic acids of Staphylococcus aureus in skin tests. Przeglad Dermatol. 55: 465.

180. Yoshida, K., Smith, M. R., and Naito, J., 1970, Biological and immunological properties of encapsulated strains of Staphylococcus aureus by the serum-soft agar technique. Infect. Immun. 3: 535.

181. Zimmerman, T. S., and Muller-Eberhard, H. J., 1971, Blood coagulation initiated by a complement mediated pathway. J. Exp. Med. 134: 1601.

IMMUNOMODULATION BY *CORYNEBACTERIUM PARVUM*

A. Ghaffar,[1] R. D. Paul,[2] M. M. Sigel,[1] W. Lichter[2] and L. L. Wellham[2]

[1]Department of Microbiology and Immunology
University of South Carolina School of Medicine
Columbia, SC
[2]Department of Microbiology
University of Miami School of Medicine
Miami, FL

Corynebacterium parvum which has recently been reclassified as a Propionibacterium (1) was initially noted for its ability to stimulate the reticuloendothelial system (RES) as manifested by increased clearance of particulate material from the circulation and increased spleen and liver weights (2-5). Since then, the ability of this organism to modify various immune functions has been extensively studied.

Among the prominent immunomodulating properties of *C. parvum* are its nonspecific antitumor effects (6, 7) which have been shown to be at least in part independent of T cell-mediated immunocompetence of the host (8). However, when the vaccine was administered intratumorally, the response of the host was dependent on the dose of the organism injected, antigenicity of the tumor and required normal component of T cell function (9, 10). It would appear from previously published data and our own observations that *C. parvum* could also modulate the resistance to a secondary tumor challenge by acting as an adjuvant in association with tumor-specific antigens administered either as nonviable tumor cells or as live tumor and subsequently treated chemotherapeutically.

Aside from enhancing tumor resistance, *C. parvum* has been shown also to modulate phagocytic and cytotoxic functions of macrophages, their lysozomal enzyme contents and their histochemical characteristics. Generally, *C. parvum* treatment *in vivo* resulted in increased phagocytic activity, increased cytotoxic potential, increased lysozomal enzyme and prostaglandin contents, and increased adherence of macrophages (11-13). Furthermore, C. parvum injected in combination with or prior to thymus-dependent antigens in an optimal dose caused an augmentation of humoral immune responses (4, 18-21). However, injected with thymus-independent antigens, C. parvum caused a time, route and dose dependent augmentation or suppression of humoral responses (19, 20, 22).

C. parvum administration has also been reported to cause suppression of certain parameters of the immune function. Thus, splenocytes from C. parvum treated mice failed to respond to various nonspecific mitogenic stimuli *in vitro* (23). This failure of responsiveness was due to macrophages which suppressed proliferative responses of T and B cells to nonspecific mitogens. *In vivo*, certain doses of C. parvum caused suppression of cell-mediated immune responses (24).

We have recently observed that, under certain conditions, C. parvum could exert very strong immunosuppressive effects on thymus-dependent humoral immune responses (25) and decrease resistance of mice to a secondary tumor challenge (26). These findings have been summarized below.

Effect on Primary Humoral Response

Young adult (8-10 weeks old) BALB/c or BDF_1 (C57Bl x DBA/2) mice were injected with 1.4 mg C. parvum* by the i.p. (or in some experiments, i.v.) route at different times in relation to immunization with 1 x 10^8 SRBC. Four days after immunization (except where stated otherwise) splenic plaque forming cells (PFC) were measured by Cunningham's technique (27). In BALB/c mice, when C. parvum was injected i.p. ten days before 1 x 10^8 SRBC, there was over 90% suppression of anti-SRBC response (Table 1). This suppression was evident with both PFC per spleen and PFC per 10^6 levels indicating that the suppression was not merely a reflection of alteration in the cellularity of the spleen. Similar suppression was observed when the effect of C. parvum on the immune response of BDF_1 mice was examined. As indicated in Fig. 1, C. parvum injected 1-16 days before SRBC caused significant suppression of anti-SRBC IgM and IgG PFC responses. By contrast, when injected on the day of immunization, C. parvum significantly augmented IgM and IgG responses. It is clear from Fig. 2 that the suppressive effect of C. parvum does not merely indicate a delay in the onset of the PFC response. Our previous observations also indicated that the suppressive effect of C. parvum is not due to overstimulation of the RE system by a very large dose of the vaccine. Thus, as little as 56 μg C. parvum

* Kindly supplied by Burroughs Wellcome Co., Research Triangle Park, North Carolina

TABLE I

Suppression of primary IgM response by *C. parvum*[a]

Treatment	IgM PFC[b] per 10^6	IgM PFC[b] per spleen
Saline	1,284	234,447
C. parvum	53[c]	29,682[c]

[a]1.4 mg *C. parvum* or saline injected i.p. 10 days before i.p. immunization with 1 x 10^8 SRBC. PFC measured 4 days post immunization

[b]Geometric mean of groups containing 5 mice.

[c]Significant suppression ($p < 0.001$)

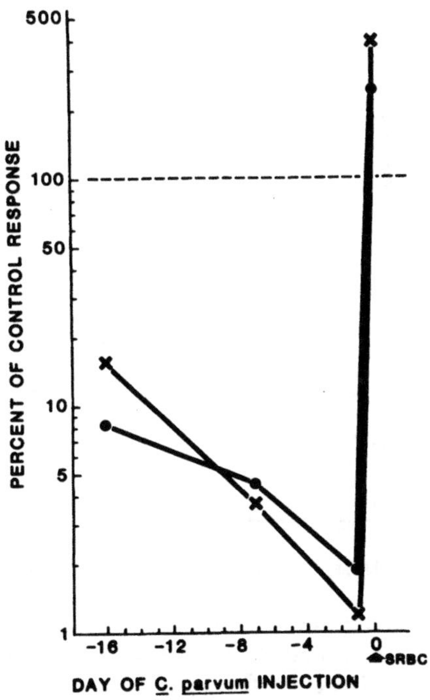

Fig. 1. Time-dependent suppression and augmentation of anti-SRBC responses by *C. parvum* in BDF_1 mice. 1.4 mg *C. parvum* injected i.p. 16, 7, 1 or 0 days before i.p. immunization with 1 x 10^8 SRBC, ●——● IgM and X——X IgG PFC. Percent response was calculated from PFC per spleen data. Dotted line represents control response. (Based on previously published data, reference 25).

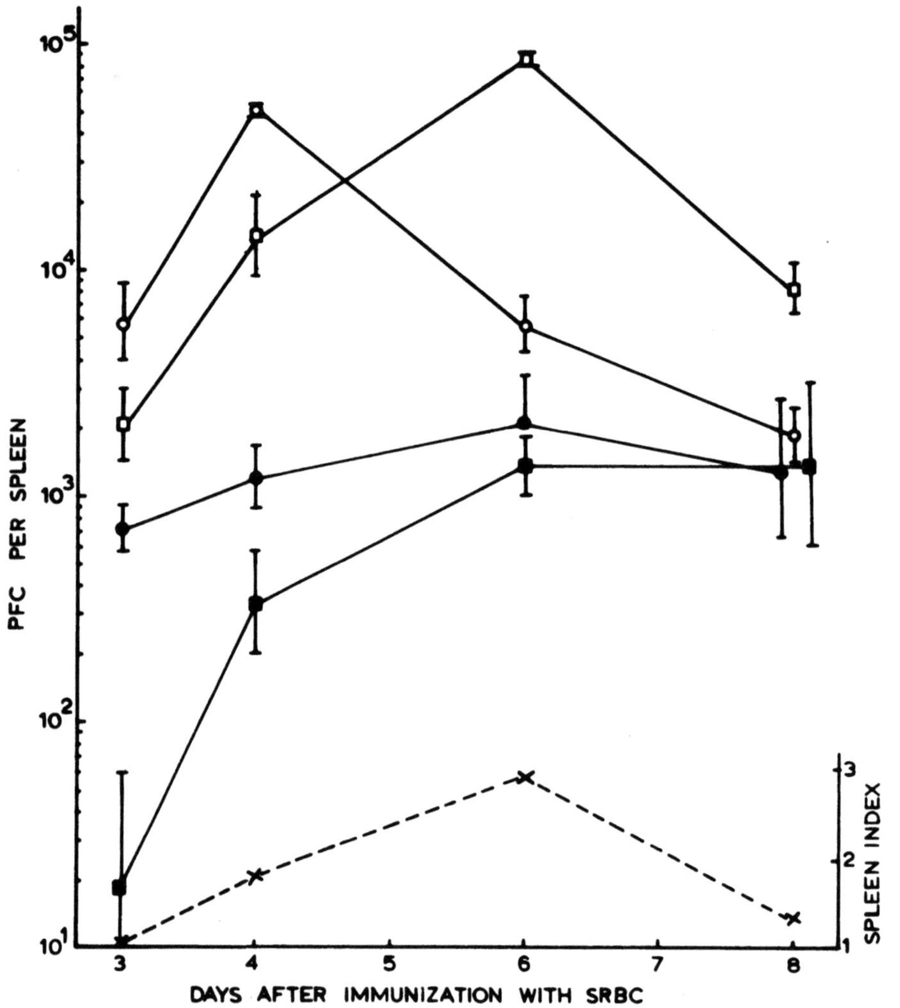

Fig. 2. Suppression of anti-SRBC responses in BDF_1 mice by 1.4 mg C. parvum injected 1 day before 1 x 10^8 SRBC. (○), IgM in control mice; (●), IgM in C. parvum-treated mice; (□), IgG in control mice; (■) IgG in C. parvum-treated mice; (x) Mean spleen weight in C. parvum-treated mice/ Mean spleen weight in control mice. (Data published in reference 25).

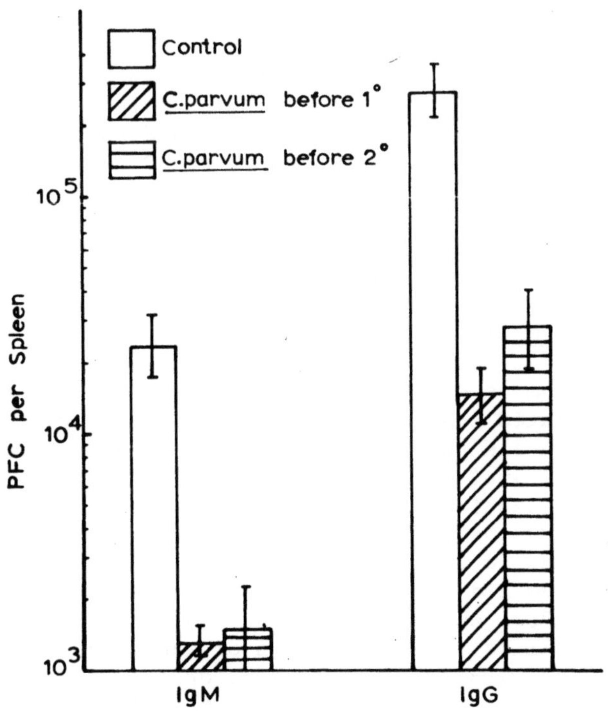

Fig. 3 Suppression of secondary anti-SRBC response by C. parvum in BDF_1 mice. 1.4 mg C. parvum injected 1 day before priming or before 2° challenge with 1 x 10^8 SRBC. (Based on previously published data, reference 25).

caused a significant suppression (25). The immunomodulating effect of C. parvum was, however, dependent on the route of treatment. Thus, C. parvum injected i.p. caused a suppression when SBC were injected i.p. but it augmented the response to i.v. administered SRBC (25). Furthermore, i.v. administration of C. parvum always augmented the response to SRBC whether injected i.p. or i.v. (25).

Effect on Secondary Response

In addition to suppressing primary anti-SRBC responses, C. parvum also suppressed secondary anti-SRBC IgM and IgG PFC responses. The suppression of secondary responses were equally marked when C. parvum was injected on day before priming or one day before the secondary challenge given 16 days after priming (Fig. 3). This indicated that C. parvum injected before SRBC did not only preempt the development of a primary response reported above, but it also inhibited the development of memory cells. Moreover, injection of C. parvum prior to secondary challenge also suppressed the development of a secondary response indicating that this organism could also interfere with the expression of memory cells.

Postulated Mechanisms Involving Suppression of Humoral Responses

Since C. parvum is one of the most powerful stimulants of the RES, it was postulated that the suppression caused by this agent might be related to its ability to alter the clearance rate and localization of the antigen. Results indicated that C. parvum did alter the localization of SRBC in the spleen. In mice injected with C. parvum by the i.p. route, relatively smaller amounts of antigen localized in the spleen (Fig. 4). In contrast, i.v. injection of C. parvum led to a several-fold increase in the splenic localization of SRBC. While the altered distribution of the antigen in the spleen parallels the suppression or augmentation of the immune response associated with respective (i.p. or i.v.) routes of administration of C. parvum, the magnitudes of the effects do not coincide. Thus, the striking increase in the splenic uptake of mice injected with C. parvum by the i.v. route is disproportionately high in comparison to the modest augmentation of PFC responses in similarly treated mice. Conversely, the profound suppression by i.p. injection of C. parvum is incompatible with the small reduction of splenic uptake of SRBC in such animals.

In search of another mechanism for the reduced response in C. parvum injected mice, we investigated the possibility that C. parvum might shift the balance of regulatory cells towards suppressor cells in response to optimal doses of SRBC. Two groups of BDF_1 mice were injected with either saline or C. parvum and one day later each group was subdivided into two subgroups, one receiving 1 x 10^8 SRBC and the other being treated with saline. Fourteen days after the SRBC injection, mice were sacrificed and their splenocytes (4×10^7 cells) were transferred into normal recipients together with 1×10^8 SRBC. The response of recipients measured 4 days later has been summarized in Table 2. Responses of mice receiving splenocytes from donors treated with C. parvum were similar to those receiving control untreated splenocytes. Splenocytes from donors previously immunized with 1×10^8 SRBC were slightly suppressive in one experiment (statistically not significant). The striking observation was that when donor mice were injected with 1.4 mg C. parvum one day before 1×10^8 SRBC, their splenocytes caused a significant suppression in recipient mice in both experiments. It is clear from the results that recipient animals, although they received primed splenocytes, did not give a typical secondary response. This is reflected by the ratio of IgM to IgG response.

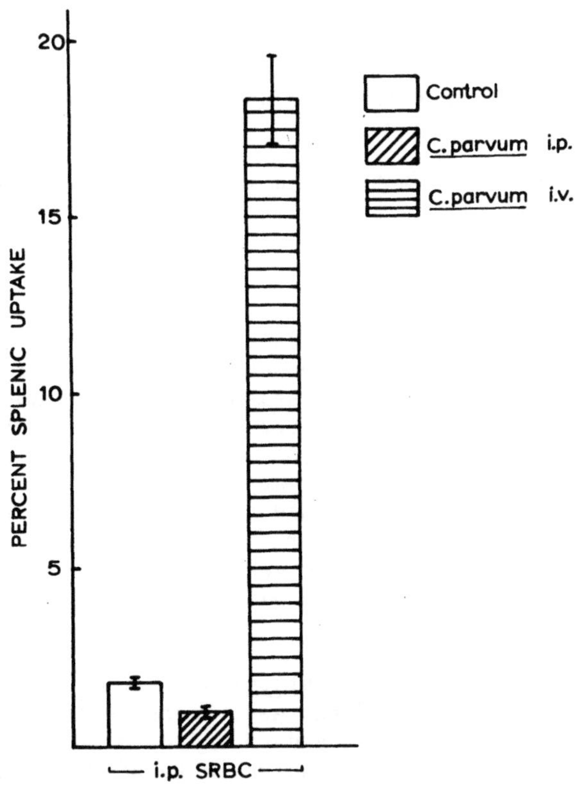

Fig. 4. Effect of C. parvum on the splenic uptake of SRBC in BDF_1 mice. (Data published in reference 25).

TABLE II

Induction of suppressor cells by C. parvum[a]

Donor Treatment	Mean[b] PFC per 10^6			
	Expt. I		Expt. II	
	IgM	IgG	IgM	IgG
Nil, saline	1,061	314	649	106
C. parvum	1,466	355	846	169
1×10^8 SRBC	874	396	317	307
C. parvum + 1×10^8 SRBC	424	220	88[c]	71[c]

[a] 1.4 mg C. parvum injected i.p. 1 day before immunization of spleen cell donors with 1×10^8 SRBC. Fourteen days after immunization, 40×10^6 splenocytes were transferred i.v. into normal syngeneic BDF_1 mice. Recipients also received 1×10^8 SRBC i.p. at the time of cell transfer. PFC measured 4 days later.

[b] Geometric mean of PFC per 10^6 nucleated spleen cells for groups containing a minimum of 5 mice.

[c] Significantly lower ($p < 0.01$) than group injected with splenocytes from donor treated with SRBC alone.

Normally, an IgG response on day 4 after a secondary challenge with SRBC is far greater than the IgM response. Thus, suppression of IgM response in mice receiving immune splenocytes could not be due to a feedback suppression by IgG produced by the donor cells. Furthermore, in the second experiment splenocytes from donors treated with C. parvum and SRBC caused a significant suppression of not only IgM but also of IgG responses. It should be stressed that IgG responses in these experiments were not measured at the optimal time of primary IgG response and, hence, there was a tremendous variation in the response of individual mice and differences between groups were often not significant.

These data indicate that C. parvum, when combined with a normally optimal immunizing dose of antigen, leads to the induction of suppressor cells. Our preliminary data indicate that when C. parvum was combined with a supraoptimal antigen dose of SRBC which consistently induced suppressor cells, such combination resulted in the alleviation of suppressor cells. Thus, C. parvum could play a dual role: in response to optimal antigen dose it leads to induction of suppressor cells, whereas in response to supraoptimal antigen dose it causes relief from suppression. These findings are in concordance with our earlier observations showing that C. parvum, while suppressive when injected with optimal or suboptimal doses of SRBC, was augmentative when administered prior to a supraoptimal dose of SRBC (25).

Effect on Tumor Growth

It is well established that C. parvum injected systemically can moderately retard the growth of various types of subcutaneous tumors. The antitumor effect of this organism injected systemically (i.p. or i.v.) is equally apparent in immunologically intact and thymus-deprived immunodeficient mice (8). By contrast, however, the antitumor effect of C. parvum injected intratumorally is extremely dependent on an intact T cell function (8, 10). Thus, C. parvum can exert its antitumor effect by nonspecifically modulating the host RES as well as by acting as an adjuvant and augmenting the immunity to tumor-specific antigens. The results reported here indicate that effects of C. parvum could be variable depending on the type of tumor studied.

The effect of C. parvum on the growth of two lymphocytic leukemias was compared. Tumors studied were P388 lymphocytic leukemia of DBA/2 origin and Gardner lymphosarcoma (GL) of C3H origin. P388 (1×10^4) or GL (5×10^4) tumor cells were inoculated i.p. into BDF_1 or C3H mice, respectively. Four days after tumor inoculation, some of the mice were injected i.p. with 1.4 mg C. parvum. The survival time of these mice was monitored. Results, summarized in Table 3, clearly indicate that C. parvum caused significant prolongation of life of mice bearing P388 tumor. By contrast, C. parvum treatment resulted in a small but significant reduction in the survival of mice bearing the GL tumor.

The effect of C. parvum was also studied in tumor-bearing mice which received chemotherapy with the nitrosourea, MeCCNU. Mice were injected with 30 mg/kg MeCCNU 2 or 6 days following tumor inoculation. Some mice also received 1.4 mg C. parvum 4 days after tumor injection. Results, summarized in Table 4, indicated that chemotherapy with MeCCNU administered 2 days after P388 or GL tumor completely cured over 90% of mice (survival beyond 42 days for P388 and beyond 52 days for GL), whereas delayed treatment on day 6 was less effective and only 25-30% of mice survived beyond 52 days. Combination of C. parvum with delayed chemotherapy on day 6 in mice bearing P388 tumor had a synergistic effect and resulted in 100% cure of the mice. By contrast, when C. parvum was combined with MeCCNU in C3H mice bearing GL tumor, the vaccine produced an antagonistic effect and reduced the survival time from 35 days to 17.5 days. It is clear that combination of C. parvum with chemotherapy on day 2 did not have any effect on the survival time of mice bearing P388 tumors.

TABLE III

Effect of C. parvum[a] on survival of mice with two different tumors[b]

Tumor	Mean Survival Time (MST) ± 1 S.E.[c] Control	*C. parvum*	p values[d]
P 388	16.6 ± 0.5 (16)	25.7 ± 1.0 (15)	<0.001
Gardner	15.1 ± 0.3 (36)	13.8 ± 0.3 (39)	<0.005

a
1.4 mg C. parvum injected i.p. 4 days after tumor.

b
BDF_1 mice injected with 1×10^4 viable P388 lymphocytic leukemia cells and C3H/HeN mice injected with 5×10^4 viable Gardner lymphosarcoma cells.

c
Figures in parentheses are number of mice in each group; no survivors beyond 28 days.

c
C. parvum caused significant prolongation of MST in mice bearing P388 tumor but caused a small although significant reduction in the MST of mice bearing the GL tumor.

Mice surviving the primary tumor following chemotherapy (MeCCNU on day 2) or chemoimmunotherapy (MeCCNU on day 2 and C. parvum on day 4) were rechallenged with a second load of the respective tumor and the resistance of these mice to second tumor challenge was assessed. It is clear from data in Table 5 that mice cured of P388 leukemia by treatment with MeCCNU alone 2 days following the primary tumor were not resistant to the second tumor challenge. However, if chemotherapy on day 2 was followed by C. parvum treatment 4 days after P388 inoculation, the survivors were significantly more resistant to the second tumor challenge than mice which received chemotherapy alone. By contrast, combination of immunotherapy with chemotherapy did not improve the resistance of mice to the second challenge with GL. The suppression of resistance to a secondary tumor challenge following chemotherapeutic elimination of the primary tumor described above has been observed also with a chemically-induced fibrosarcoma in CBA mice (26). Mice immunized with 1×10^6 irradiated tumor cells were resistant to a challenge with 1×10^5 live fibrosarcoma cells (2/24 tumor-free survivors). When the challenge inoculum was increased, all mice developed tumor although the growth rate in preimmunized mice was slower than the rate in control mice (42% reduction in the growth rate). However, if immunization with irradiated cells was preceded (0-5 days) by

TABLE IV

Modulation chemotherapeutic effect of MeCCNU by C. parvum[a]

MeCCNU[b] (day)	P388[c] Control	P388[c] C. parvum	p	Gardner[c] Control	Gardner[c] C. parvum	p
None	16.6 (0/16)	25.7 (0/16)	<0.001	15.1 (0/8)	13.2 (0/8)	<0.025
+2	39.5 (11/12)	39.5 (6/8)	n.s.	49.9 (7/8)	49.7 (7/8)	n.s.
+6	34.1 (2/7)	42.0 (8/8)	<0.001	35.0 (2/8)	17.5 (0/7)	<0.001

[a] 1.4 mg C. parvum injected i.p. 4 days after 1 x 10^4 P388 or 5 x 10^4 Gardner lymphosarcoma cells.

[b] 30 mg/kg MeCCNU injected i.p. 2 and 6 days after tumor.

[c] Mean survival time in days. Numbers in parentheses represent number of survivors/number of mice injected. P values were calculated by the Student's t-test; n.s. = not significant ($p > 0.05$). Data obtained on day 42 after the initial injection of P388 and day 52 after the injection of GL tumor.

700 μg C. parvum injected s.c., the protective effect of x-irradiated tumor cells was abrogated and 100% of mice grew tumor. This observation of abrogation of resistance was dependent on the dose of C. parvum injected and lower doses of C. parvum caused reducing degrees of abrogation: 90 μg C. parvum did not at all reduce the resistance conferred by x-irradiated cells. On the contrary, it acted synergistically with x-irradiated tumor cells as indicated by lower incidence of tumor in mice challenged with larger numbers of live tumor cells (92% in mice treated with x-irradiated cells alone *vs*. 67% in mice pretreated with x-irradiated cells plus 90 μg C. parvum) (26).

CONCLUSIONS

It has been demonstrated that C. parvum (Propionibacterium acnes) can modulate humoral immune responses against thymus-dependent and thymus-independent antigen (19, 22, 25). The augmentation of the thymus-dependent responses has been shown to be mediated by macrophages which require an obligatory role of T cells (27, 28). Thus, macrophages from C. parvum injected mice caused an

TABLE V

Resistance of Mice Against Tumor Following Chemotherapy of the Primary Tumor and its Modulation by _C. parvum_

Previous Exposure to Tumor	MeCCNU[a]	P388[b]			Gardner[b]		
		Control	_C. parvum_[c]	p[d]	Control	_C. parvum_[c]	p[d]
No	No	17.4 (0/8)	n.t.		14.2 (0/10)	n.t.	
Yes	Yes	15.7 (0/11)	23.2 (0/6)	<0.001	14.0 (1/7)	14.0 (0/7)	n.s.

[a] 30 mg/kg MeCCNU injected 2 days after the first tumor inoculation (see Table 4). All survivors were rechallenged with 1×10^4 P388 or 5×10^4 Gardner lymphosarcoma cells 42 days after the primary tumor inoculation.

[b] Mean survival time calculated 42 days after the second challenge. Numbers in parentheses are survivors/numbers challenged.

[c] 1.4 mg _C. parvum_ injected 4 days after the primary tumor inoculation (see Table 4); n.t. = not tested.

[d] P values calculated by the Student's t-test; n.s. = not significant ($p > 0.05$).

augmentation of normal response to SRBC (27). However, if mice were deprived of T cells before the inoculation of C. parvum their macrophages failed to improve a normal anti-SRBC response (28). The suppression of immune response to SRBC might be partly due to altered localization of the antigen in lymphoid organs and partly due to induction of suppressor cells. These suppressor cells could not be induced in mice treated with C. parvum alone and required exposure of mice to SRBC as well as C. parvum. At present, the nature of suppressor cells is not established in these studies. Although suppressor cells induced with high doses of SRBC have been shown to be T cells (29), the role of other cells (e.g., macrophages) as suppressor cells cannot be excluded.

It is clear that antitumor effects of C. parvum may vary from tumor to tumor. Depending on the tumor, C. parvum may act synergistically or antagonistically with chemotherapy. In addition, C. parvum may abrogate immunity against tumor-specific antigens. The mechanism by which C. parvum abrogates tumor-specific immunity and promotes tumor growth is currently under investigation. It is likely that C. parvum might promote the induction of suppressor cells in response to tumor-specific antigens (30).

The immunomodulating activities of C. parvum may be summarized as follows: It causes enhancement of humoral responses when injected with or prior to antigen by the i.v. route or when injected by the i.p. route with antigen injected by the i.v. route. By contrast C. parvum suppresses antibody responses when injected i.p. before immunization by the i.p. route. The suppressive activity of C. parvum is, however, not reflected when antigen is supraoptimal. Furthermore, C. parvum can augment, under optimal immunization conditions, the induction of suppressor cells.

In tumor immunotherapy C. parvum can either inhibit or promote the growth of tumor depending on the tumor model system and the promotion of tumor growth is due to suppression of antitumor resistance and, hence, might depend on the immunogenicity of the tumor. Although the mechanisms of tumor promoting effect of C. parvum are currently not understood, implications of this finding are very significant in the selection of patients with various tumors for immunotherapy with this agent (31).

Portions of this work were supported by USPHS Contract No. NO1-CM-57041 from the National Cancer Institute.

REFERENCES

1. Johnson, J. L., and Cummins, C. S., 1972, J. Bacteriol. 109: 1047.

2. Halpern, B. N., Prevot, A. R., Biozzi, G., Stiffel, C., Mouton, D., Morard, J. C., Bouthillier, Y., and Decreusefond, C., J., 1964, Reticuloendothel. Soc. 1: 77.

3. Adlam, C., and Scott, M. T., 1973, J. Med. Microbiol. 6: 261.

4. O'Neill, G. J., Henderson, D. C., and White, R. G., 1973, Immunol. 24: 977.

5. McBride, W. H., Daws, J., Dunbar, N., Ghaffar, A., and Woodruff, M. F. A., 1975, Immunol. 28: 49.

6. Woodruff, M. F. A., and Boak, J. L., 1966, Br. J. Cancer. 20: 345.

7. Scott, M. T., 1974, Semin. Oncol. 1: 367.

8. Woodruff, M. F. A., Dunbar, N., and Ghaffar, A., 1973, Proc. Roy. Soc. Lond. B. 184: 97.

9. Scott, M. T., 1974, J. Natl. Cancer Inst. 55: 65.

10. Woodruff, M. F. A., and Dunbar, N., 1975, Br. J. Cancer. 32: 34.

11. McBride, W. H., Jones, J. T., and Weir, D. M., 1974, Br. J. Exp. Path. 55: 38.

12. White, R. G., 1975, In: Corynebacterium parvum: Applications in Experimental and Clinical Oncology (B. Halpern,) (ed.), pp. 148-161. Plenum Press, New York.

13. Farzad, A., Penneys, N. S., Ghaffar, A., Ziboh, V. A., and Schlossberg, J., 1977, Prostaglandin 14: 829.

14. Nussenzweig, R. S., 1967, Exp. Parasitol. 21: 224.

15. Adlam, C., Broughton, E. S., and Scott, M. T., 1972, Nature, New Biol. 235: 219.

16. Morahan, P. S., Glasglow, L. A., Crane, J. L., Jr., and Kern, E. R., 1977, Cell. Immunol. 28: 404.

17. McBride, W. H., Weir, D. M.,Kay, A. B., Pearce, D., and Cladwell, J. R., 1975, Clin. Exp. Immunol. 19: 143.

18. Nebeu, T., Branellec, A., and Biozzi, G., 1964, Ann. Inst. Pasteur. 106: 771.

19. Howard, J. G., Scott, M. T., and Christie, G. H., 1973, In. Immunopotentiation (G. E. W. Wolstenholme and J. Knight) (eds.), Associated Scientific Publishers, Amsterdam, Ciba Foundation Symposium 18: 101.

20. Warr, G. W., and Sljivic, V. S., 1974, Clin. Exp. Immunol. 17: 519.

21. Greenberg, C. S., and Dimitrov, N. V., 1976, Clin. Immunol. Immunopath. 5: 264.

22. Howard, J. G., Christie, G. H., and Scott, M. T., 1973, Cell. Immunol. 7: 290.

23. Scott, M. T., 1974, Cell. Immunol. 13: 251.

24. Allwood, G. G., and Asherson, G. L., 1972, Clin. Exp. Immunol. 11: 579.

25. Ghaffar, A. and Sigel, M. M., 1978, Immunol. 35: 685.

26. Woodruff, M. F. A., Ghaffar, A., Dunbar, N. and Whitehead, V. L., 1976, Br. J. Cancer, 33: 491.

27. Watson, S. R., and Sljivic, V. S., 1976. Clin. Exp. Immunol. 23: 149.

28. Sljivic, V. S., and Watson, S. R., 1977, J. Exp. Med. 145: 45.

29. Whisler, R. L., and Stobo, J. D., 1976, J. Exp. Med. 144: 398.

30. Fujimoto, S., Greene, M. I., and Sehon, A. H., 1976, J. Immunol. 116: 791.

31. Rao, B., Wanebo, J., Ochoa, M., Lewis, J. L., and Oettgen, H. F., 1977, Cancer, 39: 514.

IMMUNOMODULATION BY BCG AND SYNTHETIC BACTERIAL-LIKE ADJUVANTS

Louis Chedid
Groupe de Recherche n° 31 du CNRS, Immunothérapie expérimentale, Institut Pasteur, 28 rue du Dr. Roux
75724 Paris cedex 15, France

Various substances extracted from animal sources and also from plants, bacteria, viruses or parasites, have been shown capable of regulating the immune response. However the most studied and probably the strongest exogenous immunomodulators are bacteria and their products (25). Attempts at isolating chemically well-defined agents are justified and timely as they may lead to preparations that retain the therapeutic values which are required yet cause less toxicity. Indeed although BCG and *C. parvum* have been shown to be dramatically effective in certain experimental models, investigators are well aware of the fact that they contain a great variety of heterogeneous antigens, some of which could cross-react to host's tissues (8, 10, 52) or produce certain side effects, or even, following dose and mode of administration, unexpected immune responses (for instance tumor enhancement instead of rejection (54)). The recent development of synthetic immunomodulators of low molecular weight has renewed interest to the field of adjuvants. What is particularly appealing is the possibility that one can now tailor the structure of these molecules in such a way as to use them effectively to influence pre-selected components of the immune system. Certain of these molecules such as polynucleotides (25), peptide analogs of tuftsin (51) or thymic factors (34), have been synthesized because of their analogy to host products. Others have been produced because they represent analogy with microbial products (11). It is our purpose today to select in this vast arsenal synthetic mycobacterial-like adjuvants. These derivatives can be distributed according to their structure in the following classes:

a) glycolipids such as cord factor;
b) glycopeptides such as muramyl peptides;
c) glyco-peptidolipids;

d) peptidolipids.

In our laboratory we have tested compounds of these four classes, but because of time limitation we will refer only to MDP glycopeptides and to some derivatives of MDP of class c) and d).

BCG and other mycobacteria have been intensively studied for their non-specific effects on immunity against tumors and against infectious challenges. They have also received a great deal of attention since the original observation of Jules Freund on the effect of paraffin oil and mycobacteria on antibody formation and sensitization. Such adjuvants have been considered as the most potent enhancing agents of the immune response. However, the utilization of the remarkable activity of Freund's complete adjuvant (FCA) other than in experimental procedures has been restricted by the toxic reactivity of mycobacteria which can induce various side effects (increased susceptibility to endotoxin, granuloma formation and lymphoid hyperplasia, adjuvant arthritis, sensitization to tuberculin, etc...) related to their content in cord factor, PPD and probably also to yet non-identified components. Last but not least clinical applications have been greatly limited by the presence of non-metabolizable oil in FCA.

In his early studies, Freund suggested the existence of a rather widely dispersed common adjuvant unit when he wrote: "It would be of great interest to identify the fraction or fractions which exert the adjuvant effect of mycobacteria and to know whether the effect could be produced without sensitizing to tuberculin" (19). It is now possible to answer that the fraction has been identified, synthesized and that it does not sensitize to tuberculin.

In recent years, the pioneering studies of Dr. Lederer and his colleagues have permitted the identification and synthesis of two biologically active components of the mycobacterial cell wall: trehalose dimycolate (TDM) or cord factor and muramyl dipeptides (MDP) such as N-acetyl-muramyl-L-alanyl-D-isoglutamine and its derivatives (1, 17, 33, 37).

MDP was the first adjuvant analogous to a bacterial cell wall to be synthesized and to be shown by A. Adam and E. Lederer to substitute to mycobacteria in FCA. Shortly after similar findings were reported by Dr. Kotani and his colleagues (5, 29). The various aspects of biological activity of MDP and its derivatives have been reviewed recently (11) and mechanisms of action studied in various systems. Since its synthesis in 1974 (17, 37) multiple analogs of MDP have been synthesized in Europe, in the US and in Japan with minor modifications (more than 150 have been tested in our laboratory) and correlations between biological activity and chemical structure are beginning to be understood. To illustrate, certain derivatives such as MDP stereoisomer where D-alanine were substituted for the L form, were capable of inhibiting the immune response, suggesting their possible use as immunosuppressors (11). It is also of importance that certain of these synthetic adjuvants were shown to stimulate phagocytosis and to increase non-specific resistance to infection (12). These derivatives were active by various routes including oral administration both in adult and in newborn mice. More recent experiments have shown that muramic acid is required for adjuvant activity but not for enhancement of non-specific resistance to infection (39).

Although most of the data obtained when this synthetic adjuvant was administered in saline concerns systems involving humoral antibody production, it must be recalled that when administered in Freund's incomplete adjuvant (FIA), MDP can induce delayed hypersensitivity and even autoimmune diseases (50, 38). In a very recent report it was shown that autoimmune encephalomyelitis can be induced by a synthetic auto-antigen (a tryptophan nonapeptide) administered either with FCA in guinea pigs or with MDP in FIA. This antigen has been shown to be the shortest active encephalitogen peptide when administered with FCA. However autoimmune disease was also induced by a tryheptapeptide administered with MDP in FIA but not with FCA. Administration with either adjuvant of even shorter peptides (containing six or less aminoacids) had no effect, showing how critical is the presence of a single aminoacid in this system. These experiments are remarkable not only because they demonstrate a maximal amplification of the immune response under the influence of a synthetic antigen and of a synthetic adjuvant but also because they provide a most interesting model for cell-mediated autoimmune reactions since such haptenic synthetic peptides cannot induce antibody production (38).

As stated previously, in contrast to other bacterial or cell wall adjuvant fractions, MDP and several derivatives were found to be very effective when injected in an aqueous medium. Humoral antibody titers were markedly enhanced under these conditions. Moreover this activity was demonstrable by various routes including the oral administration (3). These glycopeptides can also stimulate *in vitro* specific (32, 35, 45, 46) and non-specific (14, 15, 26, 48) immune responses, such as polyclonal stimulation or macrophage activation. Other responses have been measured *in vitro*, showing that adjuvant active derivatives of MDP incubated with peritoneal exudate macrophages could increase bactericidal activity, lymphocyte activating factor synthesis, enzyme production and levels of prostaglandins (23, 49, 53). The profile of these synthetic adjuvants is rather unique since several of the side effects inherent to mycobacteria are not elicited by them. Thus, these compounds do not sensitize to tuberculin, do not induce adjuvant polyarthritis or increase susceptibility to endotoxins (11). Moreover, although they can stimulate the RES as measured by carbon clearance (48), their administration is not followed by lymphoid hyperplasia and hepatosplenomegaly. It must also be noted that the molecule is removed very rapidly from the host as was shown in studies using ^{14}C-labelled MDP (41). Indeed, MDP can be very effectively labelled on the C_1 of the lactyl group starting from DL-bromo-2-propionic acid ^{14}Cr (figure 1). The results of in vivo administration of ^{14}C-MDP showed that the synthetic glycopeptide is eliminated extremely rapidly when administered to mice in saline. Furthermore most of the radioactivity recovered in the urine was excreted without modifications and only a very small amount was detectable in the liver and degraded to a smaller product containing Mur-NAc. The in vivo activity of MDP in saline must therefore be explained either because this molecule has an immediate effect at the cellular level or because minute amounts are effective in vivo.

We would like to discuss now various procedures which can be used to potentiate the activity of MDP. MDP effectively increased host resistance to Trypanosoma cruzi after repeated injections to mice or continuous subcutaneous administration in an osmotic minipump (27). Retardation of release of MDP could also be obtained by inclusion in liposomes and by conjugation on synthetic carriers.

There is a general consensus that in many cases an adjuvant capable of increasing T cell activity in the absence of non-metabolizable oil component will be required (30). Most studies dealing with MDP in vivo have shown that this molecule was not capable of increasing cell-mediated responses when it was administered with the antigen in an aqueous medium. However, positive results have been reported when the hydrophobicity of these molecules was increased (fatty acid derivatives) and when they were incorporated in liposomes (28, 36). Thus, enhancement of immunity was reported with a Plasmodium falciparum merozoite antigen administered with an MDP derivative in liposomes to Aotus monkeys. Protection was measured by survival and by parasitemia after infectious challenge (44).

Several separate reports have also shown that cell-mediated immunity can be enhanced when lipophilic derivatives were administered in saline. This was studied in vivo and in vitro using various test systems such as allogenic cytotoxicity or protection against murine tumors (6, 24, 55). In these assays MDP was weaker or inactive as compared to its fatty acid derivatives.

The immunostimulant properties of a new MDP derivative bearing a lipophilic moiety on the C-terminal end of the peptide chain has been recently described (39). This 1-O(AcMur-L-Ala-D-isoGln-L-Ala)-glycerol-3-mycolate (MDP-L-Ala-glycerol mycolate) had an increased immunostimulant activity in comparison with MDP. It induced hypersensitivity even when administered with an antigen in saline and gave a higher protection against bacterial infections than MDP.

MDP

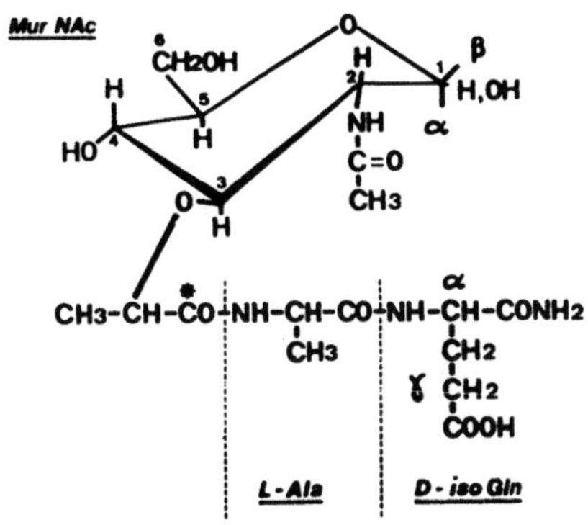

Fig. 1. Muramyl dipeptide formula. Certain samples of synthetic N-acetyl muramyl-L-alanyl-D-isoglutamine were ^{14}C-labeled on C_1 of the lactyl residue.

A quite unexpected finding was obtained with the corresponding des-muramyl compound 1-O(L-Ala-D-isoGln-L-Ala)-glycerol-3-mycolate which was not pyrogenic, had no activity in producing humoral antibodies, but was just as active as the muramic acid containing compound in stimulating non-specific resistance to bacterial infections. Modifications of the peptide moiety or the lipid moiety of this peptidolipid lead to decrease, or even loss of activity (39).

As stated above these results showed the importance of the N-acetyl-muramyl moiety in MDP for humoral antibody production.

Adjuvant activity of MDP derivatives can be poteniated by conjugating glycopeptides and synthetic antigen on a synthetic carrier A--L (multipoly-DL-alanyl-poly-L-lysin). The synthetic antigen comprises the fragment P_2 of the coat protein of the MS_2 polyphage. The glycopeptide represented a small molecular weight glycopeptide prepared from Bacillus megaterium. When injected in PBS or FIA, P_2-A--L without the glycopeptide did not elicit antisera possessing anti-phage activity. However, when the adjuvant was chemically linked to the P_2-A--L conjugate, it had a marked effect if administered in FIA (31). As was reported by M. Sela et al. recently, when synthetic adjuvants were conjugated to synthetic antigens increased antibody response was observed even in the absence of FIA (16bis).

Polymerization of MDP has also been shown to potentiate its immunostimulant properties. The β-D-ρ-aminophenyl glycoside of

MDP (PAP-MDP) does not have most of the biological activities of MDP (in vivo humoral antibody response, in vitro stimulation of spleen cells, increased resistance to infection). A remarkable finding was that following cross-linkage with glutaraldehyde, this oligomer protected mice against a Klebsiella challenge and stimulated thymidine uptake more effectively than MDP (40). A marked enhancement of activity was also observed when MDP or MDP derivatives were conjugated to synthetic multi-poly (DL-Ala)-poly (L-Lys) and referred to as the A--L chain. However, several of the active MDP derivatives which can activate macrophages and enhance non-specific resistance to infection, can also elicit fever (16, 29). In contrast, the N-acetyl-muramyl-D-Ala-D-Glu-NH_2 derivative referred to as MDP(DD) is devoid of biological activities and of pyrogenicity. A recent study has demonstrated that macromolecularization of MDP by attachment of several units to the A--L chain potentiates the anti-infectious activity of MDP but also its pyrogenicity and its immunogenicity. Surprisingly, MDP(DD), after conjugation under the same conditions, became capable of increasing non-specific immunity although its lack of pyrogenicity was not greatly modified. Moreover, the MDP(DD) conjugate was capable of activating macrophages in vitro but still remained devoid of adjuvant, sensitizing or eliciting activity (13, 22). As shown previously with the peptidolipid MDP derivative, it therefore appeared that there exists no strict correlation between the structure required for adjuvant activity and the structure required for macrophage activation or for enhancement of non-specific immunity.

MDP has also been conjugated to various proteins either in view of rendering this small synthetic molecule immunogenic (4) by linkage to a carrier or in view of increasing its adjuvant activity toward this protein. In such studies, in view of obtaining a good immunogen without loosing adjuvant activity, care must be taken to conjugate an optimal number of haptenic groups per carrier molecule without altering the active site (42).

Conjugation procedures by binding antigens to MDP also provides an interesting model for the future since adjuvant action could be focused on the immunocompetent cells responsive to the antigen thus minimizing stimulation of unwanted cell clones. Moreover recent experiments allow us to hope that certain derivatives will be less multifocal and conform better to a hormone target cell model.

CONCLUSION

Besides microorganisms such as Pertussis, Corynebacteria or BCG, various heterogenous and complex materials have been repeatedly used in view of enhancing the immune response. FCA has been successfully used for decades with various vaccines, including living Plasmodium antigen (1, 18, 20, 21). Its utilization was however greatly restricted by the presence of mineral oil and of the "side effects" induced by mycobacteria. Although until recently the prevailing idea concerning adjuvants was that they were "foreign" and even "aggressive" or "insulting" substances, it has now been clearly established that synthetic small molecular weight materials show this activity. MDP, a synthetic bacterial-like glycopeptide, administered in an aqueous medium by parenteral or oral route can enhance humoral antibody response to various antigens or vaccines (2, 16bis). Under these conditions, however, and in contrast to FCA, immunity cannot be raised in many situations such as malaria. The adjuvant requirement of this and probably other vaccines may be even possible in a not too distant future to obtain derivatives capable of increasing cell-mediated immunity even in the absence of liposomes or of oily vehicles. Besides their use in the area of classical vaccines for parasitic or bacterial infections and perhaps some day for tumor immunity, adjuvants seem to have a potential in totally unrelated fields. Thus, studies are being performed in view of controlling fertility and enhancing antibodies against a synthetic peptide representing part of the β-HCG subunit (47). Such an antigen has the advantage of being devoid of hormonal activity and of cross-reactivity with other endogenous hormones. Another model of synthetic "viral" antigen combined to a synthetic adjuvant has also been described recently (16bis). Since purified and synthetic antigens of the future shall most probably be weak immunogens, the need for immunopotentiation by adjuvants will therefore be increased.

Whatever the choice of the future adjuvants for vaccines, it is reasonable to believe that they will be synthetic molecules and reasonable to hope to potentiate them by procedures such as those that have been described above. Care must be taken however to make sure that these procedures do not increase hazards of their utilization. New toxicological critieria will have to be found such as measuring autoimmune or allergic reactions inherent to the administration of agents with great immunological potency.

Besides their clinical potential, synthetic compounds analogous to bacterial immunoregulating agents should also constitute useful tools for various studies in different areas of basic immunology. The chemical structure of lymphokines and other immunologically active endogenous molecules is difficult to identify and therefore to synthetize. It has been suggested that these fine biological probes may represent an easier way for the characterization of natural agents. "An interesting example of a bacterial product serving as a regulator molecule in a mammalian system is N-acetyl-muramyl-L-alanyl-D-isoglutamine (MDP). The γ glytamyl function of isoglutamine is essential for the adjuvant action of this molecule. Does the sugar dipeptide, synthetic or derived from the bacterial cell wall, do its job because it mimics a regulator molecule of the immune response?" (7).

A great deal of attention has been focused on new techniques such as genetic engineering or monoclonal antibodies obtained by cell fusion. However the production of large series of analogs by peptide synthesis should remain an additional approach of great interest. In this respect, D-isoglutamine, which is essential for the activity of MDP, is not hydrolyzable by enzymes of mammalian hosts and thus cannot be degraded easily. Substitution of the L-isomere results in the inactive product. One might speculate that the former non-degradable form may be a distinct asset as compared to natural mediators which have probably short biological half-lives. It is interesting to note that recently synthetic pentapeptides related to Met-enkephalin were shown to have prolonged parenteral and oral analgesic activity. In these molecules, D-alanine had been substituted to the glyceryl residue in position 2 (43).

REFERENCES

1. Adam, A., Ciorbaru, R., Petit, J. F., and Lederer, 1972, Isolation and properties of a macromolecular, water-soluble, immunoadjuvant fraction from the cell wall of Mycobacterium smegmatis. Proc. Natl. Acad. Sci. USA. 69: 851.

2. Audibert, F., Chedid, L., and Hannoun, C., 1977, Augmentation de la reponse immunitaire au vaccin grippal par un glycopeptide synthetique adjuvant (N-acetyl-muramyl-L-alanyl-D-isoglutamine). C. R. Acad. Sc. Paris 285D: 467.

3. Audibert, F., Chedid, L., Lefrancier, P., and Choay, J., 1976, Distinctive adjuvanticity of synthetic analogs of mycobacterial water-soluble components. Cell. Immunol. 21: 243.

4. Audibert, F., Heymer, B., Gros, C., Schleifer, K. H., Seidl, P. H., and Chedid, L., 1978, Absence of binding of MDP, a synthetic immunoadjuvant, to anti-peptidoglycan antibodies. J. Immunol. 121: 1219.

5. Azuma, I., Sugimura, K., Taniayama, T., Yamawaki, M., Yamamura, Y., Kusumoto, S., Okada, S., and Shiba, T., 1976, Adjuvant activity of mycobacterial fractions: adjuvant activity of synthetic N-acetylmuramyl dipeptide and related compounds. Infect. Immun. 14: 18.

6. Azuma, I., Sugimura, K, Yamawaki, M., Uemiya, M., Kusumoto, S., Okada, S., Shiba, T., and Yamamura, Y., 1978, Adjuvant activity of synthetic 6-O-"mycoloyl"-N-acetyl-muramyl-L-alanyl-D-isoglutamine and related compounds. Infect. Immun. 20: 600.

7. Barksdale, L., and Kim, K. S., 1977, Mycobacterium. Bact. Rev. 41: 217.

8. Borsos, T., and Rapp, H. J., 1973, Antigenic relationship between Mycobacterium bovis (BCG) and a guinea pig hepatoma. J. Nat. Cancer Inst. 51: 1085.

9. Brown, K. N., Brown, I. N., and Hills, L. A., 1970, Immunity to malaria. I. Protection against Plasmodium knowlesi shown by monkeys sensitized with drug-suppressed infections or by dead parasites in Freund's adjuvant. Exptl. Parasit. 28: 304.

10. Bucana, C., and Hanna, Jr., M. G., 1974, Immunoelectron microscopic analysis of surface antigens commont to Mycobacterium bovis (BCG) and tumor cells. J. Nat. Cancer Inst. 53: 1313.

11. Chedid, L., Audibert, F., and Johnson, A. G., 1978, Biological activities of muramyl dipeptide, a synthetic glycopeptide analogous to bacterial immunoregulating agents. Progress in Allergy 25: 63.

12. Chedid, L., Parant, M., Parant, F., Lefrancier, P., Choay, J., and Lederer, E., 1977, Enhancement of non-specific immunity to Klebsiella pneumoniae infection by a synthetic immunoadjuvant (N-acetyl-muramyl-L-alanyl-D-isoglutamine) and several analogs. Proc. Natl. Acad. Sci. USA 84: 2089

13. Chedid, L., Parant, M., Parant, F., Audibert, F., Lefrancier, P., Choay, J., and Sela, M., 1979, Enhancement of certain biological activities of muramyl dipeptide derivatives after conjugation to a multi-poly (DL-alanine)--poly(L-lysine) carrier. Proc. Natl. Acad. Sci. USA. 76: in press.

14. Damais, C., Parant, M., and Chedid, L., 1977, Nonspecific activation of murine spleen cells in vitro by a synthetic immunoadjuvant (N-acetylmuramyl-L-alanyl-D-isoglutamine). Cell. Immunol. 34: 49.

15. Damais, C., Parant, M., and Chedid, L., 1978, In vitro spleen cell responsiveness to various analogs of MDP (N-acetylmuramyl-L-alanyl-D-isoglutamine), a synthetic immunoadjuvant, in MDP high responder mice. Cell. Immunol. 35: 173.

16. Dinarello, C. A., Elin, R. J., Chedid, L., and Wolff, S. M., 1978, The pyrogenicity of the synthetic muramyl dipeptide and two structural analogues. J. Infect. Dis. 138: 760.

16bis. Edelman, R., Hardegree, C., and Chedid, L., 1979, Summary of the Int. Symposium on Potentiation of the Immune Response to Vaccines. J. Infect. Dis.: in press.

17. Ellouz, F., Adam, A., Ciorbaru, R., and Lederer, E., 1974, Minimal structural requirements for adjuvant activity of bacterial peptidoglycan derivatives. Biochem. Biophys. Res. Comm. 59: 1317.

18. Freund, J., 1956, The mode of action of immunologic adjuvants. In Adv. Tuberc. Res. 7: 130 (Karger, Basel).

19. Freund, J., 1947, Some aspects of active immunization. A. Rev. Microbiol. 1: 291.

20. Freund, J., Sommer, H. E., and Walter, A. W., 1945, Immunization against malaria: vaccination of ducks with killed parasites incorporated with adjuvants. Science 102: 200.

21. Freund, J., Thomson, K. J., Sommer, H. E., Walter, A. W., and Pisani, T. M., 1948, Immunization of monkeys against malaria by means of killed parasites with adjuvants. Am. J. Trop. Med. 28: 1.

22. Galelli, A., Le Garrec, Y., Chedid, L., Lefrancier, P., Derrien, M., and Level, M. Macrophage stimulation in vitro by an inactive MDP derivative after conjugation to a multipoly(Dl-alanyl)--poly(L-lysine) carrier. Submitted for publication.

23. Hadden, J., Englard, A., Sadlik, J. R., and Hadden, E. M., 1979, The comparative effects of Isoprinosine, Levamisole, Muramyl Dipeptide and SM 1213 on lymphocyte and macrophage proliferation and activation in vitro. Int. J. Immunopharmacol. 1:17.

24. Igarashi, T., Ikada, M., Azuma, I, and Yamamura, Y., 1977, Adjuvant activity of synthetic N-acetylmuramyl-L-alanyl-D-isoglutamine and related compounds on cell-mediated cytotoxicity in syngeneic mice. Cell. Immunol. 34: 270.

25. Johnson, A. G., Audibert, F., and Chedid, L., 1978, Synthetic immunoregulating molecules: a potential bridge between cytostatic chemotherapy and immunotherapy of cancer. Cancer Immunol. Immunother. 3: 219.

26. Juy, D., and Chedid, L., 1975, Comparison between macrophage activation and enhancement of non-specific resistance to tumors by mycobacterial immunoadjuvants. Proc. Natl. Acad. Sci. USA. 72: 4105.

27. Kierszenbaum, F., and Ferraresi, R. W., 1979, Enhancement of host resistance against Trypanosoma cruzi infection by the immunoregulatory agent muramyl dipeptide. Infect. Immun. 25: 273.

28. Kotani, S., Kinoshita, F., Morisaki, I., Shimono, T., Okunaga, T., Takada, H., Tsujimoto, M., Watanabe, Y., Kato, K., Shiba, T., Kusumoto, S., and Okada, S., 1977, Immunoadjuvant activities of synthetic 6-O-acyl-N-acetyl-muramyl-L-alanyl-D-isoglutamine with special reference to the effect of its administration with liposomes. Biken J. 20: 95.

29. Kotani, S., Watanabe, Y., Shimono, T., Harada, K., Shiba, T., Kusumoto, S., Yokogawa, K., and Taniguchi, M., 1976, Correlation between the immunoadjuvant activities and pyrogenicities of synthetic N-acetylmuramyl peptides or -amino acids. Biken J. 19: 9.

30. The Lancet, Editorial: Immunological adjuvants: less alchemy and more science? July 30, vol. II for 1977, 230.

31. Langbeheim, H., Arnon, R., and Sela, M., 1978, Adjuvant effect of a peptidoglycan attached covalently to a synthetic antigen provoking anti-phage antibodies. Immunology 35: 573.

32. Leclerc, C., Löwy, I., and Chedid, L., 1978, Influence of MDP and some analogous synthetic glycopeptides on the in vitro mouse spleen cell viability and immune response to sheep erythrocytes. Cell. Immunol. 38: 286.

33. Lederer, E., 1979, Cord factor and related synthetic trehalose diesters. Springer Semin. Immunopathol. 2: 133.

34. Low, T. L. K., and Goldstein, A. L., 1979, Thymosin and other thymic hormones and their synthetic analogues. Springer Semin. Immunopathol. 2: 169.

35. Lowy, I., Bona, C., and Chedid, L., 1977, Target cells for the activity of a synthetic adjuvant: muramyl dipeptide. Cell. Immunol. 29: 195.

36. Masek, K., Zaoral, M., Jezek, J., and Straka, R., 1978, Immunoadjuvant activity of synthetic N-acetylmuramyl-dipeptide. Experientia 34/10: 1363.

37. Merser, C., Sinay, P., and Adam, A., 1975, Total synthesis and adjuvant activity of bacterial peptidoglycan derivatives. Biochem. Biophys. Res. Comm. 66: 1316.

38. Nagai, Y., Akiyama, K., Kotani, S., Watanabe, Y., Shimono, T., Shiba, T., and Kusumoto, S., 1978. Structural specificity of synthetic peptide adjuvant for induction of experimental allergic encephalomyelitis. Cell. Immunol. 35: 168.

39. Parant, M., Audibert, F., Chedid, L., Level, M., Lefrancier, P., Choay, J., and Lederer, E., Immunostimulant activities of a lipophilic muramyl dipeptide derivative, and of des-muramyl peptidolipid analogs. Submitted for publication.

40. Parant, M., Damais, C., Audibert, F., Parant, F., Chedid, L., Sache, E., Lefrancier, P., Choay, J., and Lederer, E., 1978, In vivo and in vitro stimulation of nonspecific immunity by the β-D-ρ-aminophenyl glycoside of N-acetylmuramyl-L-alanyl-D-isoglutamine (MDP) and an oligomer prepared by cross-linking with glutaraldehyde. J. Infect. Dis. 138: 378.

41. Parant, M., Parant, F., Chedid, L., Yapo, A., Petit, J. F., and Lederer, E., 1979, Fate of the synthetic immunoadjuvant, muramyl dipeptide (^{14}C-labelled) in the mouse. Int. J. Immunopharmac. 1: 35.

42. Reichert, C. M., Carelli, C., Jolivet, M., Audibert, F., Lefrancier, P., and Chedid, L., 1979, Synthesis of conjugates containing N-acetylmuramyl-L-alanyl-D-isoglutaminyl (MDP). Their use as hapten-carrier systems. Molecular Immunol. in press.

43. Roemer, D., Buescher, H. H., Hill, R. C., Pless, J., Bauer, W., Cardinaux, F., Closse, A. M., Hauser, D., and Huguenin, R., 1977, A synthetic enkephalin analogue with prolonged parenteral and oral analgesis activity. Nature. 268: 547.

44. Siddiqui, W. A., Taylor, D. W., Kan, S. C., Kramer, K., Richmond-Crum, S. M., Kotani, S., Shiba, T., and Kusumoto, C., 1978, Vaccination of experimental monkeys against Plasmodium falciparum: a possible safe adjuvant. Science 201: 1237.

45. Specter, S., Cimprich, R., Friedman, H., and Chedid, L., 1978, Stimulation of an enhanced in vitro immune response by a synthetic adjuvant muramyl dipeptide. J. Immunol. 120: 487.

46. Specter, S., Friedman, H., and Chedid, L., 1977, Dissociation between the adjuvant vs. mitogenic activity of a synthetic muramyl dipeptide for murine splenocytes. Proc. Soc. Exp. Biol. Med. 155: 349.

47. Stevens, V. C., 1975, Female contraception by immunization with HCG. Prospects and status. In Immunization with hormones in reproduction research, pp. 217-231 (Neschlag ed.), North-Holland, Amsterdam.

48. Tanaka, A., Nagao, S., Saito, R., Kotani, S., Kusumoto, S., and Shiba, T., 1977, Correlation of stereochemically specific

structure in muramyl dipeptide between macrophage activation and adjuvant activity. Biochem. Biophys. Res. Comm. 77: 621.

49. Togawa, A., Oppenheim, J. J., Mizel, S. B., Kirkpatrick, C., and Chedid, L., 1978, Transfer factor (TF) and other stimulants activate human macrophages to produce lymphocyte activation factor (LAF). Fed. Proc. 37: 1589.

50. Toullet, F., Audibert, F., Voisin, G. A., and Chedid, L., 1977, Production d'une orchiepididymite aspermatogenetique auto-immune chez le cobaye, a l'aide de differents adjuvants hydrosolubles. Ann. Immunol. (Inst. Pasteur) 128C: 267.

51. Tzehoval, E., Segal, S., Stabinsky, Y., Fridkin, M., Spirer, Z., and Feldman, M., 1979, Immunostimulation by an Ig derived tetrapeptide, tuftsin. Springer Semin. Immunopathol. 2: 205.

52. Vandenbard, A. A., Burger, D. R., and Vetto, R. M., 1975, Cell-mediated immunity in experimental allergic encephalomyelitis. Cross reactivity between myelin basic protein and mycobacteria antigens. Proc. Soc. Exp. Biol. Med. 148: 1233.

53. Wahl, S. M., Wahl, L. M., McCarthy, J. B., Chedid, L., and Mergenhagen, S. E., 1979, Macrophage activation by mycobacterial water soluble components and synthetic muramyl dipeptide. J. Immunol. 122: 2226.

54. Werner, G. H., Maral, R., Floc'h, F., and Joyanne, M., 1977, Toxicological aspects of immunopotentiation by adjuvants and immunostimulating substances. Bull. Inst. Pasteur 75: 5.

55. Yamamura, Y., Azuma, I., Sugimura, K., Yamawaki, M., Uemiya, M., Kusumoto, S., Okada, S., and Shiba, T., 1976, Adjuvant activity of 6-O-mycoloyl-N-acetyl-muramyl-L-alanyl-D-isoglutamine. Gann. 67: 867.

IMMUNOSTIMULATION BY LPS AND ITS DERIVATIVES

U. H. Behling and A. Nowotny

University of Pennsylvania
Philadelphia, PA

Of the vast number of biological properties attributed to endotoxins, their unique capacity to stimulate the body's natural defenses in an immunologically non-specific way is unquestionably their most important property. That the effect of endotoxin on the immune system is not a singular, well-defined interaction becomes obvious from studies *in vivo* and *in vitro*. The non-specific effects of endotoxin upon resistance to various pathogens have been reported by many investigators (7, 18, 26, 44) and are attributed to many different cellular and non-cellular mechanisms (3). Alterations of the hemopoietic system include an early appearance of leukopenia followed several hours later by marked leukocytosis (20, 25). The histological picture of the bone marrow, spleen, thymus, and lymph nodes also follows a bi-phasic response which is initially characterized by intensely degenerative-appearing tissue, hypocellularity and loss in size and weight. Within 24 to 48 hours, cell-rich foci appear, giving rise to hyperplasia several days thereafter (44, 20, 50). This is the result of increased production of granulocytes, lymphocytes, myelocytes, and macrophages. Functional changes are also evident during this time.

Likewise it has been demonstrated that the administration of endotoxin induces biphasic histological and functional changes in the reticuloendothelial system, as indicated by the rapid clearance of foreign substances from the blood (2, 5, 15). This increased phagocytic activity following the initial depression and lasting for almost one week closely parallels the non-specific resistance to infection and is thought to be a major contributing factor. In addition, the influence on the production, release, or interaction of endotoxin on humoral factors involving opsonins (4), complement (17), interferon (51), properdin (27), histamine (19) and serotonin

(14) have all been implicated in directly or indirectly affecting immunity.

The Relationship of Structure to Function in Bacterial Endotoxin

For all the extensive studies involving endotoxin-induced bioeffects, their precise mode of action remains poorly understood. Not even the primary cellular or sub-cellular targets of endotoxic action have been clearly established. One can readily appreciate the complexity of this problem when the chemical heterogeneity of endotoxins is realized. It is clear that different bacterial strains produce chemically dissimilar bacterial products including their serologically immunospecific endotoxins.

Before discussing specific immuno-stimulatory effects of LPS and their relationship to the chemical-structural compositions, it seems appropriate to briefly review and reference our most basic understanding of this complex biological product. For the benefit of the reader several very extensive literature reviews covering the chemical and biological aspects of endotoxin are available (13, 29, 30, 35, 36).

The endotoxins of Gram-negative bacteria consist of two major regions, the larger of which is the polysaccharide (PS) moiety. This consists of an O-antigen component which is responsible for the unique serological specificity and a "core" polysaccharide whose structure is common to most bacteria. The core polysaccharide is linked through the 2-keto-3 deoxy octonate trisaccharide to the lipid component designated as "lipid A". This lipid A component is characterized by a phosphorylated glucosamine disaccharide unit with ester- and amide-linked fatty acids. A small and variable percentage of bound peptides constitute the third but minor component of most purified LPS preparations. Although their pharmacological significance is not firmly established, their structural importance may be that of linking the endotoxic LPS to the bacterial cell wall (36).

Mild acid hydrolysis was first used by Boivin and associates in 1933 (6) for the separation of the lipid moiety from the polysaccharide portion of the parent LPS molecule. It was principally the work of Westphal, Lüderitz, and their associates that led to the recognition that the biologically active part of the endotoxic lipopolysaccharide is its lipid moiety (47, 48, 46, 24, 23). Subjecting LPS to 1N HCl at 100 degrees C for 30 minutes yielded an insoluble lipid precipitate and the acid-soluble partially degraded non-toxic polysaccharide moiety.

Endotoxic Activity of Lipid A

Continued investigations in our laboratory have focused attention on the structure-function relationship of these two major components of endotoxin. Our findings confirm these earlier observations which implicate the intact lipid moiety in the elicitation of most of the characteristic endotoxic reactions (46, 33, 32, 22, 34, 40, 11). The work of Nowotny and associates regarding the significance of the lipid moiety in endotoxicity reactions comes from three major groups of experiments.

1. Chemical detoxification. The aim of this approach was to destroy selectively certain functional groups in the endotoxin structure and to observe changes in the biological activities. The detoxification procedures involved (a) trans-esterification with boron trifluoride, (b) deacylation with potassium methylate and (c) treatment with equimolar mixture of pyridine and formic acid. Our observations clearly indicate that those procedures which cleave ester-bound carboxylic acids lead to detoxification of the endotoxin preparation; however the beneficial effect of the endotoxin-induced adjuvancy remained unaffected. The data originally reported by Johnson and Nowotny (22) are summarized in Table I. Detoxification of LPS with potassium methylate also produced marked hyperplasia of granulocytes in bone marrow and demonstrated strong protection against whole-body irradiation in mice (25, 31).

2. Immunological detoxification. Rabbit hyper-immune O-antiserum was adsorbed with chemically detoxified endotoxins. This treatment removed antibodies reacting specifically with the polysaccharide moiety of the LPS molecule. The residual supernatant which no longer reacted with detoxified endotoxin or with the acid-hydrolysis breakdown product (PS) still could neutralize endotoxicity of the untreated endotoxin (46).

Residual toxicity was measured when endotoxin was neutralized or partially neutralized by varying the Ag to Ab ratio. Less than optimal ratios increasingly tended to restore endotoxicity (Table II). When optimal Ab neutralized endotoxin was tested for nonspecific resistance to infection, it proved to be as effective as the control LPS (Table III). Of interest is that human serum - antiserum Ag-Ab precipitate showed no significant protection.

3. Endotoxins of the heptose-less Re mutants. The use of rough mutants of Gram negative bacteria which were first isolated by Dr. Otto Lüderitz and associates have provided an invaluable tool in structure-function relationship studies of endotoxin. These mutant strains lack certain enzyme functions which subsequently prevents synthesis of the complete polysaccharide structure of the "smooth" parent strain. Independent studies by Reisman (41) and White (49) describe that "smooth" to "rough" conversion of certain bacterial strains is characterized by partial or complete loss of the polysaccharide moiety of the O-antigens in these bacterial endotoxins. Current studies in our laboratory involve the chemical

TABLE I

The Biologic Effect of Detoxified Endotoxin[1]

Treatment of LPS	Mouse lethality[2] µg	Shwartzman reactivity[3] to 10 µg	Non-specific Resistance[4] (% survival)	Adjuvant effect to HGG[5] (titer)
Untreated LPS	180	50%	80	320
Boron trifluoride treated-LPS	2000	0	90	5120
Potassium methylate treated LPS	4000	0	90	1280
Pyridinium formate treated LPS	2000	0	90	2560
Control: no LPS	-	-	30	2560

1 This table is a summary of data presented by A. G. Johnson and A. Nowotny, J. Bact. 87: 809-814, 1964.

2 Swiss albino mice were injected i.p.; death occurred within 3 days.

3 New Zealand white were injected with 10 µg i.d. with the preparations; 20 hrs later the animals were injected with 100 µg of the parent LPS to provoke the reaction.

4 Swiss Webster mice were given 2 µg i.p. of the preparation; 24 hrs later they were chellenged with 7 x 10^8 bacterial cells of Salmonella typhosa 0-901.

5 Balb/c mice were injected simultaneously with 50 µg of the endotoxic preparation and 3 mg of HGG. Serum anti-HGG titers were determined 12 days later.

and biological characterization of the R-5 and R-7 endotoxins. Although chemical analysis has shown only minor differences, preliminary data suggest significant differences in their biological potency.

From the above data one can conclude that an intact lipid moiety is essential for the expression of endotoxicity. Both chemical and immunological neutralization of the lipid component reduced its endotoxicity. In contrast, such detoxified products possessed the

TABLE II

Neutralization of Endotoxic Effects by O-Antiserum

Ab/Ag ratio	% of optimal amount of Ab added	Shwartzman reactivity	Mouse Lethality LD_{50} (mg)	Pyrogenicity* 1 hr	3 hrs
6.60	100	neg.	>>2.0	0.6	0.0
2.20	33	neg.	>2.0	0.6	0.3
1.10	17	+	~2.0	0.7	0.5
0.20	3	++	1.0	1.3	0.7
0.00	0	++++	0.3	1.7	2.8
Controls:					
N.R.S.°+ endotoxin		++++	0.3	1.6	2.9
N.H.S.°°+ N.H.S. anti-serum ppt		neg.	non-toxic	0.0	0.0

* Elevation of the body temperature in degrees C.

° N.R.S. - normal rabbit serum.

°° N.H.S. - normal human serum.

TABLE III

Inducement of Non-specific Resistance in Mice with Endotoxin and with Antibody+Endotoxin Complex

Pretreatment	Dose of Endotoxin in the Pretreatment	Number of Survivors/ Number of Total
Saline	None	3/20
Endotoxin in Saline	1 μg	18/20
Endotoxin + O-Antibody ppt	1 μg	17/20
Human + anti-human ppt	none	2/20

ability to increase non-specific resistance in mice equal to that elicited by the parent endotoxin. These detoxified preparations also showed immune enhancement to a foreign protein antigen. It appears that the ability to impart non-specific resistance and immune adjuvancy can be dissociated from the toxic nature of endotoxin as well as its antigenic stimulus.

Role of the Polysaccharide Moiety in Endotoxic Activity

It has been firmly established that the major immunogenic component for the endotoxic LPS lies in the polysaccharide moiety (28). Subsequently it was reported that the acid soluble, partially degraded hydrolytic product of endotoxin is rich in carbohydrates and does not show any residual toxicity. Although this preparation was able to react with homologous antibodies it could not elicit their production.

Colony Stimulation of Bone-marrow Cells (CSF)

In recent years, studies conducted in our laboratories indicated that the same hydrolytic product (PS) is active in bone marrow colony stimulation (10). Lipid preparations obtained after acidic hydrolysis or by using the endotoxic glycolipid (GL) extracted from rough Re mutants were either inactive or showed a grossly reduced activity (Table IV)

Further studies of the CSF inducing component in the PS fraction showed that (a) it was not readily dialyzable, (b) the majority of

TABLE IV

Serum CSF Induced by Various Fractions of *S. minnesota* LPS

Preparation Injected i.p.	Number of Colonies
LPS[a]	262 ± 14
PS[b]	250 ± 15
"Lipid A"[c]	96 ± 10
GL[d]	48 ± 8
Saline	45 ± 5

[a]Lipopolysaccharide form smooth *S. minnesota* 1114.
[b]Water-soluble hydrolytic products of *S. minnesota* 1114 LPS.
[c]Precipitated hydrolytic products of *S. minnesota* 1114 LPS.
[d]Endotoxic glycolipid of *S. minnesota* R595 heptoseless mutant.

activity within this mixture was of molecular weight greater than 10,000 and (c) that by composition 54% consists of carbohydrates with no detectable levels of fatty acids. In addition, treatment of the PS preparation with metaperiodate at cold room temperature for 24 hours completely abolished its CSF activity. All of the above findings indicate that carbohydrate components of the PS preparation are responsible for CSF activity (Table V).

As a logical continuation other immuno-stimulatory effects of such PS (and lipid) preparations were tested. Table VI summarizes the results of the standard endotoxicity measurement which were reported in 1975 (37). Although endotoxic LPS and GL preparations were fully active in all these test assays, including B-cell mitogenisis, the PS preparations from S. minnesota and Serr. marcescens were nearly inert.

Radio-protective Effect.

That endotoxin should protect against the deleterious effects of ionizing radiation which differentially affects hemopoietic and cellular components of the immune system is a logical expectation and has been amply documented (1, 39, 43).

During the first three days following whole-body irradiation, the hemopoietic tissues of endotoxin-treated animals do not significantly differ histologically from controls. While continued degenerative processes and immune paralysis lead to death between the first and second week following irradiation of control animals,

TABLE V

Effect of Acid Hydrolysis and Periodate Oxidation on CSF Inducing Activity

Serum	Number of Colonies
Normal	73 ± 5
LPS[a]	383 ±15
Dialyzed PS[b]	286 ±14
Dialyzed IO_4 treated PS	82 ± 4

[a] Lipolysaccharide from smooth S. marcescans.

[b] Water-soluble hydrolytic products of S. marcescans LPS

TABLE VI

Endotoxicity Measurements of LPS, PS and GL

Preparations	Mouse LD_{50}[a]	Chick Embryo LD_{50}[b]	Local Schwartz- man	B cell mito- genesis[d]	Limulus lysate clotting[e]
LPS (S. minnesota)	450-500	0.015	80	25.1	10^{-9}
PS (S. minnesota)	>4000	>10.0	0	1.8	$>10^{-5}$
GL (S. minnesota)	1100	0.018	110	34.2	10^{-8}
LPS (S. marcescens	350-450	0.003	130	18.4	10^{-9}
PS (S. marcescens)	>4000	>10.0	0	0.9	$>10^{-5}$

[a] LD_{50} expressed in μg/mouse.

[b] LD_{50} expressed in μg/embryo.

[c] Size of skin hemorrhage elicted by 10 μg given i.d. The figure is the product of two diameters measured in millimeters.

[d] Stimulation index, measured by the incorporation of ^{3}H thymidine.

[e] Lowest concentration of the preparation in g/ml which still gave positive clotting.

regenerative foci of developing erythrocytes and leukocytes are scattered throughout the bone marrow as early as the fifth day. By the tenth day hemopoietic cells are visibly present and continue to increase in number leading to temporary hypercellularity and dividing cells.

The radio-protective effects of endotoxin and its derivatives against a lethal exposure dose of 700r was measured by survival of mice treated with 10 μg (i.p.) 48 hours before irradiation (Fig. 1). The results clearly indicate that although the LPS and PS demonstrated significant protection, the lipid A showed no significant enhanced survival at this dose level.

Immune Adjuvancy

Since the first report of immune adjuvancy of endotoxic LPS (12,21), large numbers of such preparations have proven to be

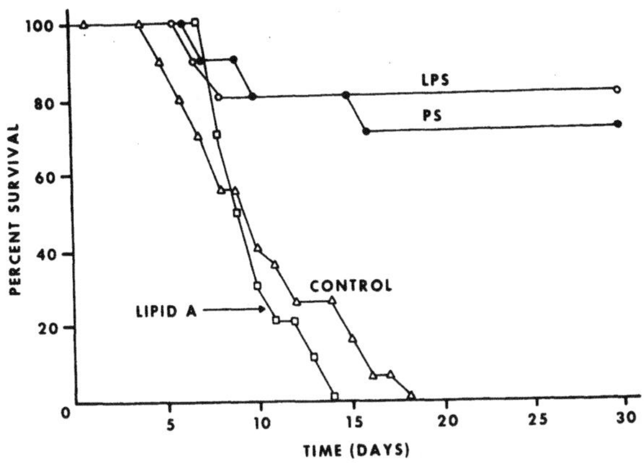

Fig. 1. The radio-protective effect of 10 µg of LPS, Lipid A and PS in ICR mice when administered i.p. 48 hours before 700 r whole body x-irradiation.

effective adjuvants for both soluble and cellular immunogens in a host of laboratory animals (see review by Neter (30)). Similarly, in vitro studies of spleen cell cultures treated with bacterial endotoxins have shown an increase in number of antibody producing cells (38, 42, 45). When we initially tested our PS preparation by administering it simultaneously with SRBC, it showed no adjuvant effect in the hemolytic plaque-forming cell assay (37). However, when PS was subsequently administered at various time intervals prior to antigenic challenge with SRBC, we observed several cycles of alternating enhancement and suppression of the immune response. A similar but shifted time-dependent oscillation was observed when LPS was used (Table VII). Although lipid A provided no adjuvancy it must be mentioned that the endotoxic glycolipid from _S. minnesota_ R 595 exhibeted good enhancement of antibody forming cells to SRBC. _In vitro_ adjuvancy of the same LPS and PS preparations were also demonstrated in collaboration with Dr. Friedman and associates (16).

Endotoxic Mediators

Post LPS and PS Serum

The above described positive effects of LPS and its non-toxic PS derivative principally involve the direct injection of either of these two preparations into a living host. Only in the CSF stimulation in which the sera of previously LPS- or PS-treated mice is added to the tissue culture of marrow cells do we have evidence that the biological activity does not necessarily involve the direct interaction of these preparations and the various cell populations which are ultimately affected. In studying the anti-tumor resist-

TABLE VII

The Time-dependent Effect of LPS and PS Treatment on the Immune Response to SRBC

Days		-18	-16	-14	-12	-10	-9	-8	-7	-6	-5	-4	-3	-2	-1	-0
Treatment	PS	.80*	1.0	1.1	1.7	4.2	.61	1.9	2.2	5.6	2.2	1.2	.74	11	.65	.48
	LPS	.11	.19	1.2	3.9	1.8	.18	.40	.48	9.8	.55	9.3	5.9	.10	4.6	7.2

* Value represent stimulation index which is the ratio of PFCs/10^6 spleen cells in treated groups to the number of PFCs/10^6 spleen cells in control group.

TABLE VIII

Adjuvancy, Radio-protection, and Colony Stimulation of Post LPS/PS Sera

Treatment	PFCs/spleen	S.I.	Colonies/plate	S.I.	Irradiation (% survival)
Normal mouse serum	495 ± 99	4.5	5 ± 3	1	40
Post Etox serum	2021 ± 202	18.3	157 ±14	31.4	80
Post PS serum	4248 ± 418	38.6	99 ± 8	19.8	70
None	110 ± 113	-	-	-	0

ance effect of endotoxin, we reported that CSF-rich post endotoxin serum can passively transfer non-specific resistance to normal recipients (8). Particularly active were sera produced by LPS and PS in previously BCG infected mice (9).

We subsequently tested the sera of mice 3 hours following 5 μg i.v. injection of either LPS or PS for their ability to confer radioprotection and immune enhancement. Mice were injected with 0.5 ml sera i.p. 24 hours before exposure to lethal irradiation of 750r . For immune enhancement 0.5 ml of serum was administered i.p. with 1×10^7 SRBC. Bone marrow colony stimulation was also tested by adding 50 μl of serum to each culture dish containing 5×10^5 cells. The results of these three test assays for post-LPS and post-PS sera are given in Table VIII. The immune stimulating activity is readily evident for both sera. It must be pointed out that repeatedly we observed moderate stimulation by normal serum.

Mediators of Lung Culture Filtrates (LCF)

Most recently we have investigated the ability of LPS and PS to affect in vivo major organs which when subsequently placed in culture may release mediators capable of inducing the above described endotoxic immune stimulation when passively transferred to a normal recipient.

Organ culture titrates were prepared according to the method of Sheridan and Metcalf (17, 18). Mice were injected with 5 μg of endotoxin or PS intravenously. Three hours later their lungs were removed under sterile conditions. Each pair of lungs was cut into several small pieces and incubated for 48 hours (37 degrees C - 5% CO_2) in 6 ml of serum-free Dulbecco Modified Eagle's medium. Following centrifugation (10,000 x g for 30 min), the supernatant was inactivated at 56 degrees C for 30 min. and dialyzed against distilled water for 3 days. The dialysate was again centrifuged (10,000 x g for 15 min.) and lyophilized. For the determination of radiation protection and adjuvancy, mice were treated with a 100 μg dose (i.p.) of lyophilized LCF. For CSF activity 50 μl of the liquid LCF was added to each culture dish. The results summarized in Table IX show that the lung culture of previously LPS- or PS-treated mice had stimulatory effects which closely paralleled the activity of sera of similarly treated animals. As was the case with normal serum, moderate radio-protection and immune enhancement was observed for normal LCF.

SUMMARY

From these observations several conclusions can be drawn: The most obvious conclusion is that certain biological activities attributed to endotoxin are the result of specific endotoxin induced mediator(s); that the whole endotoxic molecule is not necessary for the production or release of mediator(s) inasmuch as the non-toxic PS component can be shown to induce similar effects; that at least one or more of the target cells of endotoxin and PS resides in the lung; and finally that these mediators are released within a short period of time into the blood stream where they rise to a maximum level in approximately 3 hours. No ready explanation can be offered for the reduced but still apparent adjuvant and radio-protective effect induced by passive transfer of normal serum and lung culture filtrate. One can only speculate that these mediators are normally present in the mammalian organism and are produced and/or released by cells in larger quantities when properly stimulated.

TABLE IX

Adjuvancy, Radio-protection, and Colony Stimulation of Post LPS/PS Lung Culture Filtrates (LCF)

Treatment	PFCs/spleen	S.I.	Colonies/plate	S.I.	% survival
Normal mouse LCF	825 ± 123	7.5	124 ± 11	31.4	30
PostEtox LCF	3190 ± 328	29.0	204 ± 17	40.8	80
Post PS LCF	1595 ± 191	15.4	178 ± 13	35.6	60
Control	110 ± 113	1.0	5 ± 3	1	0

REFERENCES

1. Ainsworth, E. J., and Chase, H. B., 1959, Proc. Soc. Exptl. Biol. Med. 102: 483.

2. Andre-Schwartz, J., Rubenstein, H. S., and Coons, A. H., 1968, Am. J. Path. 53: 33.

3. Austen, K. F., and Cohn, Z. A., 1963, New Eng. J. Med. 268: 933.

4. Benacerraf, B., 1960, Bacteriol. Rev., 24: 35.

5. Biozzi, G., Benacerraf, B., and Halpern, B. N., 1963, Proc. Soc. Exptl. Biol. Med. 112: 78.

6. Boivin, A., Mesrobeanu, I., Mesrobeanu, L., 1933, C. R. Seances Soc. Biol. 113: 490.

5. Biozzi, G., Benacerraf, B., and Halpern, B. N., 1963, Proc. Soc. Exptl. Biol. Med., 112: 78.

6. Boivin, A., Mesrobeanu, I., Mesrobeanu, L., 1933, C. R. Seances Soc. Biol. 113: 490.

7. Box, E. D., and Briggs, N. T., 1961, J. Immunol. 87: 485.

8. Butler, R. C., and Nowotny, A., 1976, IRCS Med. Sci. 4: 206.

9. Butler, R. C., Abdelnoor, A., and Nowotny, A., 1978, PNAS 75: 2893.

10. Chang, H., Thompson, J. J., and Nowotny, A., 1974, Immunol. Comm. 3: 401.

11. Chang, C. M., and Nowotny, A., 1975, Immunochemistry, 12: 19.

12. Condie, R. M., Zak, S. J., and Good, R. A., 1955, Proc. Soc. Exp. Biol. Med. 90: 355.

13. Davis, D. A. L., 1960, Adv. Carbohydrate Chem. 15: 271.

14. Des Pres, R. M., Horowitz, H. I., and Hook, E. W., 1961, J. Exptl. Med., 114: 857.

15. Forbes, I. J., 1965, J. Immunol. 94: 37.

16. Frank, S., Specter, S., Nowotny, A., and Friedman, H., 1977, J. Immunol. 119: 855.

17. Gewurz, H., Mergenhagen, S. E., Nowotny, A., and Phillips, J. K., 1968, J. Bacteriol. 95: 397.

18. Gledhill, A. W., 1959, Brit. J. Exp. Path. 40: 195.

19. Greisman, S. E., 1960, Proc. Soc. Exptl. Biol. Med. 103: 628.

20. Herion, J. C., Walker, R. I., Herring, W. B., and Palmer, J. G., 1965, Blood. 25: 522.

21. Johnson, A. G., Gaines, S., and Landy, M., 1956, J. Exp. Med. 103: 225.

22. Johnson, A. G., and Nowotny, A., 1964, J. Bacteriol. 87: 809.

23, Kasai, N., and Nowotny, A., 1967, J. Bacteriol. 94: 1824.

24. Kim, Y. B., and Watson, D. W., 1967, J. Bacteriol. 94: 1320.

25. Kinosita, R., Nowotny, A., and Shikato, T., 1963, Blood. 21: 779.

26. Landy, M., and Pillemer, L., 1956, J. Exp. Med. 104: 383.

27. Landy, M., and Weldanz, W. P., 1964, In Bacterial Endotoxins. M. Landy and W. Braun, eds., Rutgers Univ. Press, New Brunswick, J. J. p. 275.

28. Luderitz, O., Staub, A. M., and Westphal, O., 1966, Bacteriol. Rev. 30: 192.

29. Luderitz, O., Jann, K., and Wheat, R., 1968, Comprehensive Biochem. 26A: 105.

30. Neter, E., 1969, Curr. Top. Microbiol. Immunol. 47: 82.

31. Nowotny, A., Wein, J., Shikata, T., and Kinosita, R., 1962, Abstract VIIIth Internatl. Congress for Microbiol.

32. Nowotny, A., 1963, J. Bacteriol. 85: 427.

33. Nowotny, A., Thomas, S., Duron, O. S., and Nowotny, A., 1963, J. Bacteriol. 85: 418.

34. Nowotny, A., Cundy, K. R., Neale, N. L., Nowotny, A., Radvany, R., Thomas, S. P., and Tripodi, D., 1966, Ann. N.Y. Acad. Sci. 133: 586.

35. Nowotny, A., 1969, Bacteriol. Rev. 33: 72.

36. Nowotny, A., 1971, Naturwissenschaften, 58: 397.

37. Nowotny, A., Behling, U. H., and Change, H. L., J. Immunol. 115: 199.

38. Ortiz-Ortiz, L., and Jaroslow, B. N., 1970, Immunol. 19: 387.

39. Perkins, E. H., and Marcus, S., 1958, J. Infect. Dis. 102: 81.

40. Radvany, R., Neale, N. L., and Nowotny, A., 1966, Ann. N. Y. Acad. Sci. 133: 763.

41. Reiman, H. A., 1926, J. Exp. Med. 43: 107.

42. Sjoberg, O., Andersson, J., and Moller, G., 1972, Europ. J. Immunol. 2: 326.

43. Smith, W. W., Alderman, I. M., and Gillespie, R. E., 1957, Am. J. Physiol. 191: 124.

44. Smith, W. W., Alderman, I. M., and Gillespie, R. E., 1958, Am. J. Physiol. 192: 263.

45. Stevens, K. M., and McKenna, J. M., 1958, J. Exp. Med. 107: 537.

46. Tripodi, D., and Nowotny, A., 1966, Ann. N. Y. Acad. Sci. 133: 604.

47. Westphal, O., Nowotny, A., Luderitz, O., Hurni, H., Eichenberger, E., and Schonholzer, G., 1958, G. Pharm. Acta. Helv. 33: 401.

48. Westphal, O., 1960, Ann. Inst. Pasteur. 98: 789.

49. White, P. B., 1927, J. Path. and Bact. 30: 113.

50. Yoshida, M., Hiratu, M., Satodate, R., and Shiba, T., 1974, Jap. J. Med. Sci. 27: 114.

51. Younger, J. S., and Stinebring, W. R., 1966, Virology. 29: 310.

INDUCTION OF IMMUNOMODULATORY FACTORS BY LPS AND NONTOXIC DERIVATIVES

R. Christopher Butler, Alois Nowotny and Herman Friedman

The Arlington Hospital, Arlington, VA; University of Pennsylvania, Philadelphia, PA; and University of South Florida Medical College, Tampa, FL

ABSTRACT

Bacterial lipopolysaccharide (LPS) has been demonstrated to produce immunostimulatory effects on a wide variety of immunologic responses. Many cellular mechanisms have been proposed to explain these phenomenona. However, only recently has it become apparent that many of the immune response enhancing activities of LPS involve the induction of immunoregulatory factors. We have studied several of these factors in an attempt to establish a unified concept of their role in the mechanism of action of LPS on immune functions. The LPS-induced factors which are examined here include such lymphokines as myeloid colony stimulating factor (CSF) and migration inhibition factor (MIF). Antitumor effects of LPS were demonstrated to be mediated by a tumor resistance enhancing factor and by tumor necrotizing factor (TNF). The enhancement of specific antibody responses by LPS was also mediated by a macrophage-derived helper factor. In addition to studying the induction of each of these factors by LPS, we attempted to determine which position of the LPS molecule was responsible for these activities. A nontoxic polysaccharide-rich LPS hydrolytic product (PS) was able to induce the production of all of these factors to a degree similar to that of whole LPS. Thus, the PS moiety contained an active site for the induction of immunomodulatory factors.

Bacterial lipopolysaccharides (LPS) are well known for their toxic and potentially lethal effects to both animals and individual cells. These toxic effects have been conclusively shown to be due to the Lipid A moiety of the LPS. However, most of the recent investigations into the mechanisms of LPS activity have focused upon ways in which LPS can nonspecifically enhance a broad variety of immune responses so as to produce a broad range of potentially beneficial effects (1-9). LPS has been demonstrated to regulate many of these immunostimulatory effects through the induction of lymphokines, monokines and other immunoregulatory factors. Effects of LPS which may be mediated through the production of these factors include the adjuvant effect upon *in vitro* antibody responses (1, 2), tumor resistance enhancement (3, 4, 5), tumor necrotizing activity (3, 4, 6, 7), *in vitro* myeloid colony stimulation (5, 8, 9), as well as a wide variety of other activities.

In spite of all these potentially beneficial effects of LPS, the toxic effects of LPS continue to make it unacceptible for general use as an immunostimulatory therapeutic agent for humans. Clearly, before considering widespread clinical trials, the LPS would have to be treated in a manner such as to remove its toxic activity while maintaining the immunostimulatory activity. We have attempted to produce a product with these qualifications through the partial acid hydrolysis of LPS and the removal of the toxic Lipid A component. The resultant polysaccharide-rich (PS) fraction is completely nontoxic (8). This PS fraction contains active sites for the induction of many of the stimulatory effects of LPS including *in vivo* (10) and *in vitro* (11) adjuvant activity, colony stimulating factor (CSF) production (5, 8), protection from lethal irradiation (10), and some antitumor effects (5).

This paper reviews many of our studies into the immunomodulatory effects of LPS, with emphasis on demonstrating the ways in which the nontoxic PS fraction can parallel the activity of the whole LPS in the stimulation of these immune responses. A central theme of these studies has been the demonstration of the ability of both LPS and PS to induce the production of immunomodulatory factors which mediate the cellular interactions which are essential for enhanced immunologic responsiveness. The PS-induced factors which will be discussed include myeloid colony stimulating factor (CSF), tumor resistance emhancing factor, tumor hemorrhagic factor (TNF), leukocyte migration inhibition factor (MIF), and antibody response helper factor.

MATERIALS AND METHODS

Experimental Animals

Female ICR and C57Bl/6J mice were obtained from the Skin and Cancer Hospital, Temple University, Philadelphia, PA. Male BALB/c mice were obtained from Cumberland View Farms, Clinton, TN. All animals were housed in groups of 6 to 10 and fed Purina mouse pellets and water *ad libitum*. Mice were 6 to 10 weeks old at the time of initial treatment.

LPS and PS Preparations

Lipopolysaccharide (LPS) was obtained from *Serratia marcescens* 08 by trichloroacetic acid extraction as previously described (12). Polysaccharide-rich preparations (PS) were prepared from *Serratia marcescens* 08 LPS by hydrolysis with 1M HCl at 100° for 30 minutes, as described elsewhere (8). The PS fraction consisted of approximately 65% carbohydrate, 10% protein, 0.1% nucleic acid, and less than 0.5% lipid. It has a molecular weight of approximately 10,000 daltons. PS preparations contained no measurable endotoxicity when tested by the *Limulus* lysate assay, chick embryo lethality assay and rabbit pyrogenicity test (8).

Cell Lines

The nonspecific TA3-Ha ascites tumor was originally a spontaneous mammary adenoma isolated from strain A mice and then converted to the ascites form. It was kindly provided by S. Friberg, Karolinska Institute, Stockholm, Sweden and has been maintained intraperitoneally in female A/J mice. Sarcoma 37 tumor was maintained by passage as an ascites tumor in female ICR mice. The P388D1 transformed macrophage cell line was kindly donated by D. Rosenstreich, NIDR, Bethesda, MD. The cells were passaged in RPMI 1640 plus 10% fetal bovine serum and antibiotics.

Antigen

Sheep red blood cells (SRBC) in Alsevers solution were obtained from Baltimore Biological Laboratories, Baltimore, MD. The erythrocytes were washed several times in medium and resuspended to a 0.1% concentration.

In Vitro Immunization

Covered plastic Linbro plates were used as culture chambers. Spleen cells from normal mice were washed in media and the numbers of viable nucleated cells determined by the trypan blue exclusion technique with a hemacytometer. A suspension of 8 x 10^6 viable splenocytes suspended in 2.0 ml of complete tissue culture medium enriched with a standard nutrient cocktail and 20% fetal bovine serum were cultured in the Linbro plate wells as described elsewhere (13). For *in vitro* immunization 0.1 ml of the 0.1% suspension of SRBC was added to each culture (approximately 2 x 10^6 erythrocytes). All cultures were incubated for 5 day at 37° under CO_2.

Assay for Antibody-forming Cells

The numbers of direct hemolytic plaque forming cells (PFC) to SRBC were determined by the micromethod of Cunningham and Szenburg (14).

The numbers of PFC were enumerated for at least 8 to 24 cultures prepared from 2 to 4 spleen cell preparations, and the average number of PFCs per million cells calculated. In all cases only direct non-facilitated plaques were enumerated and these were considered due to 19 S IgM antibody producing cells.

Post-LPS Serum

Mice were injected i.p. with 20 μg of LPS or PS and exsanguinated two to four hours later. For some experiments the post-LPS serum was obtained from mice which had been pretreated by i.p. injection of 10^7 viable BCG 14 days earlier as previously described (5).

Fractionation of Splenocyte Populations

Splenocytes were fractionated into adherent and nonadherent cell populations by incubating 5 x 10^7 splenocytes per ml in plastic tissue culture flasks for one hour at 37°. The nonadherent cells were successively transferred for two additional one hour incubations to remove residual adherent cells. The adherent cell monolayers were washed repeatedly to remove nonadherent and weakly adherent cells. Microscopic examination revealed that greater than 90% of the adherent cells were macrophages.

In Vitro Factor Production

Suspensions of 10^7 splenocytes per ml were incubated in RPMI 1640 plus 10% FCS and antibiotics at 37° under CO_2. Experimental cultures received 10 μg/ml LPS at the time of culture initiation. Supernatants were collected after various time intervals and either stored on ice or frozen at -70° until tested.

Enhancement of Resistance to Tumor

Female ICR mice were treated with intraperitoneal injections of 20 μg of LPS or PS one day prior to i.p. challenge with 1600 TA3-Ha tumor cells. Mice were monitored for the development of a lethal tumor load. Native hapten was delivered in multiple daily doses before and/or after the time of tumor challenge. Post-LPS and post-PS sera were administered in doses of 0.3 to 0.5 ml i.p. 2 hours prior to tumor challenge.

Tumor Hemorrhage Assay

Sarcoma 37 tumor was harvested from the ascites form and washed with sterile saline. Female ICR mice received 0.1 ml of a 50% suspension of cells subcutaneously. After 7 days the mice received i.v. injections of either LPS or post-LPS or post-PS serum. One day after treatment the tumors were observed for areas of acute hemorrhage extending over 25% or more of the surface of the tumor.

Determination of Colony Stimulating Factor (CSF) Levels

The CSF content of the post-LPS and post-PS serum preparations was determined by bone marrow colony formation in semisolid agar by the method described by Bradley and Metcalf (11).

Assay for MIF

To assay the MIF levels in supernatants from LPS and PS treated cultures, capillary tubes were filled with a suspension of 5×10^7 normal splenocytes per ml in medium 199 containing 10% heat inactivated fetal calf serum as described by Bloom and Bennett (15). The capillaries were centrifuged at 500 x g and then cut at the cell-fluid interface. The cell-bearing tubes were placed in Sykes-Moore chambers together with the supernatants being tested. The test chambers were incubated for 24 hr at 37° and the area of migration from each capillary tube was measured.

RESULTS

The first effect of LPS which can be mediated by the nontoxic PS fraction is the enhancement of nonspecific resistance to tumor. Table 1 demonstrates that the pretreatment of mice with LPS one day before i.p. challenge with approximately 2 - 3 TD_{50} of the TA3-Ha ascites tumor strongly enhanced the rejection of this tumor as evidenced by an increased rate of survival. In a similar manner the treatment of mice with PS also significantly enhanced the rate of survival.

As an independent confirmation that lipid-free preparations rich in LPS polysaccharide components can enhance tumor resistance, we tested a preparation of "native hapten". This "native hapten" is a lipid-free metabolic precursor of LPS which contains the polysaccharide antigenic sites. As demonstrated in Table 2, repeated

TABLE I

Enhancement of Tumor Resistance by LPS and PS

Treatment (Day -1)*	% Survival (p)
Saline	16%
20 μg PS	43% (< .01)
20 μg LPS	70% (< .001)

* ICR mice were challenged with 1600 TA3-Ha cells i.p. on day 0.

TABLE II

Effect of Native Hapten on Resistance to TA3-Ha Tumor

Treatment* (20 μg/dose)		Days of Administration	% Survival (p)
I	Saline		8%
	Native Hapten	(-5,-4,-3,-2,-1)	70% (<.001)
	Native Hapten	(-2,-1,0,1,3,5,7,9)	25% (<.05)
II	None		5%
	Native Hapten	(-1)	10%
	Native Hapten	(-3,-1)	35% (<.005)

* Mice were challenged with 1600 TA3-Ha cells i.p. on day 0.

pretreatment with "native hapten" could also stimulate tumor resistance.

Table 3 demonstrates that the tumor resistance enhancing effect of LPS is mediated through the production of soluble factors. This factor (or factors) is released into the serum of mice within 2 hours of i.p. injection of LPS.

TABLE III

Post-LPS Serum Enhances Resistance to Tumor

Species	Pretreatment (-2 hr)	Challenge Dose	% Survival (p)
C57Bl/6J	0.3 ml Saline	7×10^4	10%
"	0.3 ml Normal Serum	7×10^4	10%
"	0.3 ml Post-LPS Serum*	7×10^4	45% (<.025)
"	10 μg LPS	7×10^4	70% (<.005)
ICR	0.5 ml Saline	1.6×10^3	30%
"	0.5 ml Normal Serum	1.6×10^3	40%
"	0.5 ml Post-LPS Serum*	1.6×10^3	100% (<.05)

* Post-LPS serum was collected from either C57BL/6J or ICR mice 2 hr after injection of 20 μg of *Serratia marcescens* LPS.

The treatment of either inbred or random bred mice with relatively small amounts of post-LPS serum strongly enhanced tumor resistance. Normal sera had no such activity. This effect was not due to residual endotoxin in these sera because these levels were less than 1 ng/ml which was 1000-fold lower than the dose of LPS required to produce the effect directly (5).

Table 4 demonstrates that post-PS serum was only slightly less active than post-LPS serum in transferring tumor resistance, with 75% of post-LPS and 66% of post-PS serum treated mice surviving. Pre-infection of serum donors with BCG 2 weeks prior to serum collection primed the response of mice to both LPS and PS. The post-LPS and post-PS sera from these animals conferred very strong resistance to the recipients. Also demonstrated here are the colony stimulating factor (CSF) titers of each of these sera. These CSF titers also increased in BCG treated mice and the CSF levels closely paralleled the serum antitumor activity.

A second antitumor effect of LPS is the hemmorrhage and necrosis of solid subcutaneous tumors. Table 5 shows the results of an assay in which LPS or different pretreated sera were injected i.v. into mice bearing subcutaneous Sarcoma 37 tumors. Twenty-four hours later the tumors were visually examined for areas of acute hemorrhage. Again, both the post-LPS and the post-PS sera mediated the effects of LPS.

Similar to the resistance enhancing activity, the production of tumor hemorrhaging activity in post-LPS and post-PS sera was increased by BCG pretreatment as shown in Table 6.

TABLE IV

BCG Preinfection of Serum Donors Increases the Potency of Post-LPS Serum in Tumor Protection

Treatment (0.5 ml)[a]	% Survival (p)	CSF Titer[b]
Saline	33	22
Normal Serum	40	36
Post-PS Serum	66 (< .01)	169
Post-LPS Serum	75 (< .01)	192
BCG Serum[c]	50	66
Post-PS + BCG Serum	95 (< .001)	316
Post-LPS + BCG Serum	100 (< .001)	344

a Post-LPS and post-PS sera were collected 2 hr after i.p. injection of either LPS or PS from Serratia marcescens.

b Colony forming units per 10^5 cells.

c BCG sera were obtained from mice 18 days after infection with 2×10^7 BCG.

TABLE V

Induction of Hemorrhage of Sarcoma 37 Tumors by Post-LPS and Post-PS sera

Treatment (0.5 ml i.v.)	% of Tumors Hemorrhaged[a] (p)
Saline	7
Normal Serum	13
Post-PS Serum	35 (<.05)
Post-LPS Serum	36 (<.05)
20 μg LPS	71 (<.005)

[a] Mice bearing subcutaneous Sarcoma 37 tumors received i.v. injections of post-LPS or post-PS serum. After 24 hr the tumors were examined for areas of acute hemorrhage covering 25% or more of the surface.

The third factor that we have studied which is induced by PS is migration inhibition factor (MIF). Table 7 demonstrates the *in vivo* production of MIF by LPS and PS. The results are expressed

TABLE VI

BCG Preinfection Increases the Potency of Post-LPS and Post-PS Sera in the Sarcoma 37 Hemorrhage Assay

Treatment (0.5 ml i.v.)	% of Tumors Hemorrhaged[a] (p)
Saline	0
Normal Serum	0
Post-PS Serum[b]	40 (< .025)
Post-LPS Serum[b]	40 (< .025)
BCG Serum	0
Post-PS + BCG Serum	80 (< .001)
Post-LPS + BCG Serum	95 (< .001)

[a] Based on the number of subcutaneous Sarcoma 37 tumors with extensive areas of acute hemorrhage within 24 hr after treatment.

[b] Post-LPS and post-PS sera were collected 2 hr after i.p. injection of either LPS or PS from *Serratia marcescens*.

as a percent of control migration. Supernatants from LPS and PS treated splenocytes moderately inhibited leukocyte migration. The

TABLE VII

Production of MIF by Splenocytes Cultured *In Vitro* with LPS, PS, and BCG for 2 Days

Treatment of Donor Cultures[a]	% Control Migration ± S.E. (p)[b]
None	100 ± 12
20 μg LPS	65 ± 16
20 μg PS	76 ± 10
10^5 BCG	114 ± 5
10^5 BCG + 20 μg LPS	34 ± 12 (<.05)
10^5 BCG + 20 μg PS	43 ± 6 (<.02)
20 μg LPS direct[c]	97 ± 11
20 μg PS direct[c]	93 ± 9

a Supernatants from cultures of 10^7/ml normal splenocytes incubated for 2 days with LPS, PS or BCG.

b "p" values were determined by the Student's "t" test.

c As a control, LPS and PS were added directly to the chambers at the time of assay.

incubation of splenocytes with BCG did not generate MIF. However, combined treatment with BCG and LPS or PS induced the highest level of MIF production. As a control, direct treatment of leukocytes with LPS or PS did not affect their migration, thus ruling out the possibility of inhibition due to toxicity.

Finally, the fourth stimulatory activity of LPS which can also be induced by the PS fraction is the adjuvant effect. Table 8 shows that both LPS and PS can stimulate the antibody response to sheep erythrocyte antigens *in vitro*.

These adjuvant effects of both LPS and PS can be mediated by soluble factors as shown in Table 9. At low serum concentrations both post-LPS and post-PS sera contained factors which increased the antibody response level, whereas normal serum had no effect. It was also noted that high doses of mouse sera were suppressive for this assay.

The next set of experiments was an initial attempt to identify the cell types producing and responding to these adjuvant factors. Table 10 shows that these post-LPS serum factors appeared to selectively bind to a bone marrow cell population. Normal serum and post-LPS serum were each absorbed extensively with either thymo-

TABLE VIII

Dose-Response for Stimulation of the *In Vitro* PFC Response to SRBC by *Serratia marcescens* LPS or PS

Treatment (μg/culture)[a]	% Control[b] (p)
None (control)	100
0.1 μg LPS	104
1.0 μg LPS	139 (<.005)
10.0 μg LPS	267 (<.001)
20.0 μg LPS	181 (<.005)
0.1 μg PS	102
1.0 μg PS	120 (<.05)
10.0 μg PS	231 (<.001)
20.0 μg PS	169 (<.005)

a Indicated dose of LPS or PS was added to cultures of 8×10^6 normal spleen cells sensitized *in vitro* with 2×10^6 SRBC.

b Average PFC response for 8 cultures/treatment 5 days after sensitization.

TABLE IX

Effects of Post-LPS and Post-PS Sera on Antibody Responses *In Vitro*

Treatment[a]	Volume (ml)	% Control[b] (p)
None (control)		100
Normal Serum	0.001	110
	0.01	109
	0.1	106
	0.5	52 (<.001)
Post-PS Serum	0.001	128 (<.05)
	0.01	196 (<.001)
	0.1	160 (<.001)
Post-LPS Serum	0.001	121
	0.01	213 (<.001)
	0.1	150 (<.005)
	0.5	25 (<.001)

Table IX continued next page

TABLE IX (continued)

[a] Cultures of normal splenocytes were treated with indicated amounts of normal mouse serum or sera collected 2 hr after i.p. injection of LPS or PS.

[b] Average PFC response for 8 - 24 cultures per group after 5 days of culture

TABLE X

Absorption of Post-LPS Serum Helper Factors by Bone Marrow Cells

Culture Treatment[a]	% Control PFCs[b] (p)
None (Control)	100
Normal Serum	101
Normal Serum Absorbed with Thymocytes[c]	104
Normal Serum Absorbed with Bone Marrow[c]	94
Post-LPS Serum	224 (<.005)
Post-LPS Serum Absorbed with Thymocytes[c]	168 (<.05)
Post-LPS Serum Absorbed with Bone Marrow[c]	109

[a] Cultures of 8×10^6 splenocytes from normal BALB/c mice were treated with 0.01 ml of normal or post-LPS sera and immunized *in vitro* with 2×10^6 SRBC.

[b] Average PFC response for 8 cultures assayed 5 days after sensitization.

[c] Sera were absorbed with 10^8/0.1 ml bone marrow or thymus cells for 1 hr at 37°

cytes or bone marrow cells. The post-LPS serum absorbed with thymocytes was still active, but helper factor activity was removed from the serum by bone marrow cells.

In addition, we have determined that the T cell is not involved in the production of this LPS-induced factor. Table 11 shows the *in vivo* production of helper factors by athymic nude mice. Post-LPS sera from nude and normal mice were equally active in enhancing the antibody response of normal splenocytes, and were also quite active in stimulating nude cells.

Going a step further, Table 12 shows the production of factors *in vitro* by nude mouse splenocytes. These supernatants enhanced the responses of both nude and normal splenocytes to similar degrees. Fractionation of these cells into nonadherent and macrophage-rich

TABLE XI

Production of Helper Factors by Athymic BALB/c nu nu Mice

Culture Treatment[a]	Source of Responding Cells	% Control PFCs (p)
None	BALB/c	100
BALB/c Normal Serum	"	113
Nude Normal Serum	"	116
BALB/c Post-LPS Serum[b]	"	213 (<.01)
Nude Post-LPS Serum[b]	"	182 (<.02)
None	BALB/c nu nu (Nude)	100
BALB/c Normal Serum	"	150
Nude Normal Serum	"	84
BALB/c Post-LPS Serum[b]	"	419 (<.01)
Nude Post-LPS Serum[b]	"	447 (<.01)

a. Cultures of 8 x 10^6 normal BALB/c or BALB/c nu nu Nude mouse splenocytes were treated with 0.01 ml of normal or post-LPS sera and immunized *in vitro* with 2 x 10^6 SRBC.

b Serum was collected from either BALB/c or Nude mice 4 hr after injection of 25 µg LPS i.p.

adherent cell populations indicated that the macrophage was probably the cell type producing this factor.

To confirm this hypothesis we examined the P388D1 transformed macrophage cell line for production of this factor. Table 13 shows the stimulatory effects of 3 and 5 day supernatants from normal and LPS-treated macrophages. LPS greatly enhanced the production of helper factor activity in these cells.

DISCUSSION

These studies have demonstrated the ability of PS preparations to parallel the activity of whole LPS in the induction of a variety of immunomodulatory effects. As previously reported (4, 5, 16), both LPS and PS are capable of enhancing host resistance to tumor. Here we have demonstrated that direct pre-treatment of mice with PS improved the rate of survival following tumor challenge. While this enhancement of tumor resistance by PS has been both significant and reproducible (4, 16), the PS preparations have been generally somewhat less effective than whole LPS in inducing this effect. This could be due to a number of factors related to size, solubility, and clearance time, but could also indicate that the lipid A moiety

TABLE XII

Production of Helper Factors by Nude Mouse Adherent Splenocytes

Source of Supernatants for Culture Treatment[a]		Source of Responding Cells[b]	% Control PFCs (p)
Splenocyte Population	Treatment		
None		BALB/c	100
Whole	None	"	107
Whole	LPS	"	185 (<.01)
Nonadherent	None	"	87
Nonadherent	LPS	"	109
Adherent	None	"	119
Adherent	LPS	"	159 (<.02)
None		BALB/c nu nu	100
Whole	None	"	123
Whole	LPS	"	201 (<.02)
Noneadherent	None	"	112
Nonadherent	LPS	"	114
Adherent	None	"	107
Adherent	LPS	"	171 (<.02)

[a] Supernatants from 5 day cultures of 10^7/ml of normal or LPS-stimulated whole, nonadherent, or adherent spleen cells.

[b] Splenocyte cultures from normal BALB/c or athymic BALB/c nu nu mice were treated with 0.1 ml of spleen cell culture supernatants and immunized *in vitro* with SRBC.

contains additional active sites, such as the site for mitogenicity, which enhance the immune mechanism of tumor rejection.

The presence of some of these active sites in the lipid fraction is consistent with our previous studies in which several heptose-less *E. coli* Re mutant glycolipids were very effective in enhancing survival (17). In contrast, studies of a series of *Salmonella minnesota* LPS mutants ranging from smooth to Re mutants indicated that the resistance-enhancing effect decreased with decreasing polysaccharide chain length (17).

The reasons for these apparently conflicting results in which both the purified glycolipid preparations and the lipid-free PS preparations stimulated resistance mechanisms is unclear. The existance of multiple active sites residing in both the polysaccharide and the lipid moiety is the most tantalizing explanation. The

TABLE XIII

Helper Factor Production by the P388D1 Macrophage Cell Line

Culture Treatment[a]	% Control PFCs (p)
None	100
10 μg LPS	298 (<.005)
3d P388D1 sup'n	125
3d P388D1 + LPS sup'n	113
4d P388D1 sup'n	172 (<.025)
4d P388D1 + LPS sup'n	229 (<.001)
5d P388D1 sup'n	210 (<.01)
5d P388D1 + LPS sup'n	443 (<.0005)

[a] Splenocyte cultures were treated with 0.1 ml of P388D1 culture supernatants collected after 3, 4, or 5 days of culture from untreated cells or cultures incubated with 10 μg/ml LPS.

observations that the PS and the glycolipids each stimulate some effects such as tumor resistance enhancement and the induction of CSF (5), but that they differ in the ability to induce other effects such as lymphocyte transformation indicates the presence of at least 2 different active sites.

Previous studies on the induction of CSF by PS have demonstrated that the active fraction of the PS preparation was periodate sensitive (18), thereby indicating that the active site was either a polysaccharide or polysaccharide-linked. Supporting the polysaccharide nature of this active LPS component was the observation that the native hapten preparation could also enhance tumor resistance. This native hapten was a lipid-free precursor of the LPS "O" antigenic portion of the molecule. So LPS polysaccharide fractions prepared by two totally different isolation procedures were both active in inducing elevated resistance to tumor.

The mechanism of action of both LPS and PS in enhancing resistance involved the production of intermediary regulatory factors which could be passively transferred by post-LPS or post-PS sera. Preinfection of serum donors with BCG enhanced the production of these factors in response to both LPS and PS.

We have previously discussed (5) the strong correlation which exists between the resistance enhancing capacity of post-LPS sera and the serum myeloid colony stimulating factor (CSF) levels. However, the exact role of CSF in the elevation of resistance levels is still not clear. The studies presented in this report indicate that the post-LPS and post-PS sera also contain other immunomodulatory factors in addition to CSF. One or more of these factors such as MIF or antibody response helper factors may ultimately prove to be responsible for a significant portion of this enhancement.

In addition to enhancing resistance to tumor challenge, the post-LPS and post-PS sera contained a second antitumor factor which mediated the tumor hemorrhaging effect of LPS (3, 4). This second factor was most likely the tumor necrotizing factor (TNF) described by Carswell et al. (7) which induces tumor hemorrhage followed subsequently by tumor necrosis. Whether the tumor hemorrhaging activity of post-LPS serum really represents an immunologic function as opposed to a vascular or clotting mechanism is yet to be determined.

Another stimulatory effect of LPS which could also be induced by the PS fraction was the adjuvant effect upon the in vitro antibody response to sheep erythrocyte antigens. As with the antitumor effects, the adjuvant activities of both LPS and PS were mediated through the induction of soluble mediators. LPS and PS were equally active in stimulating the release of this factor into the serum in vivo.

In an attempt to determine the cell type directly responding to these serum factors, post-LPS sera were absorbed with either thymocytes or bone marrow cells. If the factor responsible for this adjuvant effect were lymphocyte activating factor (LAF), then the absorption of serum with thymocytes should remove this activity To date this has not been demonstrated. In contrast, the incubation of sera with bone marrow cells completely removed the helper activity, presumably by binding to a bone marrow cell population. The nature of the cell type binding the factor is under investigation.

These and previous studies (4) have demonstrated that the T-cell is not involved in the production of this helper factor and may also not be required for its function. Athymic nude mice produced normal factor levels in response to LPS. In addition, nude mouse splenocyte antibody responses could be strongly enhanced by these serum factors.

The helper factor activity could also be induced in vitro from cultures of nude or normal splenocytes. Fractionation of the splenocytes into adherent and nonadherent cell populations indicated that factor production was a function of the macrophage-rich adherent cell population. To confirm that the macrophage was the cell type producing this factor the P388D1 transformed macrophage-like cell like was examined for factor production. Stimulation of these cells with LPS induced factor production, thereby confirming that the macrophage produces the factor in direct response to LPS.

ACKNOWLEDGEMENT

This investigation was funded in part by grant number 7R23CA26415-01, awarded by the National Cancer Institute, DHEW.

REFERENCES

1. Butler, R. C., Nowotny, A., Friedman, H., 1977, J. Reticuloendothel. Soc. 22: 28.

2. Butler, R. C., Nowotny, A., Friedman, H., 1979, Annals of N.Y. Acad. of Sci. 332: 564.

3. Butler, R. C., Nowotny, A., 1976, IRCS Med. Science 4: 206.

4. Nowotny, A., Butler, R. C., 1980, Adv. Exp. Med. Biol.121: 455.

5. Butler, R. C., Abdelnoor, A. M. Nowotny, A., 1978, Proc. Natl. Acad. Sci. 75: 2893.

6. O'Malley, W. E., Achinstein, B., Shear, M. J., 1962, Jr. Natl. Cancer Inst. 29: 1169.

7. Carswell, E. A., Old, L. J., Kassel, R. L., Green, S., Fiore, N., Williamson, B., 1975, Proc. Natl. Acad. of Sci. 72: 3666.

8. Nowotny, A., Behling, U. H., Chang, H. L., 1975, Jr. Immunol. 115: 197.

9. Bradley, T. R., Metcalf, D., 1966, Australian Jr. of Biol. Med. 44: 287.

10. Behling, U. H., Nowotny, A., 1977, Jr. Immuno. 118: 1905.

11. Frank, S., Specter, S., Nowotny, A., Friedman, H., 1977, J. Immunol. 119: 855.

12. Nowotny, A., Cundy, K. R., Neale, N. L., Nowotny, A. M., Radvany, P., Thoas, S. P., Tripodi, D. J., 1968, Annals of the N.Y. Acad. of Sci. 133: 586.

13. Kamo, I., Pan, S-H, Friedman, H., 1976, J. of Immunol. Meth. 11: 55.

14. Cunningham, A. J., Szenberg, A., 1968, Immunol. 14: 599.

15. Bloom, B. R., Bennet, B., 1971, In. In Vitro Methods in Cell-mediated Immunity. B. R. Bloom and P. Glade (eds.). p. 285. Plenum Press, N.Y.

16. Butler, R. C., Nowotny, A., Eur. J. Immunopath. Immunother. (in press).

17. Ng, A-K, Butler, R. C., Chen, C. H., Nowotny, A., 1976, J. Bact. 126: 511.

RIBOSOMAL VACCINES AS IMMUNOMODULATORS

T. K. Eisenstein, C. R. Angerman, and L. W. Deakins

Department of Microbiology and Immunology
Temple University School of Medicine
Philadelphia, PA 19140

INTRODUCTION

"Ribosomal vaccines" can be defined as ribosome-rich subcellular extracts of microorganisms used as vaccines. Extracts of this sort have been shown to be highly protective against a number of experimental bacterial and fungal infections, but their mechanisms of protection are still under investigation (1). This paper is concerned with protection induced by such subcellular extracts prepared from *Salmonella typhimurium*. Experiments have been carried out using a murine model of salmonellosis in which animals were immunized intraperitoneally and challenged three weeks later, intraperitoneally. Survival of vaccinated and control animals was followed for 30 to 40 days post-challenge.

Three models will be considered with regard to the possible mechanisms of action of ribosomal vaccines (Fig. 1). In the first model it is assumed that ribosomal vaccines induce immunity by some unique mechanism. Youmans and Youmans have proposed such a unique mechanism of action with regard to ribosomal extracts of *Mycobacterium tuberculosis* (2). Previous work from our laboratory and from other laboratories has provided evidence that O antigens are present in ribosomal extracts of Salmonella (3) and that they are partly responsible for the protection engendered by such subcellular extracts (3, 4, 5). These observations have raised the question whether all of the protection induced by ribosomal extracts of Salmonellae is due to surface antigens which contaminate the ribosomes, or whether the ribosomal extracts have a degree of immunogenicity that exceeds levels that could be expected by merely combining surface antigens. These alternatives are presented in Models 2 and 3, also shown in

Fig. 1. Model 2 presents the hypothesis that ribosomal extract consists of multiple protective antigens, including the O antigen of lipopolysaccharide, outer membrane proteins, and possibly other as yet undefined antigens, including perhaps ribosomal antigens. In this model, protection would be equal to the sum of the protective capacities of each of the individual components. The third model presents the hypothesis that the ribosome acts as a carrier, to which is complexed lipopolysaccharide, outer membrane proteins, and possibly outer membrane fragments. In this model, protection would be greater than the sum of the parts due to factors such as the three-dimensional configuration of the antigens, their hydrophobicity, or the size of the immunogenic complex. It is noteworthy that at present we are still defining the protective antigens involved in immunity to Salmonella infection and trying to establish their relative importance for host defenses (6, 7). Furthermore, immunity to Salmonella infection can be mediated by both the humoral and the cellular arms of the immune system (8, 9) and the protective antigens for the two arms of the immune system may be different (10). Since overall immunity may be a summation of the humoral plus the cellular arms of the immune system, and since we may be dealing with a presently undefined number of unknown antigens, it can be appreciated that the

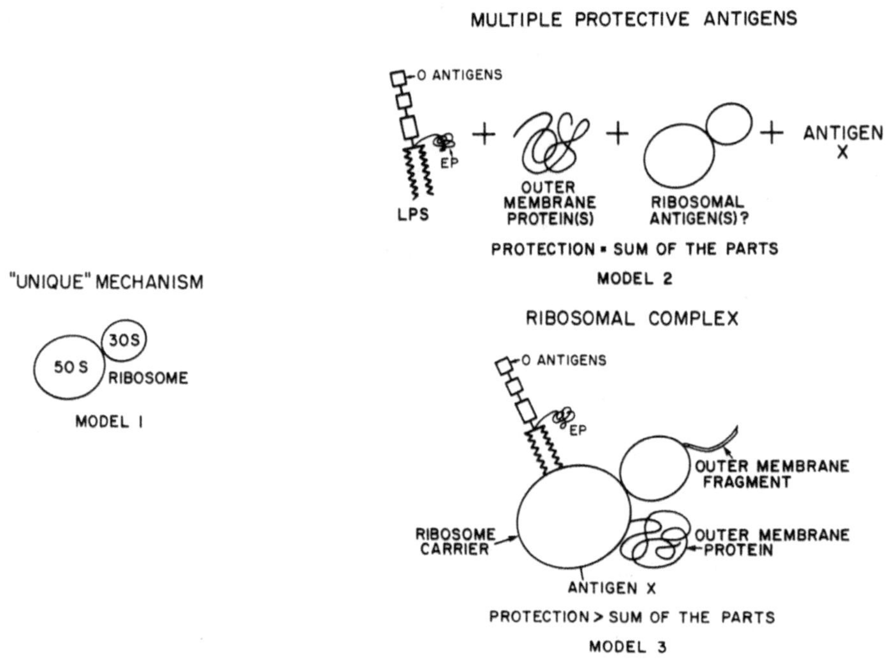

Fig. 1. Three possible models to explain the mechanism of action of ribosomal vaccines. LPS = lipopolysaccharide; EP = endotoxic protein.

problem of dissecting Model 2 from Model 3 will not be an easy task.

To investigate these questions, we have carried out studies designed to establish whether Salmonella ribosomal vaccines are really superior to other nonliving vaccines in their ability to induce short- and long-term protection. To look for an adjuvant effect, protection has been correlated with humoral immune responses. In addition, we have looked at these vaccines as protective agents in C3H/HeJ mice, a strain which is known to be nonresponsive mitogenically to phenol-water extracted lipopolysaccharide (11) and to give poor immune responses to this highly purified LPS (12, 13).

MATERIALS AND METHODS

Animals

Female CD-1 mice, 18-21 g, were purchased from Charles River Mouse Farm, Wilmington, MS. Female C3H/HeJ mice were purchased from Jackson Laboratories, Bar Harbor, ME. Animals were housed in plastic disposable cages with Absorb-Dri for bedding. Purina Mouse Chow was available ad libitum, and fresh water was provided in plastic sterilizable bottles. In each experiment, mice of the same age were used.

Organisms

Salmonella typhimurium, strain W118-2, was obtained from Dr. Samuel Formal, Walter Reed Army Institute of Medical Research. This strain has been used previously in our laboratory (4). Its intraperitoneal LD_{50} is 1 x 10^4 organisms for CD-1 mice and <6 cells for C3H/HeJ mice. Characteristics of strain TA1659, a rough mutant, have already been described (3).

Bacterial Storage and Culture

Stock cultures were stored lyophilized at -20°C. Organisms used for antigen preparation or challenge were obtained from lyophils rehydrated with brain heart infusion broth (BHI), and grown as previously described (4). For challenge, the bacteria were counted in a Petroff-Hausser chamber and the culture diluted in saline to the desired concentration. The actual number of viable bacteria in the culture was determined by duplicate plate counts.

Vaccines

Ribosomal vaccine, acetone-killed cells, and phenol-water purified lipopolysaccharide (PW-LPS) were prepared as previously described (4). Trichloroacetic acid-extracted LPS (TCA-LPS), endotoxic protein (EP) and $PW\text{-}LPS_{bs}$ were prepared by the methods of Sultzer and Goodman (11) and generously provided for these studies by Dr. Sultzer (Downstate Medical Center, Brooklyn, NY). Vaccine dosages were standardized on a dry weight basis. For the ribosomal vaccine 1 O.D.$_{260}$ unit is equal to 78 μg, dry weight.

Immunization and Challenge

Mice were immunized with one intraperitoneal injection of vaccine in a volume of 0.5 ml. When appropriate, vaccines were suspended in sterile, nonpyrogenic saline (Abbott or Cutter Laboratories) or in sterile phosphate-buffered saline. Control mice received saline. Unless otherwise indicated, mice were challenged intraperitoneally with the desired dosage of live W118-2 in 0.5 ml saline three weeks after immunization. Cells were grown, and the inoculum standardized and verified, as described above. Protection was assessed by survival.

Serological Studies

Serum was collected from separate groups of four or six control mice or from four or six immunized mice before immunization (pre) and 12 and 21 days post-vaccination. Pre and 12-day sera were obtained from the retro-orbital plexus, and 21-day serum by heart puncture. Equal amounts of serum from each mouse were pooled. Passive hemagglutination titers were carried out as previously described (14). Whole-cell agglutination titers were determined in tubes or round-bottomed microtiter plates. For tubes, 0.5 ml of serum was serially diluted and 0.5 ml of 5×10^8 acetone-killed cells was added to each tube. Tubes were incubated at 36°C for 2 h and then overnight at 4°C. For microtiter plates, .05 ml of serum or dilutions was used with 3.8×10^7 acetone-killed cells added in a volume of .05 ml. Incubation times and temperatures were the same as those used for tubes. In both assays the titer was read as the last tube or well with 2+ agglutination.

Mitogenicity Assay

Spleens of three mice were teased together in cold RPMI 1640 with L-glutamine, pH 7.2 (MBA, Maryland), to which had been added Penicillin-Streptomycin Mixture (MBA) (100 U penicillin and 100 μg streptomycin/ml, final concentration). Cells were transferred to conical centrifuge tubes and large clumps were allowed to settle for 10 min. The supernatant cell suspension was collected and centrifuged at 1,000 rpm for 10 min in an International Centrifuge. The cell pellet was resuspended in the same RPMI medium to a final white cell concentration of 2×10^6 viable cells/ml. Assays were carried out in Linbro flat-bottomed, 96-well plates (Flow Laboratories, Hamden, CN). To each well was added 20 μl of mitogen suspended in medium, or medium alone for the background counts. Each mitogen was tested in triplicate. Two hundred μl of the cell suspension was added to each well to yield a final concentration of 4×10^5 cells/well. The plates were covered and incubated at 37°C for 42 h in a humidified atmosphere with 5% CO_2. At 42 h, 0.25 µCi of ^3H-thymidine (Amersham) was added to each well in a volume of 10 µl, and the plates were reincubated for 6 h. The contents of each well were harvested onto glass-fiber filter strips using a Bellco Micro-harvester (Vineland, NJ). Filter paper discs cut from the strips were placed in scintillation vials to which was added 3.5 ml of scintillation fluid (1 gal of toluene plus 15.2 g PPO and 190 mg POPOP). Vials were counted in a scintillation counter for 1 min each. Counts per minute for the triplicate cultures were averaged. The Stimulation Index (S.I.) was calculated by dividing mean counts for mitogen-stimulated cultures by mean background counts.

Statistics

The levels of significance for the observed frequencies were determined by Fisher's exact test for 2 x 2 tables (15). The maximum protective capacity of each vaccine was determined graphically according to the method of Nowotny (16). The log of the vaccine dose was plotted against the log of the number of surviving mice divided by the number of dead mice. The point at which data line crosses the ordinate indicates the challenge dose which would be expected to result in 50% survival in optimally immunized mice.

RESULTS

Comparative Protection by Vaccines

In a previous study, a thorough comparison was made of the relative protective capacities of several different vaccines of Salmonella in CD-1 mice. Graded doses of live cells, acetone-killed cells, ribosomal extract, and lipopolysaccharide were given to groups of mice which were then challenged three weeks post-vaccination with increasing infectious doses of Salmonella. For each vaccine an optimal immunizing dose was determined based on the ability to give good protective capacity with minimal toxicity (3). Using this optimal dose, the maximum protective capacity of each vaccine can be determined graphically. As shown in Fig. 2, lipopolysaccharide is markedly inferior to the other vaccines in its capacity to protect, whereas acetone-killed cells and ribosomal vaccine have almost identical maximal protective capacities. Both of these latter vaccines approach live cells in their ability to protect mice against as many as 5,000 LD_{50} doses. These results establish (1) that purified lipopolysaccharide is protective, although not at as high levels as the more complex vaccines, and (2) that ribosomes are not unique among nonviable vaccines in providing high levels of protection against Salmonella infection.

Duration of Protection

The four vaccines were also compared with respect to duration of protection. All animals were received in the same shipment and their vaccination time was staggered, so that all animals were challenged on the same day. Groups of 10 animals each were vaccinated with the optimal dose of the desired vaccine at intervals of three weeks, two months, four months, or six months prior to challenge. Two different challenge doses were used. The results are shown in Figs. 3 and 4. Again, it was found that lipopolysaccharide is inferior to the other vaccines, in this case with respect to duration of protection, at all times tested after the three-week time period. At six months post-immunization, ribosomal vaccines and live cells still provided significant protection against the low challenge

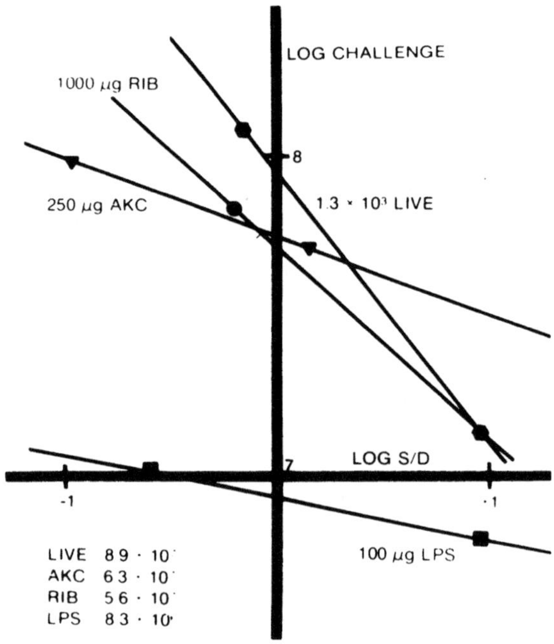

Fig. 2. Calculation of the Maximum Protective Capacity of the optimal immunizing dose of each vaccine using the intraperitoneal route of challenge. CD-1 mice were immunized with the optimal vaccine dosage ip and were then challenged ip with increasing doses of S. typhimurium W118-2. The point at which each line crosses the ordinate indicates that challenge dose which would be expected to result in 50% survival in the optimally immunized mice. LD_{50} values for each vaccine are given at the bottom of the Figure. ■ LPS = 100 μg lipopolysaccharide; ▼ AKC = 250 μg of acetone-killed cells; ● RIB = 1,000 μg ribosomal preparation; and ⬢ Live = 1.3 x 10^3 live cells.

Log S/D = log of the number of surviving mice divided by the number of dead mice.

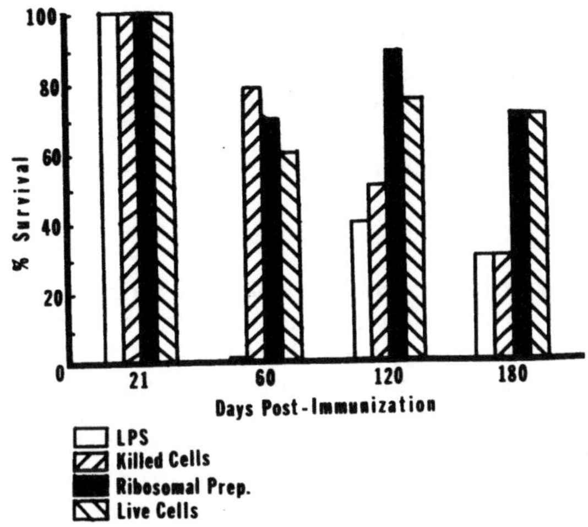

Fig. 3. Duration of protection by various vaccines. Groups of 10 mice each were all received on the same date and were immunized at staggered intervals with the optimal dose of the designatee vaccine. LPS = 100 μg of lipopolysaccharide; Killed cells = 250 μg of acetone-killed cells; Ribosomal preparation = 1,000 μg; Live cells = 1 x 10^3 cells. All animals were challenged on the same day with 4 x 10^6 live cells of W118-2.

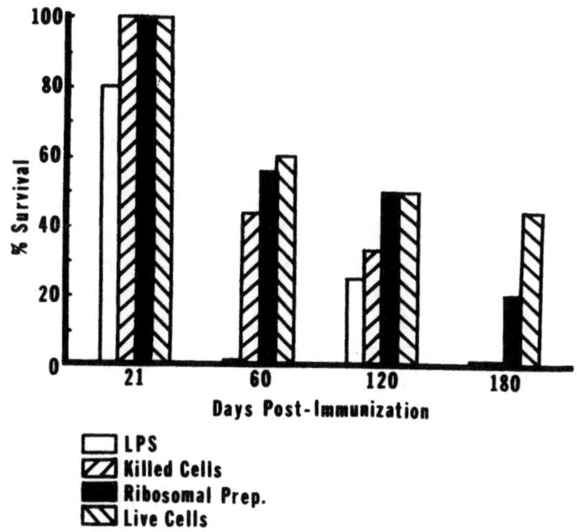

Fig. 4. Duration of protection by various vaccines. Groups of 10 mice each were all received on the same date and were immunized at staggered intervals with the optimal dose of the designated vaccine. LPS = 100 μg of lipopolysaccharide; Killed cells = 250 μg of acetone-killed cells; Ribosomal preparation = 1,000 μg; Live cells = 1 x 10^3 cells. All animals were challenged on the same day with 7.1 x 10^6 live cells of W118-2.

dose of 400 LD_{50}s, but the other nonliving vaccines were not protective (Fig. 3). When the high challenge dose was used, ribosomes and live cells protected at four months post-vaccination, while at six months, only live cells protected (Fig. 4). These results suggest that ribosomal vaccines provide a slightly enhanced duration of protection as compared with other nonliving vaccines.

Serological Studies

When antibody titers were determined in animals receiving the various vaccines and followed over the six-month time period, it was found that ribosomal vaccines and acetone-killed cells showed comparable anti-LPS hemagglutinating titers, which persisted at high levels for the six-month duration of the experiment. (Fig. 5). In contrast, lipopolysaccharide-immunized animals had high titers at three weeks post-immunization, but by two months the titers had significantly declined. When whole-cell agglutination titers were tested, (Fig. 6), mice receiving ribosomes or acetone-killed cells showed no significant differences in their titers over the six-month period. Lipopolysaccharide-immunized animals showed a marked decline in whole-cell agglutination titers, reaching negligible levels at six months. These results show that the differences in duration of protection seen between acetone-killed cells and ribosomal vaccines cannot be accounted for by differences in the serological responses measured, as serological responses of the two groups of mice are not statistically different.

Mitogenicity in C3H/HeJ Mice

To investigate further the role of factors other than LPS in ribosomal extracts, the C3H/HeJ strain of mouse was chosen. Table 1 shows a comparison of the mitogenicity of phenol-water purified lipopolysacchard (PW-LPS); endotoxic protein (EP); and TCA-extracted lipopolysaccharide, which has the endotoxic protein associated with it (TCA-LPS); and ribosomal vaccine (RIB). It can be seen that, in agreement with the literature, PW-LPS is poorly mitogenic in these animals. Endotoxic protein and TCA-LPS are potent mitogens, whereas the ribosomes are significantly inferior. At high doses ribosomes inhibit uptake of ^{3}H-thymidine.

Protection in C3H/HeJ Mice

In previous protection experiments using C3H/HeJ mice, it was shown that PW-LPS, given at several doses, was not protective and induced no passive hemagglutination titer, or whole-cell aglutination titer, in mice tested 21 days post-vaccination. However, 60 μg of acetone-killed cells or 250 μg of ribosomal vaccine induced significant prolongation of survival and an increased number of survivors 30 days post-challenge. These vaccines also resulted in appreciable antibody titers in both assays 21 days post-vaccination

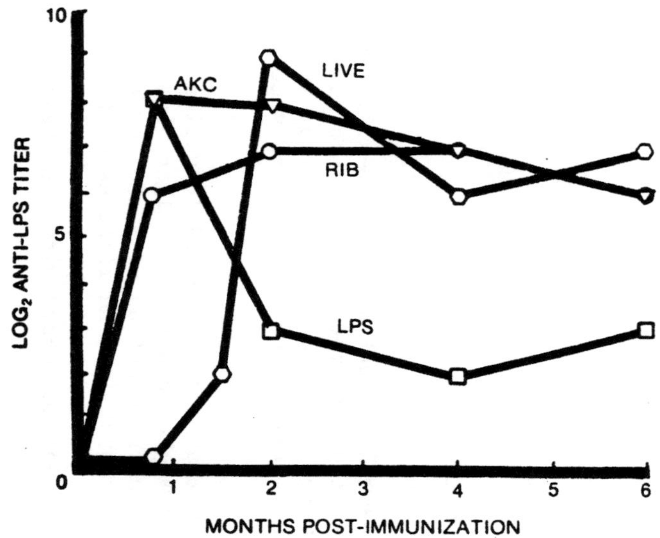

Fig. 5. Duration of the anti-LPS passive hemagglutinating antibody esponse. Groups of 6 mice each were immunized ip with the optimal dose of each vaccine. At the indicated times post-vaccination serum was collected, pooled, and titered. LPS=lipopolysaccharide; AKC=acetone-killed cells; RIB=ribosomal vaccine; Live=live-cell vaccine.

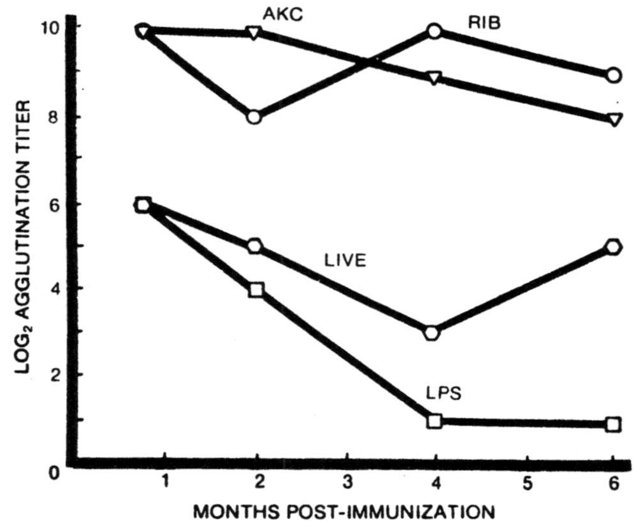

Fig. 6. Duration of the whole-cell agglutinating antibody response. Groups of 6 mice each were immunized ip with the optimal dose of each vaccine. At the indicated times post-vaccination, serum was collected, pooled, and titered. LPS=lipopolysaccharide; AKC=acetone-killed cells; RIB=ribosomal vaccine; Live=live-cell vaccine.

TABLE I

^{3}H-Thymidine Uptake by C3H/HeJ Spleen Cells

Mitogen	Dose (μg/ml)	Mean cpm ± S.D.[a]	S.I.[b]
None	-	254 ± 13	-
Con A	0.5	26,446 ± 785	104
PW-LPS$_{bs}$	0.1	403 ± 72	2
	1	738 ± 10	3
	10	1,518 ± 97	6
	100	3,527 ± 498	14
EP	0.1	8,666 ± 1,656	34
	1	22,845 ± 1,067	90
	10	29,554 ± 3,345	116
	100	23,399 ± 2,578	92
TCA-LPS	0.1	4,558 ± 226	18
	1	16,912 ± 2,054	67
	10	26,074 ± 1,649	103
	100	25,470 ± 1,433	100
RIB	0.1	823 ± 174	3
	1	4,628 ± 657	18
	10	4,792 ± 400	19
	100	81 ± 2	<1

a ^{3}H-Thymidine uptake.

b $S.I. = \frac{\text{Mean cpm of mitogen}}{\text{Mean cpm without mitogen}}$

(14). Thus, both the ribosomal extract and acetone-killed cells have the capacity to induce these nonresponder mice to make anti-O antibody, whereas phenol-water purified LPS is impotent in these capacities. For this mouse strain, then, the complex vaccines have adjuvant activity.

To test the hypothesis that protection and induction of an antibody response in these mice might require an antigen plus a mitogen, a protection experiment was carried out using phenol-water purified lipopolysaccharide, endotoxic protein, and mixtures of the two substances. Table 2 shows that the endotoxic protein by itself is not protective in these animals; and in accord with the previous results,

TABLE II

Survival and Antibody Titers of C3H/HeJ Mice Immunized with Phenol-water Extracted LPS Plus a Mitogen

Vaccine[a]	30-Day survival[b]	MTD[c]	21-Day agglutination titer
50 μg PW-LPS	0% (0/10)	12	<2
50 μg EP	0% (0/10)	11	<2
50 μg LPS + 25 g EP	0% (0/10)	13	2
50 μg LPS + 50 g EP	0% (1/10)	13	2
50 μg Acetone-killed cells	11% (1/9)	22	16
PBS	0% (0/10)	9	<2
			T.S = 32[d]

[a] Vaccines given ip in 0.5 ml.

[b] Mice injected with 17 cells of W118-2 21 days post-vaccination.

[c] MTD = mean time to death.

[d] T.S. = Typing serum.

neither is the purified lipopolysaccharide. Aqueous mixtures of these two substances did not result in protection or in antibody responses. Thus, administering a combination of a mitogen plus the O antigen to the animals is not sufficient to give protection, and does not simulate the activity of ribosomes or acetone-killed cells.

Table 3 shows the results of an experiment in which TCA-LPS was tested for its ability to protect C3H/H3J mice and to induce antibody. This preparation markedly prolonged survival time and induced agglutinating antibody.

DISCUSSION

These studies show that a Salmonella ribosomal vaccine contains O antigens and that these antigens are at least partly responsible for the effectiveness of this type of subcellular extract. Yet, when the ribosomal vaccine is compared with phenol-water purified lipopolysaccharide, the ribosomal vaccine is markedly superior and performs at levels almost equal to the level induced by live cells. The ribosomal vaccine is not unique among nonliving vaccines in giving high levels of protection, since acetone-killed cells engender levels of protection similar to those of ribosomes when

TABLE III

Survival and Antibody Titers of C3H/HeJ Mice Immunized with TCA-LPS ip

Vaccine[a]	Dose (μg)	30-Day survival[b]	MTD[c]	Agglutination titer[d]	
TCA-LPS				pre	<2
	1	0%	16	12	2
				21	4
				pre	<2
	10	0%	18	12	4
				21	4
				pre	<2
	25	40%	26	12	16
				21	8
				pre	<2
	50	40%	23	12	16
				21	16
				pre	<2
	100	10%	22	12	16
				21	16
AKC				pre	<2
	60	40%	22	12	2
				21	4
PW-LPS				pre	
	60	0%	9	12	<2
				21	
NaCl	-	0%	9		<2
				T.S. = 32[e]	

[a] Vaccines given ip in 0.5 ml.

[b] 10 mice per group. Mice challenged 21 days post-vaccination with 28 cells of W118-2.

[c] MTD = mean time to death.

[d] pre = preimmunization titer; 12 and 21 = titers on days 12 and 21 post-vaccination.

[e] T.S. = typing serum.

protection is tested three weeks post-vaccination. Ribosomes, however, do give a somewhat greater duration of protection, when compared with acetone-killed cells over a six-month period post-vaccination.

The question remains as to whether ribosomes and acetone-killed cells are superior to purified LPS because they have natural adjuvants in the preparation, because they contain multiple antigens, or for both reasons. When serological responses of animals receiving the various vaccines are compared three weeks post-immunization, it is found that animals receiving acetone-killed cells, ribosomes, or LPS have passive hemagglutination titers comparable to those of O antigens. Both acetone-killed cells and ribosomal vaccine, however, induce a significantly greater whole-cell agglutinating response, when compared with PW-LPS. To be decided is whether the agglutinating response represents induction of a different class of antibodies or is due to antibodies to antigens other than the O antigens.

It is certainly clear that the ribosomal extract is a more potent immunogen than PW-LPS in the C3H/HeJ mice, and can trigger them to make anti-O antibody, whereas the PW-LPS does not. In this sense one can say that ribosomal extracts have properties of an adjuvant, because they convert nonresponsiveness to responsiveness. At the present time it is not possible to say whether their effectiveness is a property of the ribosome, or is attributable to yet another contaminant present in the ribosomal fraction but not present in phenol-water purified LPS. It is noteworthy that acetone-killed cells and TCA-extracted LPS also prolong survival time in these mice. Since the methods used for preparing ribosomes are mild, it is reasonable to assume that the lipopolysaccharide present in these extracts would have the endotoxic protein associated with it, and thus would be more like TCA-extracted LPS than the more highly purified phenol-water product. Could all of the protection of ribosomal extracts be simulated by TCA-extracted LPS, or do ribosomal extracts have additional antigens or substances which enhance the immune response? At present we cannot say, although the fact that ribosomes are superior to the whole, acetone-killed cell vaccine, which is a more complex antigenic mixture than TCA-LPS, suggests that the answer may be, "no".

If we consider the models shown in Fig. 1, our data does not exclude a mechanism consistent with Model 1, but it offers little support for this hypothesis. The ribosomal vaccine seems to behave similarly to other nonliving vaccines, except that it outperforms them in some immunological parameters. Models 2 and 3 are viable alternatives and at present it is difficult to distinguish between them. Model 3 has some attractive features, including precedents in the literature for marked alterations in immunogenicity of molecules as a function of method of presentation. It was established by Avery and Morgan in 1925 that purified capsular polysaccharide from the type 3 pneumococcus is not immunogenic in rabbits. However, if the animals were injected with whole, smooth, killed microorganisms, they made a fine immune response to the pneumococcal polysaccharide (17). A similar situation is found in rabbits presented with purified C-carbohydrate. They do not make antibody to the purified molecule, but make an excellent immune response to C-carbohydrate when it is present in the F-polysaccharide, a lipid-rich extract of the pneumococcus (18). The polyribosephosphate (PRP) antigen of Hemophilus influenzae, type b, provides another example in which a purified antigen is nonimmunogenic in weanling rabbits, but in which an outer membrane complex containing PRP, lipopolysaccharide, and outer membrane proteins induces anti-PRP antibodies (19). The results obtained with phenol-water purified LPS and ribosomal extracts in C3H/HeJ mice fit a pattern that is similar to that of the examples cited above. It is interesting that the mixing experiments did not simulate the effects of ribosomal vaccine in CD-1 (14) or C3H/HeJ mice, perhaps suggesting that the three-dimensional configuration of the complex may be critical for immunomodulation.

At the present time there is considerable interest in preparing highly purified antigens for use in new vaccines. Older vaccines of course consisted of whole, killed microorganisms. These results discussed above suggest that whole microorganisms contain factors which produce an optimal immune response that frequently is not obtainable using the purified substances. It may be necessary or desirable to add back to the purified components additional naturally occurring bacterial products which are capable of providing optimal immunity.

ACKNOWLEDGMENT

This work was supported by Public Health Service Grants AI-11860 and AI-15613 from the National Institute for Allergy and Infectious Diseases.

REFERENCES

1. Eisenstein, T. K., 1978, Ribosomal vaccines: A review, p. 211-222. In A. Voller and H. Friedman (ed.), New trends and developments in vaccines. MTP Press, Ltd., Lancaster, England.

2. Youmans, A. S., and Youmans, G. P., 1974, The effect of metabolic inhibitors and hydroxylamine on the immune response in mice to mycobacterial ribonucleic acid vaccines. J. Immunol. 112: 271.

3. Eisenstein, T. K., 1975, Evidence for O-antigens as the antigenic determinants in "ribosomal" vaccines prepared from Salmonella. Infect. Immun. 12: 364.

4. Angerman, C. R., and Eisenstein, T. K., 1978, Comparative efficacy and toxicity of a ribosomal vaccine, acetone-killed cells,lipopolysaccharide, and a live cell vaccine prepared from Salmonella typhimurium. Infect. Immun. 19: 575.

5. Lin, J. -H., and Berry, L. J., 1978, The use of strain LT2-M1 in identifying the protective antigens in a Salmonella typhimurium-derived ribosomal vaccine. J. Reticuloendothel. Soc. 23: 135.

6. Misfeldt, M. L., and Johnson, W., 1977, Role of endotoxin contamination in ribosomal vaccines prepared from Salmonella typhimurium. Infect. Immun. 17: 98

7. Svenson, S. B., Nurminen, M., and Lindberg, A. A., 1979, Artificial Salmonella vaccines: O-antigenic oligosaccharide-protein conjugates induce protection against infection with Salmonella typhimurium. Infect. Immun. 25: 863.

8. Collins, F. M., 1970, Immunity to enteric infection in mice. Infect. Immun. 1: 243.

9. Ornellas, E. P., Roantree, R. J., and Steward, J. P., 1970, The specificity and importance of humoral antibody in the protection of mice against intraperitoneal challenge with complement-sensitive and complement-resistant salmonella. J. Infect. Dis. 112: 113.

10. Plant, J., Glynn, A., and Wilson, B., 1978, Protective effects of a supernatant factor from Salmonella typhimurium on Salmonella typhimurium infection of inbred mice. Infect. Immun. 22: 125.

11. Sultzer, B. M., and Goodman, G. W., 1976, Endotoxin protein: A B-cell mitogen and polyclonal activator of C3H/HeJ lymphocytes. J. Exp. Med. 144: 821.

12. Watson, J., and Riblet, R., 1974, Genetic control of responses to bacterial lipopolysaccharides in mice. I. Evidence for a single gene that influences mitogenic and immunogenic responses to lipopolysaccharides. J. Exp. Med. 140: 1147.

13. Rudbach, J. A., and Reed, N. D., 1977, Immunological responses of mice to lipopolysaccharide: Lack of secondary responsiveness by C3H/HeJ mice. Infect. Immun. 16: 513.

14. Eisenstein, T. K., and Angerman, C. R., 1978, Immunity to experimental Salmonella infection: Studies on the protective capacity and immunogenicity of lipopolysaccharide, acetone-killed cells, and ribosome-rich extracts of Salmonella typhimurium

in C3H/HeJ and CD-1 mice. J. Immunol. 121: 1010.

15. Fisher, R. A., and Yates, F., 1963, Statistical tables for biological, agricultural and medical research, p. 68. 6th ed. Hafner Publishing Co., New York.

16. Nowotny, A., 1969, Basic exercises in immunochemistry, p. 144. A laboratory manual. Springer-Verlag, NY.

17. Avery, O.T., and Morgan, H.J., 1925, Immunological reactions of the isolated carbohydrate and protein of pneumococcus. J. Exp. Med. 42: 347.

18. Goebel, W. F., and Adams, M. H., 1943, The immunological properties of the heterophile antigen and somatic polysaccharide of pneumococcus. J. Exp. Med. 77: 435.

19. Anderson, P., and Smith, D. H., 1977, Immunogenicity in weanling rabbits of a polyribophosphate complex from Haemophilus influenzae type b. J. Infect. Dis. 136S: S63.

THE EFFECTS OF ENDOTOXIN ON MACROPHAGES AND T-LYMPHOCYTES

David L. Rosenstreich and Stefanie N. Vogel

Departments of Medicine and Microbiology
Albert Einstein College of Medicine
Bronx, NY 10461 and,

Laboratory of Microbiology and Immunology
National Institute of Dental Research
National Institutes of Health
Bethesda, MD 20205

INTRODUCTION

The immune response is generated by a complex series of interactions between three major lymphoreticular cell types, macrophages and B and T lymphocytes (Fig. 1). This response is initiated by the interaction of an external stimulus, such as an antigen or mitogen, with each of all of these cells. The initial stimulation also results in the production of a number of soluble intercellular messengers i.e., lymphokines or monokines, that act within the system to produce a marked amplification of the response.

Bacterial lipopolysaccharides (LPS) exert potent effects on the immune system including the induction of anti-LPS antibodies, polyclonal stimulation of B lymphocytes, and a general enhancement of immunity (adjuvanticity). These effects are thought to be due in large part to the ability of LPS to act on specific cellular components of the immune system including B and T lymphocytes and macrophages. LPS acts both as a direct cell stimulatory agent, and also as an inducer of lymphokines and monokines.

The stimulatory effects of LPS on B lymphocytes are well known. In vitro, LPS induces the proliferation of these cells (mitogenic effect) and induces their non-specific differentiation into antibody forming cells (polyclonal activation). It stimulates differentiation of macrophages and induces them to secrete immunostimulatory molecules.

There is also some evidence indicating a direct effect of LPS on T lymphocytes which has not been well characterized.

Progress in endotoxin research has been especially rapid in the last 10 years because of the use of the genetically LPS-unresponsive C3H/HeJ mouse strain. These mice carry a mutation in the 4th chromosome at the endotoxin response gene locus (Lps), that renders them abnormally responsive to most of the biological effects of endotoxin (27). This defect seems to be specific for the lipid A moiety of LPS and is expressed in the cells (i.e., T and B lymphocytes, macrophages, and fibroblasts) of these mice. In contrast, the

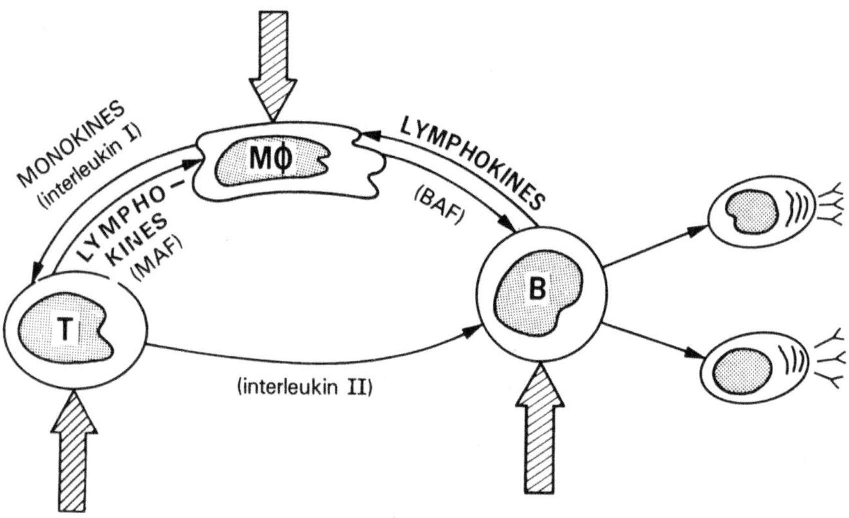

Fig. 1. Cellular Basis of the Immune Response. The immune response is produced by the interaction of three major cell types. Endotoxin can interact directly with each of these cells (large arrows). In addition, the response is enhanced by intercellular molecular messengers. Endotoxin stimulates the secretion of LAF by macrophages, MAF by B cells and TRF by T cells. Whether it also stimulates the production of a MAF-like molecule by T cells remains to be established.

effect of LPS on other humoral systems such as complement, seems to be intact (10). The nature of this defect, or conversely, the mechanism of action of the Lps gene, is not yet known. These mice have been used in a number of studies to be discussed in later sections of this report. Interpretation of some of these studies depends on the understanding that the Lps gene is expressed in cells, and that the Lps gene defect in C3H/HeJ mice is apparently specific for lipid A.

Although LPS is capable of exerting effects at many sites, we will concentrate in this report on one phase of the immune response, the limb that involves macrophages and T lymphocytes. We will discuss both the direct effects of LPS on these two cells, as well as recent work that illustrates how T cells regulate the sensitivity of macrophages to LPS. For the most part, the discussion will be limited to *in vitro* studies using murine cells.

Direct Effects of LPS on Macrophages

It has been known for many years that macrophages are involved in the adjuvant effect of LPS (1) and more recently, the role of these cells in mediating many other of its biological effects has been appreciated. For these reasons, a great deal of endotoxin research has focused on the macrophage. In this section, we will discuss some of the direct effects of LPS on these cells, i.e., those functions that require the experimental administration of LPS and that appear not to require the immediate participation of other cell types, such as lymphocytes.

LPS has two well documented effects on normal macrophages. It induces the secretion of a number of macrophage products including lymphocyte activating factor (LAF, interleukin -1), interferon, colony stimulating factor (CSF) and prostaglandins (reviewed in 15). Higher concentrations of LPS are also cytotoxic for macrophages. Finally, there are reports suggesting that LPS will induce the rapid differentiation of macrophages, most notably in the conversion of resting macrophages to activated, tumoricidal cells. These effects are all thought to result from the direct interaction of LPS with macrophages because relatively pure macrophage populations respond to LPS and because additional lymphocytes usually do not enhance these macrophage effects.

The cytotoxic effect of LPS on macrophages *in vitro* has been known for many years (29). In a more recent study, we examined the cytotoxic effect of LPS on macrophages obtained from LPS unresponsive, C3H/HeJ mice. C3H/HeJ mice are abnormally responsive to all the known effects of LPS because of a defective response to the lipid A moiety. These mice are therefore an excellent experimental tool for examining the effect of lipid A on a biological system. After

24 hrs of incubation with endotoxin *in vitro*, a high percentage of macrophages from LPS responsive C3H/HeN mice are killed (Fig. 2). In contrast, C3H/HeJ macrophages are not killed by LPS suggesting that LPS-induced cytotoxicity is a lipid A mediated event. This conclusion has been confirmed by others (14). A genetic analysis confirmed that macrophage sensitivity to LPS was controlled by the same gene (*Lps*) that controlled B cell LPS sensitivity (18).

Although the cytotoxic effect of LPS is a convenient way of determining macrophage sensitivity, we are uncertain of its biological significance for several reasons. As illustrated by the data in Fig. 2, LPS preparations vary in their cytotoxic potential without any obvious relationship to their biologic potency. We have recently found that the macrophage cytotoxic effect of LPS can be destroyed by heating at 70°C, while other biological effects are not detrimentally effected (22). This sensitivity to heat may explain the variable potency of LPS preparations, since temperature is not usually carefully controlled in hot-phenol water extractions of LPS. For the present, our evidence suggests that cytotoxicity is an event that clearly involves lipid A but whose significance and pathogenesis are incompletely understood.

The stimulation of macrophage secretion is a much more relevant immunomodulatory function of LPS. As was briefly discussed in the introduction, *in vitro* treatment with LPS will induce macrophages to produce almost all of their recognized products (Table 1) (reviewed in 15). Macrophage-produced molecules which are clearly immunoregulatory in nature include: LAF (IL-1) which acts on T-lymphocytes; interferon and colony stimulating factor, which act on macrophages; and prostaglandins, thymidine and arginase, which may function as feedback suppressors of immunity. A number of these products (interferon, CSF, and LAF) have been identified in the sera of LPS-treated animals indicating that this pathway is relevant to the immune response *in vivo* (D. Mannel - personal communication).

The phenomenon of LPS-induced LAF production by mouse macrophages is illustrated by the data in Fig. 3. Macrophage secretion of LAF is stimulated by small amounts of LPS (0.1-1 μg/ml). These quantities are below the threshold of cytotoxicity. C3H/HeJ macrophages are not stimulated to produce LAF by a protein-free LPS preparation (K235 (ph)). However, LPS extracted by butanol-water, which contains some Lipid A associated protein, induces a small, but significant stimulation of C3H/HeJ macrophages. LPS-induced macrophage secretion of other molecules is qualitatively similar, although some variation is seen depending on cell source and the nature of the stimulating LPS. Thus, resident macrophages secrete much more prostaglandins than do thioglycollate-induced cells in response to LPS, while the reverse is true with LAF.

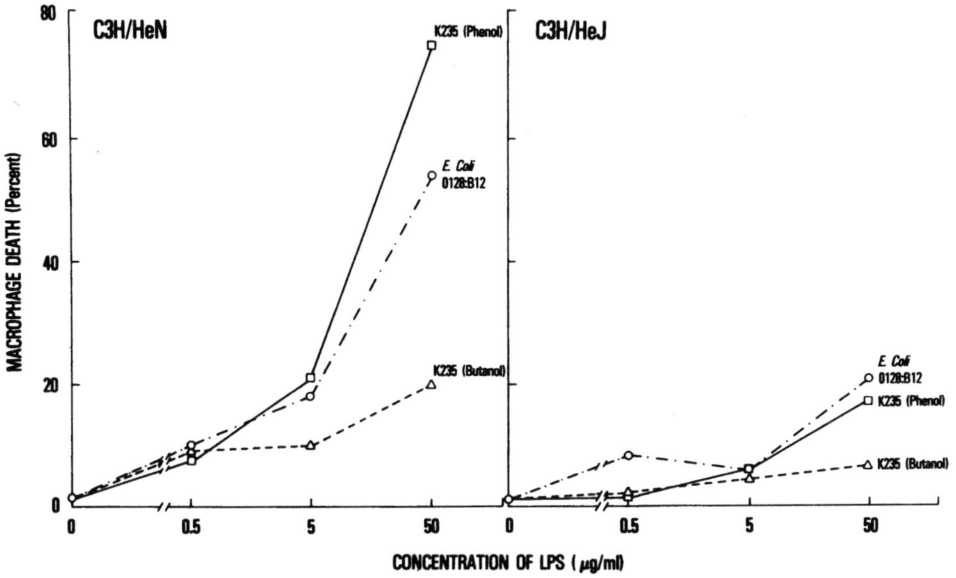

Fig. 2. Endotoxin-induced Macrophage Cytotoxicity. Thioglycollate-induced macrophages from C3H/H3N or C3H/HeJ mice were cultured 24 hrs in the presence or absence of different endotoxin preparations. Killing was measured by the failure to exclude trypan blue dye.

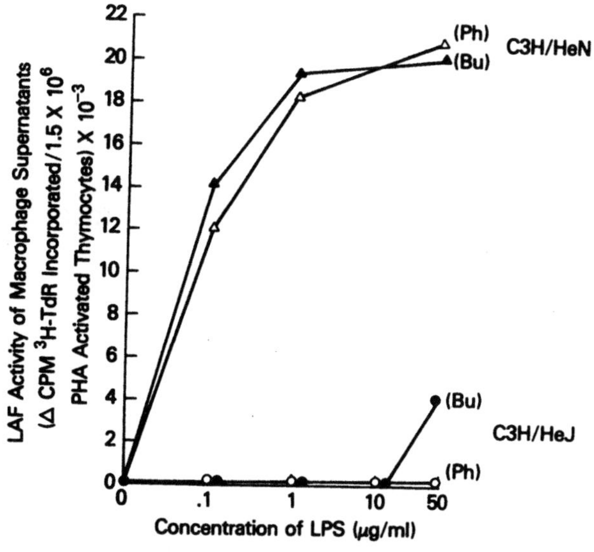

Fig. 3. EndoToxin-induced LAF Production by Macrophages. Thioglycollate-induced macrophages from C3H/HeN or C3H/HeJ mice were cultured in the presence or absence of different endotoxin preparations. After 72 hrs of culture, the macrophage supernatants were harvested and tested for LAF activity on C3H/HeJ lymphocytes.

TABLE I

Biologically Active Products of Macrophages Whose Secretion is Stimulated by Endotoxin

I. Hydrolytic Enzymes

1. Lysosomal hydrolases
2. Neutral proteinases
   - Collagenase
   - Elastase
   - Plasminogen activator

II. Cell Stimulatory Proteins

1. Colony stimulating factor (CSF)
2. Interferon
3. Immunostimulatory factors
   - Lymphocyte activating factor (LAF, Interleukin-1)
4. Immunoinhibitory factors
   - Tumor necrosis factor (TNF)
   - Thymidine
   - Arginase
5. Factors thought to act on hepatocytes
   - Glucocorticoid antagonizing factor (GAF)
   - SAA inducing protein
6. Endogenous pyrogen

III. Miscellaneous Products

Prostaglandins
Oxygen metabolites
   Superoxide anion

The process of macrophage "stimulation" involves the differentiation of a monocyte or a resident macrophage into a larger, more metabolically active, secretory cell. Endotoxin clearly plays a role in the process as indicated by its ability to stimulate secretion. However, endotoxin is also thought to play a role in the induction of other events related to the differentiation process, such as enhancement of metabolism and triggering of tumoricidal activity. However, the events leading to the fully activated state are somewhat controversial.

Endotoxin will markedly increase mouse macrophage glucose metabolism _in vitro_. However, unlike the previously discussed effects, this one is mediated at least in part by the effect of LPS on lymphocytes (21). In the guinea pig, a similar phenomenon, the enhancement of macrophage glucosamine incorporation, is totally lymphocyte dependent, and has been shown to be mediated by a lymphokine produced by LPS-stimulated B cells (30).

The exact stage at which endotoxin induces macrophages to kill tumor cells _in vitro_ is also uncertain. Some studies have indicated that LPS will cause resting macrophages to become tumoricidal, suggesting that LPS alone is inducing their differentiation to a fully "activated" state. However, in a recent study, Weinberg et al, showed very convincingly that LPS alone could not render macrophages tumoricidal (28). Instead he found that some form of macrophage "priming" was necessary. Thus, resident macrophages did not kill tumor cells even in the presence of 10 μg/ml LPS. However, proteose peptone-induced macrophages were tumoricidal in the presence of 500 ng/ml LPS. More potent priming events generated macrophages that required even less LPS to kill. After activation with a lymphokine (MAF), macrophages required only 10 ng/ml LPS to kill, and after BCG activation _in vivo_, macrophages required only 1 ng/ml to kill. In every case however, LPS was essential for killing. This elegant study strongly suggests that LPS acts as a triggering stimulus in tumor killing rather than as a true inducer of macrophage differentiation. One reasonable hypothesis that reconciles this "trigger" function with its well documented stimulatory property, is that LPS acts to induce the secretion of a tumoricidal molecule, i.e., tumor necrosis factor.

Effects of Endotoxin on T Lymphocytes.

Although the effect of endotoxin on B lymphocytes and macrophages is well known, it is not generally appreciated that endotoxin acts on T lymphocytes as well. A number of _in vivo_-studies have indicated a requirement for T cells in the adjuvant effect of LPS. More recently, several _in vitro_ studies have demonstrated this effect more clearly

Koenig et al. showed that lipid A would enhance the differentiation of relatively pure thymocyte populations in vitro, and that C3H/HeJ lymphocytes were defective in this regard (8). The role of T lymphocytes in LPS-induced adjuvanticity was recently clarified in a study by McGhee et al, who showed that in vitro adjuvanticity was mediated by an effect on T lymphocytes and macrophages, but not on B cells (9). Based on previous studies of B cell antibody production, these authors suggested that LPS stimulated macrophages to produce LAF, and T cells to produce a second immunostimulatory protein, T-cell replacing factor (TRF, interleukin II - see Fig. 1). This hypothesis has been borne out by the observation that LPS will enhance the ability of T cells to make TRF in conjunction with Con A (4). This latter observation is also consistent with a direct effect of LPS on T cells.

Macrophage Function Controlled by the Lps Gene

Very recently, evidence in several areas of biological research has been forthcoming indicating that endotoxin may exert important regulatory effects on macrophages, in ways that are not immediately apparent, or in amounts that are not ordinarily detectable. These observations are all based on the abnormal responses of C3H/HeJ mice in various biological systems that do not involve the exogenous administration of Lps, indicating a regulatory role for the Lps gene and suggesting, thereby, the involvement of LPS. These abnormal responses include a failure of their macrophages to become tumoricidal after in vivo activation with BCG (19), a failure of their macrophages to respond to the lymphokine, migration inhibitory factor (MIF) (22), and an abnormal development of macrophage surface receptors in vitro (24). In addition, this gene mutation renders mice susceptible to the lethal effects of infection with *Salmonella typhimurium*, an effect that is also presumed to be due to a macrophage defect (12).

The surface receptor abnormality of C3H/H3J macrophages is illustrated in Figure 4. Normal LPS-responsive (C3H/HeN) macrophages increase their surface Fc receptors with time in culture, here indicated by their increased ability to phagocytize antibody-coated particles (EA). In contrast, the macrophages from C3H/HeJ mice lose their surface Fc receptors over the same culture period. This same phenomenon occurs with C3b receptors (data not shown).

The relationship of all the above-mentioned defects to the Lps gene has not yet been determined. However, the tumoricidal (20) and microbicidal (12) defects have been clearly linked to the Lps gene locus, by formal genetic analyses. In view of this, and given the near congenic state between C3H/HeJ and C3H/HeN mice, it is likely that all these abnormalities are controlled by the Lps gene.

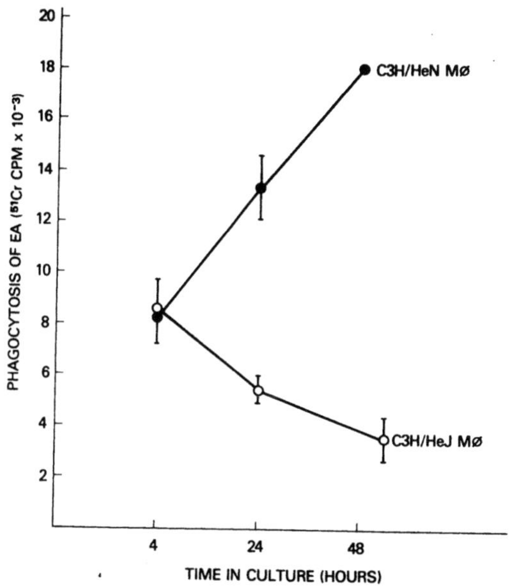

Fig. 4. Alteration of Macrophage Fc-mediated Phagocytosis with Time in Culture. Thioglycollate-induced macrophages were cultured for the specified times and then tested for the ability to phagocytose ^{51}Cr-labelled EA.

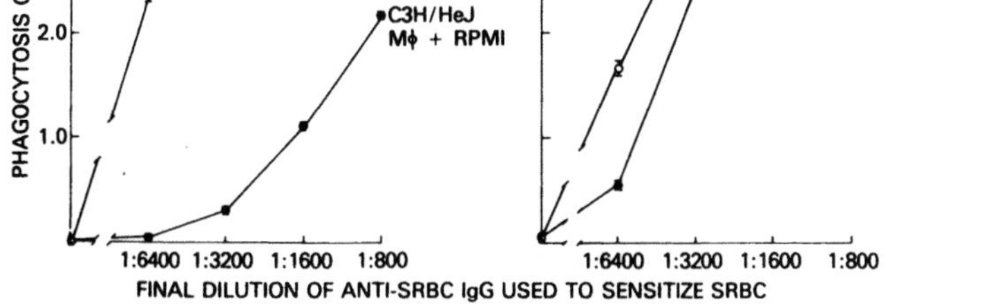

Fig. 5. Enhancement of C3H/HeJ macrophage Fc receptor function by treatment with a lymphokine-rich supernatant. Thioglycollate-induced macrophages were cultured in the presence or absence of a lymphokine derived from Con A stimulated spleen cells. After 48 hours of culture, they were tested for Fc-receptor mediated phagocytosis as specified in Figure 4.

The Internaction of Macrophages and T Lymphocytes: Relationship to Endotoxin Sensitivity

As indicated in Figure 1, the immune response consists of a cyclic interaction between macrophages and T cells, wehre T cell activation is enhanced by monokines such as MAF. In previous sections it was shown that endotoxin acted directly on macrophages and T cells. In this section we will discuss the evidence that indicates that in addition to stimulating macrophages, T cell lymphokines actually regulate and enhance macrophage sensitivity to LPS.

As was noted in the previous section, macrophages from C3H/HeJ mice lose surface Fc receptors with time in culture. However, if these cells are treated with a lymphokine-rich culture supernatant from a Concanavalin A-activated spleen cell, their abnormality is reversed, and their Fc receptor density increases in the same fashion as normal macrophages (Fig. 5). This lymphokine has been partially characterized, and very preliminary evidence indicates that it is physicochemically similar to the T cell lymphokine, MAF. It is even more interesting to note however, that in addition to reversing the Fc receptor defect of C3H/H3J macrophages, this T cell lymphokine will also render these cells sensitive to LPS *in vitro*. As illustrated in Table II, C3H/HeJ macrophages cultured in the presence of

TABLE II

Conversion of C3H/HeJ Macrophages to an Endotoxin Sensitive State by *In Vitro* Treatment with Lymphokine

Source of Macrophages	Treatment	LPS[a]-Induced LAF Production CPM ^{3}H-TdR Incorporated/ 1.5 x 10^6 thymocytes)
C3H/HeJ	Control	5,972 ± 1,177
C3H/HeJ	Lymphokine[b]-rich Supernatant	18,824 ± 5,026
C3H/HeN	Control	45,959 ± 9,557
C3H/HeN	Lymphokine-rich Supernatant	41,564 ± 8,802

[a] Results represent the arithmetic mean ± S.E.M. of 5 separate experiments. Thymocytes were tested in the presence of PHA for LAF (IL1) stimulating activity.

[b] Concanavalin A-stimulated spleen cell supernatants were used at a final concentration of 5%.

[c] A final concentration of 10 μg/ml LPS was used in these studies.

the lymphokine-rich supernatant, produce significant amounts of LAF in response to endotoxin. More recently we have found that lymphokine treatment also renders HeJ mø sensitive to the direct cytotoxic effects of LPS.

Evidence from other systems confirms that T cell derived products will enhance the sensitivity of macrophages to endotoxin. Both Ruco and Meltzer (19) and Weinberg et al (28) noted that a lymphokine-rich supernatant would enable C3H/HeJ macrophages to respond to endotoxin by killing tumor cells. As mentioned previously, similar products also enhance the endotoxin sensitivity of normal murine macrophages. More recently, Moore et al (11) demonstrated that partially purified preparations of colony stimulating factor (CSF) also enhanced C3H/HeN macrophage production of LAF in response to endotoxin.

SUMMARY AND CONCLUSIONS

Endotoxin modulates the immune response by a variety of effects on T cells and macrophages. Its direct stimulatory effects on macrophages are well established, and evidence exists for a direct effect on T cells as well. In addition, endotoxin-induced secretion of the monokine, LAF, acts to further enhance T cell reactivity. Other macrophage-derived products stimulated by endotoxin such as colony stimulating factor (CSF), interferon, and prostaglandins may also be involved in immune regulation. Finally, recent work strongly suggests that T cell products, in turn, regulate the endotoxin sensitivity of macrophages.

This latter finding raises a number of important questions concerning the role of endotoxin and the endotoxin-response gene (Lps). The first is whether the Lps gene regulates macrophage sensitivity to endotoxin or whether it regulates the general state of "activation" of the macrophage. This question has been dealt with in a number of recent papers and has not yet been settled. However, the weight of evidence favors the hypothesis that the Lps gene codes for some type of recognition of lipid A and not a more general function. Thus, the data of Weinberg et al (28), and Doe and Henson (3) indicate that the failure of C3H/HeJ macrophages to kill tumor cells is due to an abnormal response to lipid A and not to an initial global defect. Secondly, C3H/HeJ mice only exhibit increased susceptibility to LPS containing pathogens such as S. typhimurium and K. pneumoniae, and are not more susceptible to other intracellular pathogens whose killing requires activated macrophages such as R. tsutsugamushi, L. Donovani or L. monocytogenes (17).

This defect in lipid A responsiveness may secondarily contribute to a decreased state of macrophage differentiation, but may be overcome by alternative activation stimuli (BCG). However, the BCG-induced increase in macrophage activation leads to an increase in sensitivity to endotoxin. Unfortunately, this hypothesis is circular since it suggests that endotoxin is involved at two distinct sites. Clearly many more careful experiments will be required before this controversy is settled. The observation that T cells or their products can alter sensitivity of macrophages to endotoxin is extremely important, and necessitates a re-examination of the cellular basis underlying the biological effects of endotoxin. The macrophage appears to be the central cell in these effects since one can account for almost all of these activities in terms of some mediator produced by macrophages in response to endotoxin. These latest findings suggest however, that the T cell may be the primary regulator of macrophage LPS sensitivity. In addition to the in vitro studies discussed in this report, we have recently demonstrated that BCG infection will render C3H/HeJ mice sensitive to endotoxin (25). Furthermore, our data incriminates the T cell as the mediator of this increased sensitivity. Elucidating the mechanisms underlying T cell regulation of macrophage sensitivity to LPS, should prove to be important and rewarding.

REFERENCES

1. Allison, A. C., and Davies, A. J. S., 1971, Requirement of thymust-dependent lymphocytes for potentiation by adjuvants and antibody formation. Nature. 233: 330.

2. Chedid, L., Parant, M., Damais, C., Parant, F., Juy, D., and Galelli, A., 1976, Failure of endotoxin to increase nonspecific resistance to infection of lipopolysaccharide low-responder mice. Infection and Immunity 13: 722.

3. Doe, W., and Henson, P. M., 1979, Macrophage stimulation by bacterial lipopolysaccharides III. Selective unresponsiveness of C3H/HeJ macrophages to the lipid A differentiation signal. J. Immunol. 123: 2304.

4. Farrar, J. J., Mizel, S. B., Fuller-Bonar, J., Hilfiker, M. L., and Farrar, W. L., 1980, Lps-mediated adjuvanticity, effect of Lps on the production of T-cell growth factor (IL-2). In Microbiology. 1980. American Society of Microbiology, Washington, D. C. (in press).

5. Glode, L., Jacques, A., Mergenhagen, S. E., and Rosenstreich, D. L., 1977, Resistance of macrophages from C3H/HeJ mice to the in vitro cytotoxic effects of endotoxin,. J. Immunol. 119: 162.

6. Gode, L., and Rosenstreich, D. L., 1976, Genetic control of B cell activation by bacterial lipopolysaccharide is mediated by multiple distinct genes or alleles. J. Immunol. 117: 2061.

7. Green, S., Carswell, E., Old, L. J., Fiore, N., Dobriansky, A., Mamaril, F., and Schwartz, M. K., 1974, Mechanisms of endotoxin-induced tumor hemorrhagic necrosis. Proc. Am. Assoc. Cancer Res., 15: 139.

8. Koenig, S., Hoffman, M. K., and Thomas, L., 1977, Induction of phenotypic lymphocyte differentiation in Lps unresponsive mice by an Lps-induced serum factor and by lipid A-associated protein. J. Immunol. 118: 1910.

9. McGhee, J. R., Farrar, J. J., Michalek, S. M., Mergenhagen, S. E., and Rosenstreich, D. L., 1979, Cellular requirements for lipopolysaccharide adjuvanticity: A role for both T lymphocytes and macrophages in *in vitro* responses to particulate antigens. J. Exp. Med. 149: 793.

10. Moeller, G. R., Terry, L., and Snyderman, R., 1978, The inflammatory response and resistance to endotoxin in mice. J. Immunol. 120: 116.

11. Moore, R. N., Oppenheim, J. J., Farrar, J. J., Carter, C. S., and Shadduck, R. K., 1980, Macrophage activation by CSF: stimulation of LAF (IL-1) production. In Microbiology 1980. Ed. D. S. Schlesinger, American Society of Microbiology, Washington, D. C. (in press).

12. O'Brien, A. D., Rosenstreich, D. L., Scher, I., Campbell, G. H., MacDermott, R. P., and Formal, S. B., 1980, Genetic control of susceptibility to *Salmonella typhimurium* in mice: Role of the Lps gene. J. Immunol. 124: 20

13. O'Briend, A. D., Scher, I., and Formal, S. B., 1979, Effects of silica on the innate resistance of inbred mice to *Salmonella typhimurium* infection. Infection and Immunity 25: 513.

14. Peavy, D. L., Baugn, R. E., and Musher, D. L., 1978, Strain dependent cytotoxic effects of endotoxin for mouse peritoneal macrophages. Infection and Immunity, 21: 310.

15. Rosenstreich, D. L., The macrophage. In Cell Biology of Immunity and Information. Eds. J. Oppenheim, M. Potter and D. L. Rosenstreich, Elsevier-North Holland, New York (in press).

16. Rosenstreich, D. L., Gode, L. M., Wahl, L. M., Sandberg, A. L., and Mergenhagen, S. E., 1977, Analysis of the cellular defects of the endotoxin unresponsive C3H/HeJ mouse. In Microbiology 1977. Ed. D. S. Schlesinger, American Society of Microbiology, Washington, D. C., pp. 314.

17. Rosenstreich, D. L., Groves, M., O'Brien, A., and Taylor, B. A., 1979, Genetic control of natural resistance to infection in mice. In The molecular Basis of the Infective Process. Eds. H. Smith, J. J. Skehel and M. J. Turner, Berlin: Dahlem Konferenzen, Verlag Chemie GmbH. (in press).

18. Rosenstreich, D. L., Vogel, S. N., Jacques, A. R., Wahl, L. M., and J. J. Oppenheim, 1978, Macrophage sensitivity to endotoxin. Genetic control by a single codominant gene. J. Immunol. 121: 1664.

19. Ruco, L., and Meltzer, M. S., 1978, Defective tumoricidal capacity of macrophages from C3H/HeJ mice. J. Immunol. 120: 329.

20. Ruco, L. P., Meltzer, M. S., and Rosenstreich, D. L., 1978, Macrophage activation for tumor cytotoxicity: Control of macrophage tumoricidal capacity by the LPS gene. J. Immunol. 121: 543.

21. Ryan, J. L., Glode, L. M., and Rosenstreich, D. L., 1979, Lack of responsiveness of C3H/HeJ macrophages to lipopolysaccharide: The cellular basis of LPS stimulated metabolism. J. Immunol. 122: 932.

22. Tagliabue, A., McCoy, J. L., and Herberman, R., 1978, Refractoriness to migration inhibitory factor of macrophages of LPS nonresponder mouse strains. J. Immunol. 121: 1223.

23. Vogel, S. N., Marshall, S. T., and Rosenstreich, D. L., 1979, Analysis of the effects of lipopolysaccharide on macrophages: Differential phagocytic responses of C3H/HeN and C3H/HeJ macrophages in vitro. Infection and Immunity. 25: 328.

24. Vogel, S. N., and Rosenstreich, D. L., 1979, Defective Fc receptor-mediated phagocytosis in C3H/HeJ macrophages I. Correction by lymphokine-induced stimulation. J. Immunol. 123: 2842.

25. Vogel, S. N., Moore, R. N., Sipe, J. D., and Rosenstreich, D. L., 1980, BCG-induced enhancement of endotoxin sensitivity in C3H/HeJ mice. I. In vivo studies. J. Immunol. (in press).

26. Mergenhagen, S. E., 1979, Defective prostaglandon synthesis by C3H/HeJ mouse macrophages stimulated with endotoxin preparations. Infection and Immunity.23: 8.

27. Watson, J., Largen, M., and McAdam, K. P. W. J., 1978, Genetic control of endotoxic responses in mice. J. Exp. Med. 147: 39.

28. Weinberg, J. B., Chapman, H. A., and Hibbs, J. B., 1978, Characterization of the effects of endotoxin on macrophage tumor killing. J. Immunol. 121: 72.

29. Weiner, E., and Levanon, D., 1968, The *in vitro* interaction between bacterial lipopolysaccharide and differentiating monocytes. *Lab. Invest.* 19: 584.

30. Wilton, J. M. A., Rosenstreich, D. L., and Oppenheim, J. J., 1975, Requirement of bone-marrow derived lymphocytes for macrophage activation by bacterial lipopolysaccharide. *J. Immunol.* 114: 388.

IMMUNOMODULATING AND RELATED BIOLOGICAL ACTIVITIES OF BACTERIAL CELL WALLS AND THEIR COMPONENTS, ENZYMATICALLY PREPARED OR SYNTHESIZED

Shozo Kotani[1] *, Haruhiko Takada[1], Masachika Tsujimoto [1], Tomohiko Ogawa[1], Keijiro Kato [1], Takafumi Okunaga[2], Yoshitaka Ishihara[2], Akinori Kawasaki[3], Ichijiro Morisaki[4], Nagayuki Kono[4], Tsutomu Shimono[4], Tetsuo Shiba[5], Shoichi Kusumoto[5], Masaru Inage[5], Kazuhiro Harada[6], Toshiyuki Kitaura[6], Seisaburo Kano[7], Shinya Inai[8], Kazuyoshi Nagai[8], Misako Matsumoto[8], Takashi Kubo[9], Masahiko Kato[9], Zenichi Tada[9], Kanae Yokogawa[10], Shigeo Kawata[10], and Atsuo Inoue[11]

Department of Microbiology and Oral Microbiology, Osaka University Dental School, Kita-ku, Osaka, 530 Japan[1], The 2nd Department of Oral Surgery, Osaka University Dental School, Kita-ku, Osaka, 530 Japan[2], The 1st Department of Prosthetic Dentistry, Osaka University Dental School, Kita-ku, Osaka, 530 Japan[3], Department of Pedodontics, Osaka University Dental School, Kita-ku, Osaka, 530 Japan[4], Faculty of Science, Osaka University, Toyonaka, Osaka, 560 Japan[5], Laboratory of Microbiology, Osaka Prefectural Institute for Public Health, Higashinari-ku, Osaka, 537 Japan[6], Department of Pharmacology and Bacteriology, National Institute of Hygienic Sciences, Higashi-ku, Osaka, 541 Japan[7], Division of Immunology, The Center for Adult Disease, Higashi-ku, Osaka, 537 Japan[8], Kanonji Institute, The Research Foundation for Microbial Diseases, Osaka University, Kanonji, Kagawa, 768 Japan[9], Research and Development Division, Dainippon Pharmaceutical Co., Suita, Osaka, 564, Japan[10], New Product Planning Department, Daiichi Seyaku Co., Chuo-ku, Tokyo, 103 Japan[11]

BACKGROUND OF OUR STUDIES

In 1959, we isolated the cell walls of tubercle bacilli (BCG) which have long been known to have a strong immunoadjuvant activity, especially in the stimulation of cell-mediated immune responses, and elucidated the chemical and immunological properties of this cell wall fraction (32, 31). The most remarkable finding on the chemical composition of this subcellular fraction was that various lipids, especially ethanol-ether insoluble but chloroform-soluble lipids and bound lipids, which characterized tubercle bacilli were almost exclusively localized in their cell walls. It was also demonstrated that the cell walls were the most active fraction of subcellular components isolated from sonicated BCG cells, in inducing tuberculin hypersensitivity in guinea pigs and that the cell walls were involved in the development of an acquired cell-mediated resistance of mice to tuberculous infection.

In the succeeding studies (26, 27), the BCG cell walls from which free lipids were removed (cell wall skeleton) were partially solubilized by use of cell wall lytic enzymes (peptidoglycan hydrolases) different in the site of hydrolytic action, and an insoluble in water, but soluble in a mixture of chloroform-methanol-water (100:5:0.5, v/v) fraction was isolated. This fraction (bound wax D) consisted of the partially degraded peptidoglycan, mycolic acid and arabinogalactan, exhibited, like wax D isolated from human type tubercle bacilli, a marked potentiating effect on both the production of circulating antibody and the development of a delayed-type hypersensitivity against protein antigens (egg white albumin and egg white lysozyme) in guinea pigs (27). Further study (30) demonstrated that the immunopotentiating activity of the bound wax D described above was maintained even after a large proportion of arabinogalactan (and consequently mycoli acid, too) was removed by cold and hot trichloroacetic acid treatments, suggesting that a non-peptidoglycan moiety might not be directly involved in the manifestation of the immunoadjuvant activity of the bound wax D. Several years later, this finding was confirmed and extended by Azuma et al. (4). A bound lipid capable of immunopotentiation was isolated from delipidated and enzymatically digested cell walls of _Corynebacterium diphtheriae_ in a similar way (33).

In 1975, we reported that cell walls isolated from more than 20 gram-positive bacteria parasitic to mammals, and water-soluble monomers as well as polymers of peptidoglycan subunits prepared by treatment of _Staphylococcus aureus_, _Lactobacillus plantarum_ and others with cell wall lytic enzymes (endo-_N_-acetylmuramidases and endopeptidases, capable of hydrolysing glycan chains and cross bridges between the neighbouring stem peptide subunits of the peptidoglycan, respectively) showed an effect of potentiating both cellular and humoral immune responses in guinea pigs (34, 42, 43), indicating that the immunostimulating activity of bacterial cell walls was associated with the peptidoglycan moiety of the walls, and principles responsible for the activity could be made water-soluble. Further, Stewart-Tull in collaboration with us (69) revealed that a water-soluble, and strongly adjuvant-active glycolipid was obtained in large quantities from the culture supernatant fluid of Mycobacterium tuberculosis strain DT. It should be noted that similar results were reported by many workers from various laboratories and that Lederer, Chedid and their collaborators played a prominent role in this field, as reviewed by Chedid et al. (11).

We also found that the cell walls of bacteria which generally did not parasitize in mammals lacked the immunopotentiating effect (37), reflecting the fact that a chemical structure of the cell wall peptidoglycan of these bacteria differed from those of generally parasitic bacteria, as illustrated in Figs. 1 and 2 (61).

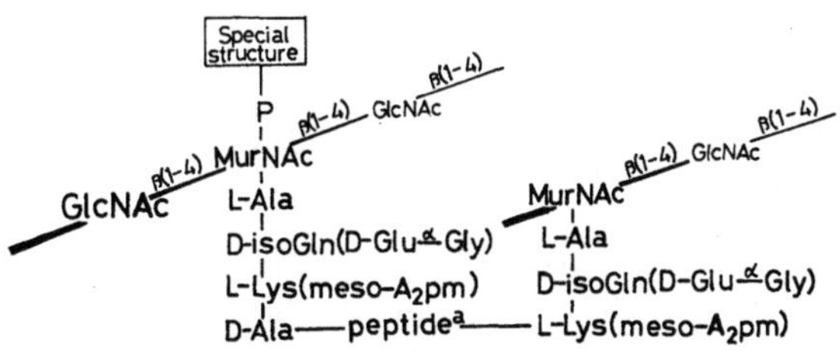

Fig. 1. A structure of a part of bacterial cell walls of group A peptidoglycan type. L-Lys type — S. aureus, Str. pyogenes etc., meso-A_2pm type — L. plantarum, Mycobacterium spp., Nocardia spp., C. diphtheriae etc, and D-Glu-Gly type — M. lysodeikticus, Arthrobacter spp. etc. [a]The neighboring stem peptides of [a]A_2pm type peptidoglycan were directly linked with each other without intervening peptides or amino acids.

Based on the achievement described above, since 1974 we have made investigations into N-acetylmuramyl peptides synthesized by mimicking the components of bacterial cell wall peptidoglycan and their structural analogues or derivatives. Thus we demonstrated, independently of Lederer and his colleagues (1, 13) that N-acetyl-muramyl-L-alanyl-D-isoglutamine (MDP) was the minimum, essential structure for the immunopotentiating activities of bacterial cell walls and the immunostimulating effect of muramyl peptides was highly dependent upon their chemical structures (29, 38, 39, 43, 77). These findings were confirmed by Azuma, Yamamura and their coworkers (5, 6), and French investigators (Chedid et al., 11).

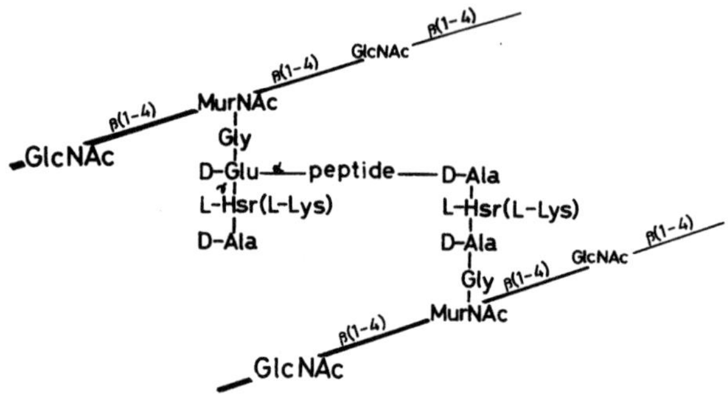

Fig. 2. A structure of a part of bacterial cell walls of group B peptidoglycan type. L-Hsr type — *C. poinsettiae*, *C. betae* etc., L-Lys type — *Microb. lacticum* etc.

GENERAL REMARKS ON CHEMICAL AND BIOLOGICAL PROPERTIES OF BACTERIAL CELL WALLS AND THEIR COMPONENTS

Bacterial cell walls are the bag-shaped, rigid structure of bacterial cell surface which protects the internal structures encased in a delicate cytoplasmic membrane from the outer environment. Cell walls are composed of two portions as shown in Table 1: One is a basal layer whose fundamental chemical structures are similar in various bacterial species, though there are considerable differences between group A and B peptidoglycan types (61), and the other is a special structure which has chemical and immunochemical features, characteristic to each of genera, species and even types or groups of the same species.

TABLE I

Chemical Composition of Bacterial Cell Walls

A. The basal layer (Peptidoglycan, Murein, Mucopeptide)
   Glycan chain: $(\text{-GlcNAc-}\beta\text{-1,4-MurNAc-})_n$
   Stem peptide: Tetra- and tri-peptide
   Cross link: Direct, amino acid, oligopeptides

B. Special components (Non-peptidoglycan moiety)
   Gram-positives: Teichoic acids, teichuronic acids, Polysaccharides, proteins
   Gram-negatives: Lipoprotein
   Outer membrane (phopholipid bilayer)
   Lipopolysaccharide (LPS)
   Acid-fast bacteria: Mycolic acid-arabinogalactan complex, polysaccharides, proteins

A peptidoglycan forming the basal layer of bacterial·species parasitic to mammalian, mostly belonging to the group A type, has the general molecular structure consisting of a variety of unique compounds, as illustrated in Fig. 1. They are muramic acid, 2,6-diaminopimelic acid, and unnatural D-isomers of amino acids such as D-glutamic acid and D-alanine. The remarkable feature of the peptidoglycan is the abundance of compounds having more than one functional group, such as 2,6-diaminopimelic acid, lysine, glutamic acid, and muramic acid. They are essential for the formation of extensive cross bridges between the neighboring stem tetra- or tripeptides and for linking the peptide portion with the glycan moiety consisting of alternative N-acetylmuramic acid and N-acetylglucosamine linked by β-1,4 glycosidic bound. The peptide linkage between the D-glutamic acid and (meso-_2,6-diaminopimelic acid or L-Lysine is an unnatural γ-type. Special structures usually connect with the peptidoglycan through phosphodiester linkages.

The peptidoglycan of group B type (Fig. 2), which is found in the cell walls of plant-pathogen corynebacteria and others, differs from the Group A type peptidoglycan in the respects that the cross bridges are formed between the α-carboxyl group of D-glutamic acid residue in one stem peptide subunit and the carboxyl group of D-alanine in the neighboring one through a dibasic amino acid or a oligopeptide containing dibasic amino acid, and that the amino acid adjacent to the muramic acid residue is generally not L-alanine, but glycine or L-serine L-homoserine or L-ornithine, in place of L-lysine or 2,6-diaminopimelic acid, often locates in the third position in stem peptide subunits.

The characteristic chemical and molecular structures described above of bacterial cell walls and their topographical feature, namely the localization in the outmost layers which makes the first contact with environmental factors, namely, various defense mechanisms of host in parasitic bacteria, allow cell walls whose peptidoglycan is group A type to exhibit a variety of immunological, pharmacological or pathological activities, as shown in Tables 2 and 3. This summary was constructed on the basis of reviews of Heymer (16) Chedid et al. (9, 10, 11, 12, 14), Parant (56), Krause (44) and Rotta (58), Yamamura (89) and on the results of studies of us and related groups (14, 15, 20-25, 31, 33-37, 39, 41-43, 50-53, 54, 55, 72-77, 79, 85) and others (8, 17, 18, 48, 57, 59, 60, 62, 63, 64, 67, 71, 82, 84).

Table 2 will show you principle biological activities of bacterial cell walls which have been detected in vivo assays: Modulation of antibody- and cell-mediated immune responses, stimulation of reticuloendothelial system, increase in non-specific natural resistance to microbial infections and tumor development, induction of experimental animal models of autoimmune diseases, pyrogenicity, induction of chromic granulomatous lesions in various tissues, increase in vascular permeability and so on.

TABLE II

Biological activities of bacterial cell walls and related compounds (in vivo)

1. Modulation (potentiation or suppression) of antibody- and cell-mediated immune responses.

2. Stimulation of reticuloendothelial system.

3. Increase of natural resistance to microbial infections and tumor development.

4. Induction of experimental, immunological diseases with or without external antigens (experimental allergic encephalomyelits, adjuvant arthritis[a] and others).

5. Pyrogenicity.

6. Epitheoloid granuloma formation[b].

7. Induction of acute inflammatory reactions and chronic granulomatous lesions in various tissues (relapsing multi-nodular lesions in the skin).

8. Increase in vascular permeability.

9. Immunogenicity[c].

a
K. Kushima, S. Nagao, and A. Tanaka, 9th Annu. Meet. Jpn. Soc. Immunol., 1979, BR 20, p. 378.

O. Kohashi, J. Kuwata, A. Ozawa, and S. Kotani, 9th Annu. Meet. Jpn. Soc. Immunol., 1979, BR 22, p. 380.

b
A. Tanaka, S. Nagao, K. Emori, K. Imai, S. Kotani, T. Shiba, O. Kohashi, and Y. Iwata, 9th Annu. Meet. Jpn. Soc. Immunol., 1979, 134, p. 267.

c
K. Maeda, K. Koga, S. Onoue, S. Kotani, and A. Sumiyoshi, Microbiol. Immunol., in press.

Bacterial cell walls and related compounds, on the other hand, can stimulate or activate _in vitro_ a variety of cells involved in natural and acquired defense functions, such as macrophages, B- and T-lymphocytes, and granulocytes. Expression of the modulation is versatile as shown in Table 3. Other biological activities of

TABLE III

Biological activities of bacterial cell walls and related compounds (in vitro)

1. Modulation of cells involved in natural and acquired immunity.

    1) Macrophages: Enhancement of adherence and spreading on solid surface[a], migration inhibition, increase of glucosamine and 2-deoxy-D-glucose, increase in superoxide[b] and glucose oxidase levels, enhancement of phagocytosis, induction of cytotoxicity on fibroblast and other cells, production of collagenase.

    2) B lymphocytes: Mitogenesis, polyclonal B cell activation[c].

    3) T lymphocytes: Mitogenesis, enhancement of helper function, induction of cytotoxic effector cells against syngeneic tumor cells, stimulation of mixed lymphocyte reaction, induction of IgE class specific suppressor T cells[d].

    4) Neutrophile leukocytes: Stimulation of phagocytosis or chemotaxis, production of endogenous pyrogen.

    5) Eosinophile leukocytes: Release of blocking factors or mediators[e].

    6) Production of lymphokines and monokines.

2. Activation of complement system through alternative and classical pathways.

3. Lysis of thrombocytes and liberation of serotonin.

4. Gelation of amoebocyte lysate of horse-shoe crab (positive Limulus reaction).

5. Contraction (or relaxation) of a strip of intestine.

6. Reactivity with antibodies (and sensitized T lymphocytes)

a
T. Tanaka, S. Nagao, K. Imai, and R. Mori, 8th Annu. Meet. Jpn. Soc. Immunol., 1978, 111, p. 219.

S. Nagao, K. Imai, M. Tomioka, A. Tanaka, T. Shiba, and S. Kotani, 9th Annu. Meet. Jpn. Soc. Immunol., 1979, 88, p. 175.

a,b
M. J. Pabst, and R. B. Johnston, personal communication.

c
T. Saito-Taki, M. J. Tanabe, H. Mochizuki, T. Matsumoto, M.

Table III (continued)

Nakano, H. Takada, M. Tsujimoto, S. Kotani, S. Kusumoto, T. Shiba, S. Kawata, and K. Yokogawa, Microbiol. Immunol., in press.

[d] T. Kishimoto, Y. Watanabe, Y. Hirai, and Y. Yamamura, 13th Joint Meet. Tuberc. Panel, U. S.-Japan Co-operative Med. Sci. Prog., 1978, p. 231.

[e] E. J. Goetzl, personal communication.

the cell walls detected by in vitro assay are as follows: Activation of complement system through pathways not always due to antigen-antibody reactions, liberation of serotonin in blood platelets, contraction or relaxation of a strip of intestine, gelation of an amoebocyte lysate of horse-shoe crab and others.

The cell walls whose peptidoglycan is group B type, on the other hand, are shown to lack a considerable part of the biological activities held by the walls with group A type peptidoglycan, such as immunopotentiating activities in vivo, a contractive effect on a strip of ileum and so on.

It is worth noting here that though MDP seems to be the essential structure responsible for the most part of biological activities summarized in Table 2 and 3, MDP often needs some additional structures or factors which act to intensify or augment the potential activities of MDP, because cell walls themselves and polymers of peptidoglycan subunits are at least seemingly devoid of some of the biological activities held by cell walls themselves (vide infra).

Hereafter, we will present recent, unpublished experimental results on the biological activities of cell walls and their components, obtained either by use of cell wall lytic enzymes or synthetic means.

TEST SPECIMEN OF CELL WALLS AND RELATED COMPOUNDS

Cell Wall Specimens

These were prepared as described in previous papers.

Water-soluble Peptidoglycan Fragments

Two specimens (SEPS and SEPS-M) which differed in the degree of polymerization of peptidoglycan subunits were prepared by enzymatic digestion of Staphylococcus epidermidis (ATCC 155) cell wall peptidoglycan: SEPS was isolated by gel filtration of a SALE (S. aureus lytic enzyme, S. Kawata and K. Yokogawa, unpublished) digest of the peptidoglycan as described in a previous paper (52). SEPS-M, on the other hand, was prepared by degradation of SEPS with the M-1 enzyme (endo-N-cethlmuramidase, 90) and by gel filtration of the M-1 digest on columns of Sephadex G50 and G25 connected in series. Chemical analyses revealed that SEPS and SEPS-M were a polymer (average glycan chain length was 10-11 disaccharide unit) and a monomer (one disaccharide unit), respectively (Fig. 3). Details of the preparation method and analytical data will be published elsewhere.

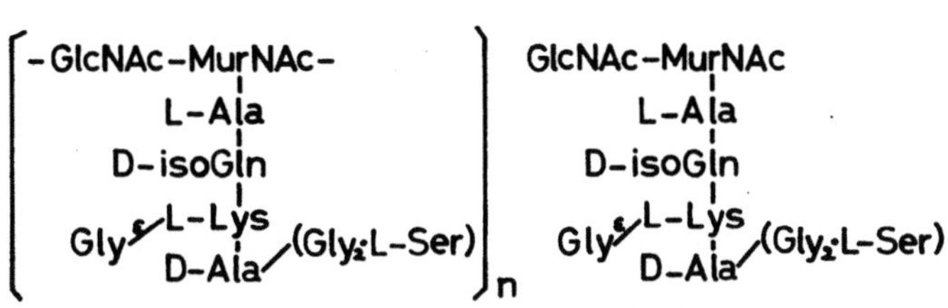

SEPS SEPS-M

Fig. 3. Possible structures of a polymer (SEPS) and a monomer (EPS-M) of the peptidoglycan subunits isolated from S. epidermidis (ATCC 155) cell walls.

6-O-acyl-muramylpeptides

Chemical structures and abbreviations of 6-O-acyl-derivatives of muramyl dipeptides used in the following studies shown in Table 4.

TABLE IV

Chemical structure of test synthetic 6-O-acyl-MDPs

6-O-Acyl derivatives of muramyldipeptides	Abbreviation
$CH_3(CH_2)_{16}CO$-MurNAc-L-Ala-D-isoGln	[L18]-MDP
$CH_3(CH_2)_{16}CO$-MurNAc-L-Ala-L-isoGln	[L18]-MDP(L-isoGln)
$CH_3(CH_2)_{22}CO$-MurNAc-L-Ala-D-isoGln	[L24]-MDP
$CH_3(CH_2)_{28}CO$-MurNAc-L-Ala-D-isoGln	[L30]-MDP
$CH_3(CH_2)_{13}$ \\ CHCO-MurNAc-L-Ala-D-isoGln $CH_3(CH_2)_{13}$ /	[B30]-MDP
$CH_3(CH_2)_{13}$ \\ CHCO-MurNAc-L-Ala-D-isoAsn $CH_3(CH_2)_{13}$ /	[B30]-MDP(D-isoAsn)
$CH_3(CH_2)_{14}CH(OH)$ \\ CHCO-MurNAc-L-Ala-D-isoGln $CH_3(CH_2)_{13}$ /	[BH32]-MDP
$CH_3(CH_2)_{21}$ \\ CHCO-MurNAc-L-Ala-D-isoGln $CH_3(CH_2)_{21}$ /	[B46]-MDP
$CH_3(CH_2)_{22}CH(OH)$ \\ CHCO-MurNAc-L-Ser-D-isoGln $CH_3(CH_2)_{21}$ /	[BH48]-MDP
$CH_3(CH_2)_{22}CH(OH)$ \\ CHCO-MurNAc-L-Ser-D-isoGln $CH_3(CH_2)_{21}$ /	[BH48]-MDP(L-Ser)
$CH_3(CH_2)_{22}CH(OH)$ \\ CHCO-MurNAc-L-Ala-L-isoGln $CH_3(CH_2)_{21}$ /	[BH48]-MDP(L-isoGln)
$CH_3(CH_2)_{22}CH(OH)$ \\ CHCO-MurNAc-L-Ala-D-isoAsn $CH_3(CH_2)_{21}$ /	[BH48]-MDP(D-isoAsn)

These test specimens were synthesized as follows: N-acetylmuramyl-L-alanyl-D-isoglutamine (MurNAc-L-Ala-D-isoGln, MDP) and its L-isoglutamine analogue were prepared as described previously (47). Many kinds of 6-O-acyl-MurNAc-L-Ala-D-isoGln (acyl-MDP) with different acyl groups were obtained via either one of the two synthetic routes already reported (2, 4, 45, 46). Thus, syntheses of stearoyl and tetracosanoyl MDP ([L18]- and [L24]-MDP) were performed by selective acylation of the 6-hydroxyl group in 1-α-O-benzyl-MDP benzyl ester followed by hydrogenolytic deprotection. On the other hand, acyl groups with more than 30 carbon atoms were introduced by means of an exchange reaction of 6-O-tosyl group in 1-α-O-benzyl-6-O-tosyl-N-acetylmuramic acid diphenylmethyl ester with potassium salts of the corresponding fatty acids. Following abbreviations were used for these acyl groups: [L30] for triacontanoyl, [B46] for 2-tetradecylhexadecanoyl, [BH32] for 3-hydroxy-2-tetradecyloctadecanoyl, [46] for 2-docosyltetracosanoyl, and [BH48] for 3-hydroxy-2-docosylhexacosanoyl. After selective removal of diphenylmethyl ester in the resulting 6-O-acyl muramic acid derivatives, coupling of the products with the dipeptide benzyl ester followed by hydrogenolysis afforded the acyl-MDPs. [BH48]-MurNAc-L-Ser-D-isoGln and [BH48]-MurNAc-L-Ala-D-isoGln-L-Lys-D-Ala were synthesized in a similar way to that for the corresponding [BH48]-MDP with the following modification. The benzyl glycoside group and the diphenylmethyl ester group were simultaneously removed prior to the introduction of the peptide moiety by catalytic hydrogenolysis. In this manner the final hydrogenolytic deprotection proceeded more rapdily than in the former method to give the acyl MDP analogues (M. Inage, S. Kusumoto, and T. Shiba, unpublished). Analogues of 6-O-acyl-MDP whose D-isoglutamine residue was replaced with L-isoglutamine or D-isoasparagine and an analogue whose L-alanine residue adjacent to muramic acid was substituted with L-serine were also synthesized in the similar manner.

The all synthetic compounds gave satisfactory elemental analyses and showed single spots on thin layer chromatography.

BIOLOGICAL ACTIVITIES DETECTED IN VIVO ASSAY

Immunopotentiating activities

Though MDP is the minimum effective structure responsible for the immunopotentiating activities of bacterial cell walls to stimulate cell-mediated as well as antibody-mediated immune responses, this water-soluble, small synthetic molecule requires the administration to subjects to be immunized with an incomplete Freund type water-in-mineral oil emulsion, to exert its full immunopotentiating activities, especially in effective stimulation of cell-mediated immuner responses.

However, MDP administered as a water-in-mineral oil emulsion causes severe irritative reactions in an injection site and the regional lymph nodes. Therefore, we have attempted to overcome this difficulty by addition of various acyl groups (linear, α-branched or α-branched and β-hydroxylated acyl groups of various chain length) at the primary hydroxyl group at C-6 position of the muramic acid residue of MDP, and by modifying physical as well as biological properties of the molecule. These 6-O-acyl-MDPs were administered in a Ribi-type squalene-in-phosphate buffered saline (PBS) emulsion, liposomes consisting of synthetic lecithin and cholesterol, and plain PBS as a vehicle. These vehicles were prepared as described previously (28,34) except that Squalene was used in place of Drakeol.

We sensitized groups of five, female albino guinea pigs by intra-footpad injection of one or two mg of ovalbumin as an antigen with indicated amounts of test adjuvants in the above mentioned vehicles (Bovine serum albumin and Keyhole limpet hemocyanin gave essentially the same results as ovalbumin as far as examined). Induction of a delayed-type hypersensitivity as a representative of the cell-mediated immunity was evaluated in terms of positive corneal reaction on the second and third week and of delayed skin reaction on the fourth week after the sensitization. Stimulation of antibody production was estimated by determination of anti-ovalbumin precipitating antibody levels in serum specimens drawn three or four days after the skin reaction (28, 34).

Fig. 4 shows the result of a control experiment where PBS-in-Drakeol emulsion (PBS/Drakeol) was used as a vehicle for the adminostration of MDP. Twenty-two nmoles (11 μg) of MDP definitely stimulated both cell- and antibody-mediated immune responses to ovalbumin in guinea pigs. However, the swelling of both the injected foot pad and regional lymph nodes was intense, even at the minimum effective dose.

Then, we investigated the combinations of 6-O-acyl-MDPs and vehicles which gave a satisfactory outcome in consideration of both the potencies of immunostimulating activity (determined in terms of the minimum effective dose) and the extent of adverse effects.

The immunopotentiating effect of [B30]-MDP administered as a Squalene-in-PBS emulsion (Squalene/PBS) are shown in Fig. 5. As little as 2.5 nmoles (2.3 μg) of [B30]-MDP exhibited a definite stimulating effect on induction of a delayed type hypersensitivity and anti-ovalbumin precipitin production, with local injurious effects which are obviously less than those caused by MDP derivative in PBS/Drakeol.

Fig. 6 shows that [BH48]-MDP and its L-serine analogue which were emulsified in Squalene/PBS were strongly active in stimulation of both cell- and antibody-mediated immune responses. The minimum effective doses of [BH48]-MDP and its L-serine analogue were 7.5 nmoles (9.0 μg) and 2.5 nmoles (3.0 μg), respectively. As a whole

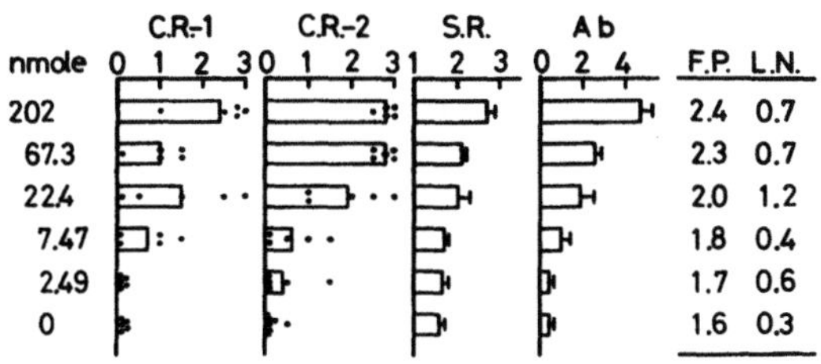

Fig. 4. Immunopotentiating activity of MDP in a phosphate buffered saline-in-Drakeol 6VR emulsion against ovalbumin. C.R.-1 and C.R.-2 – Corneal reaction (48 h reading) at the 2nd and 3rd week after the sensitization, respectively, S.R. - skin reaction (induration, 48 h reading), Ab - μg antibody nitrogen/ml serum, F.P. - footpad swelling (a ratio of the cross section of an injected footpad/that of the control foot pad), L.N. - enlargement of draining lymph nodes (a mean score; a soybean size 2, an adzuki bean size 1, and a rice grain size 0.5). the corneal reaction of an individual animal, a mean of test and control groups, and 1+ standard error. 202 nmoles of MDP are equivalent to 100 μg.

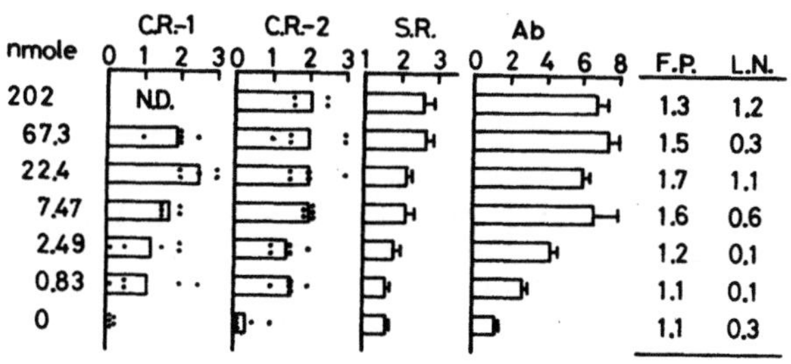

Fig. 5. Immunopotentiating activity of [B30]-MDP in a Squalene-in-phosphate buffered saline emulsion against ovalbumin. 202 nmoles of [B30]-MDP are equivalent to 188 μg. Other legends as in Fig. 4.

the L-serine type seemed to be somewhat more potent than the L-alanine type. Local injurious effects caused by these two combinations were slight.

The assay result with [B30]-MDP suspended in PBS indicate that this 6-O-acyl derivative of MDP exerts a strong immunopotentiating activity without help of oils (Fig. 7). About 7.5 nmoles (7 μg) of

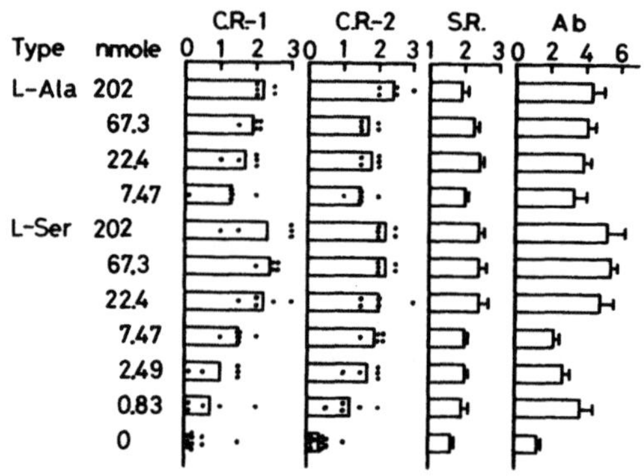

Type	nmole	F.P.	L.N.
L-Ala	202	1.3	0.9
	67.3	1.4	0.5
	22.4	1.3	0.7
	7.47	1.3	0.6
L-Ser	202	1.5	0.8
	67.3	1.3	1.1
	22.4	1.3	0.6
	7.47	1.2	0.6
	2.49	1.4	0.5
	0.83	1.3	0.4
	0	1.1	0.3

Fig. 6. Immunopotentiating activity of [BH48]-MDP in a Squalene-in-phosphate buffered saline emulsion against ovalbumin. 202 nmoles of [BH48]-MDP are equivalent to 243 μg. L-Ala type - [BH48]-MurNAc-L-Ala-D-isoGln, and L-Ser type - [BH48]-MurNAc-L-Ser-D-isoGln. Other legends as in Fig. 4.

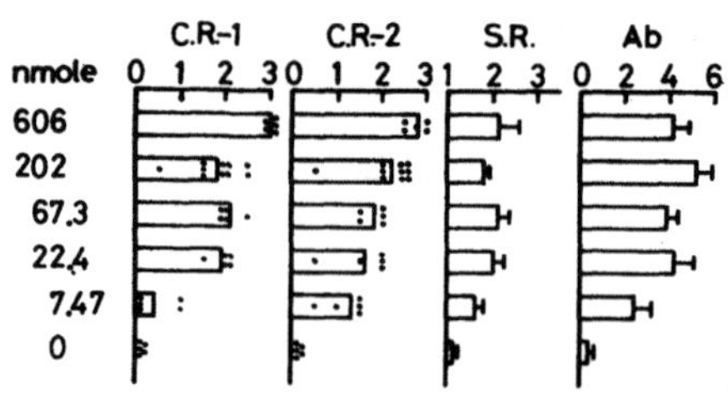

nmole	F.P.	L.N.
606	2.0	2.6
202	1.4	2.6
67.3	1.1	1.9
22.4	1.2	0.8
7.47	1.2	0.4
0	1.0	0

Fig. 7. Immunopotentiating activity of [B30]-MDP suspended in phosphate buffered saline against ovalbumin. Legends as in Fig. 4.

the specimen were found to be definitely active with only slight local adverse reactions. It should be emphasized that [B30]-MDP was the sole one among acyl derivatives of muramyl peptides examined in the present study which was proved to be immunostimulating as a PBS suspension or solution.

Usefulness of liposomes as a vehicle for the manifestation of the immunopotentiating activity of [L18]-MDP was previously reported (28). Three kinds of liposomes different in the composition were examined on their supporting effect on the immunoadjuvancy of [L18]-MDP by reference to the report of Masek et al. (48). All liposomes served as a vehicle which allowed [L18]-MDP to exert its immunopotentiating activity with the minimum local reactions (Fig. 8). Similar results were obtained with [B20]- and [BH48]-MDPs. However, the extent of immunopotentiation seemed to be lower than those achieved by combinations of [B30]-MDP with Squalene/PBS or PBS and [BH48]-MDP with Squalene/PBS.

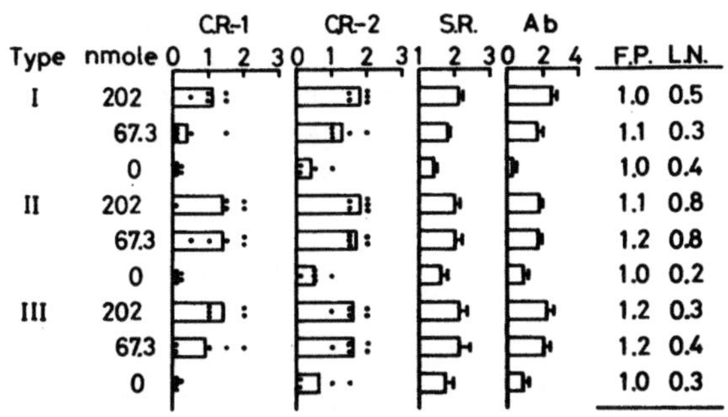

Fig 8. Immunopotentiating activity of [L18]-MDP associated with liposomes against ovalbumin. I - DL-α-phosphatidy choline (lecithin) : cholesterol = 1 : 1, II - lecithin : cholesterol = 4 : 1, and III - lecithin : cholesterol : stearylamine = 1.3 : 1 : 1 (w/w). The amount of cholesterol per injection dose was adjusted to be 1 nmole (387 μg). 202 nmoles of [L18]-MDP are equivalent to 154 μg.

Pyrogenicity

The pyrogenicity of 6-O-acyl-muramyl dipeptides was examined by injection via intravenous and intracisternal routes in rabbits (Fig. 9 and 10).

As previously reported (41), MDP, but neither its L-isoglutamine nor D-isoasparagine analogue, caused a definite febrile response in

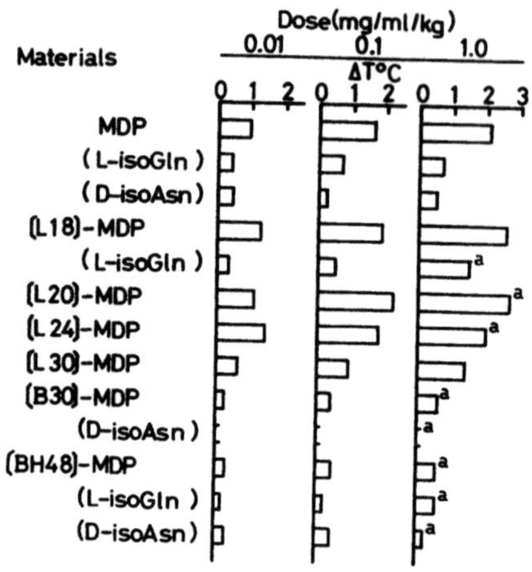

Fig. 9. Pyrogenicity of MDP, 6-O-acyl-MDPs and their analogues in rabbits by intravenous injection. Japanese domestic, male rabbits weighing 2 to 2.5 kg (2 to 6 animals per group) were intravenously injected with indicated doses of a test specimen (0.01, 0.1 and 1 mg/ml/kg). The rectal temperature was recorded continuously with an electronic recorder. The maximum temperature rise for the observation period for 6 h in each rabbit was recorded and averaged for each group. [a]Only one rabbit was submitted to the test because of limited amounts of test material.

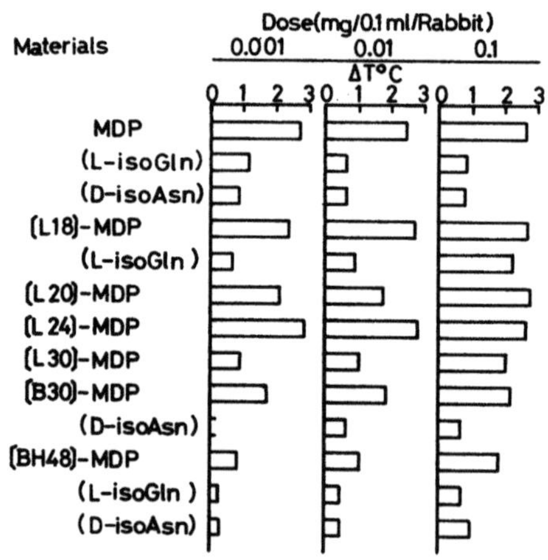

Fig. 10. Pyrogenicity of MDP, 6-O-acyl-MDPs and their analogues in rabbits by intracisternal injection. Legends are as in Fig. 9 except that 0.001, 0.01 and 0.1 mg (0.1 ml/animal) of a test specimen were injected.

rabbits by intravenous injection. Among test 6-O-acyl-muramyl dipeptides, [L18]-, [L20]- and [L24]-MDPs were found to be definitely pyrogenic, but MDP derivatives which had α-branched acyl groups of greater than thirty carbon atoms, namely [B30]- and [BH48]-MDPs, did not cause significant febrile response. [L30]-MDP whose acyl group had thirty carbon atoms, but was linear, on the other hand, seemed to have slight, but definite pyrogenicity. In this connection, an L-isoglutamine analogue of [L18]-MDP was found to be only weakly pyrogenic.

An interesting finding was that [B30]- and [BH48]-MDPs, which were not pyrogenic by intravenous injection caused a definite febrile response by intracisternal injection, while their D-isoasparagine or L-isoglutamine analogue did not cause significant increase in body temperature. These findings suggest the possibility that blood-brain barrier may participate in non-pyrogenicity of [B30]- and [BH 48]-MDPs.

Arthritogenicity

The ability to induce adjuvant arthritis of [L18]-MDP in liposomes, [B30]-MDP in PBS and [BH48]-MDP in Squalene/PBS were examined with Levis rats, as described previously (23, 25). None of the above cominations (a test dose of 6-O-acyl-MDPs as adjusted to be 67 nmoles per rat) induced any detectable arthritis.

Summary

Summary of the findings described in the foregoing sections is presented in Table 5. Taking together the minimum effective dose, the extent of resulting immunopotentiation and undesirable adverse effects into consideration, we can tentatively conclude that [B30]-MDP with Squalene-in-PBS emulsion or PBS, and [BH48]-MDP with Squalene-in PBS are the combinations of choice.

It may be added here that Azuma, Yamamura and their coworkers, along the similar line of approach, reported a number of interesting studies on the antitumor and adjuvant activities of 6-O-mycolyl-MDPs which were semi-synthesized by coupling mycolic acids isolated from mycobacteria, nocardia and others with MDP (7, 80, 81, 87, 88, Kishimoto, Y. Watanabe, Y. Hirai, and Y. Yamamura, Abst. 13th Joint Meet. Tuberc. Panel, U.S.-Japan Med. Sci. Prog., 1978, p. 231, I. Saiki, M. Uemiya, M. Yamawaki, Y. Tanino, S. Kobayashi, T. Fukuda, Y. Yamamura, and I. Azuma, Abst. 9th Annu. Meet. Jpn. Soc. Immunol., 166, 331).

Potentiation of Influenza Split Virus Vaccine

Siddiqui in a collaborative study with us recently reported that owl monkeys were effectively immunized against a human malaria

TABLE V

Summary of the Search for Combinations of Test Adjuvants and Vehicles which Exhibit Good Immunopotentiating Effects with Endurable Adverse Reactions

Test Adjuvant	Vehicle	Minimum effective dose μg(nmole)	Local Injurious Effects: Foot-pad	Local Injurious Effects: Lymph-node	Febrile response ΔT°C	Adjuvant arthritis in Lewis Rats dose : 67 nmole
MDP	PBS/Drakeol	11(22)	2.0	1.2		
	Squalene/PBS	>100(202)	1.1	0.2		
	Liposome	>131(265)	1.1	0		
	PBS	>260(525)				
[L18]-MDP	Liposome	51(67)	1.1	0.3	1.3(i.v.)[a] 1.2(s.c.)[b]	No induction
[B30]-MDP	Squalene/PBS	2.3(2.5)	1.2	0.1		
	Liposome	63(67)	1.3	0.7		
	PBS	7.0(7.5)	1.2	0.4	0.6(i.v.)[a]	No induction
[BH48]-MDP	Squalene/PBS	9(7.5)	1.3	0.6	0.5(i.v.)[a] 0.6(s.c.)[b]	No induction
	Liposome	27(22)	1.2	0.2		
	PBS	>630(528)				
[BH48]-MDP (L-ser)	Squalene/PBS	3(2.5)	1.4	0.5		

[a] Dose : 40 μg/200 μl/kg [b] Dose : 100μg/500 μl/kg

parasite, using [L18]-MDP in liposomes as an adjuvant (66). As another example of application of the above findings to potentiation of the protective activity of vaccines, a part of our recent study on potentiation of influenza split virus vaccine by synthetic muramyl peptides will be described. Groups of five, female albino guinea pigs were vaccinated by subcutaneous injection of influenza split virus vaccine for human use (a bivalent vaccine [Biken] containing A/Kumamoto/22/76 [H3N2] and B/Kanagawa/3/76) with appropriate adjuvants, and they received a booster injection of the vaccine alone about four weeks later. At five to ten days intervals, serum specimens were obtained and treated with trypsin and potassium periodate to remove non-specific inhibitors. The hemagglutination-inhibiting and virus-neutralizing antibodies of treated serum specimens were determined by the conventional method and by the plaque assay method using chick embryo (78) respectively.

Fig. 11 illustrates that [B30]-MDP, when administered as a Squalene/PBS emulsion or a PBS suspension with the vaccine, significantly enhance the hemagglutination-inhibiting antibody production to B/Kanagawa/3/76 virus (50 CCA per animal) contained in the test bivalent vaccine, especially in the primary immune response. It is noteworthy that the potentiating effect of [B30]-MDP in either vehicle seems to be apparently better than that of MDP as a PBS/

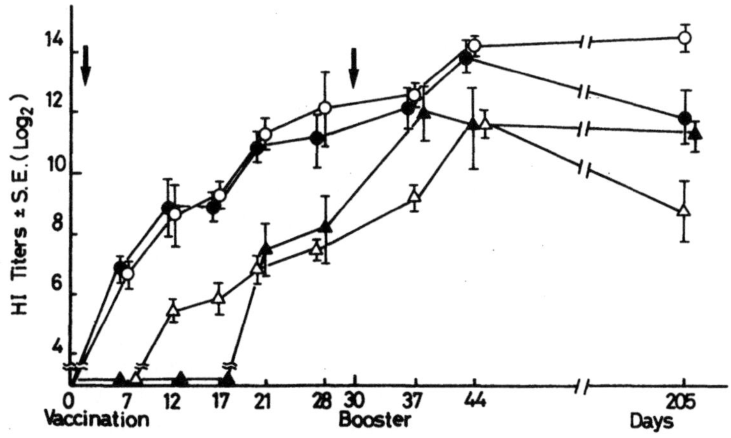

Fig. 11. Hemagglutination inhibiting antibody production of guinea pigs immunized by influenza split virus vaccine ([Biken], containing A/Kumamoto/22/76 (H3N2) 66.7 CCA and B/Kanagawa/3/76 50 CCA) with or without 6-O-acyl-MDPs and MDP in various vehicles. ○ [B30]-MDP 63 μg - Squalene/PBS, ● [B30]-MDP 63 μg - PBS, △ MDP 33 μg - PBS/Drakeol 6VR, and ▲ none. The antibody titers against B/Kanagawa/3/76 were plotted.

Drakeol emulsion. Though data are not shown, similar results were obtained on the assay with A/Kumamoto/22/76 virus (66.7 CCA per animal) contained in the test vaccine.

Determination of virus-neutralizing antibody also demonstrated the efficacy of [B30]-MDP in Squalene/PBS or PBS as an immunoadjuvant. The results with A/Kumamoto/22/76 virus are shown in Fig. 12. Here too [B30]-MDP in either vehicle gave better production of the neutralizing antibody than MDP in PBS/Drakeol. Essentially the same results were obtained with B/Kanagawa/3/76 virus.

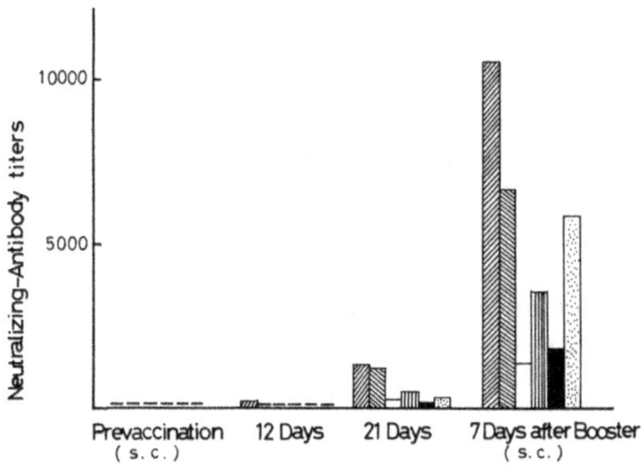

Fig. 12. Neutralizing antibody production of guinea pigs immunized by influenza split virus vaccine ([Biken], containing A/Kumamoto/22/76 (N3N2) 66.7 CCA and B/Kanagawa/3/76 50 CCA) with or without 6-O-acyl-MDPs and MDP in various vehicles. ▨ [B30]-MDP 63 μg - Squalene/PBS, ▧ [B30]-MDP 63 μg - PBS, ▥ [L18]-MDP 51 μg - liposome (I in Fig. 8), ▦ MDP 33 μg - PBS/Drakeol 6VR, and ■ , □ none. The antibody titers againstKumamoto/22/76 were shown.

Potentiation of the immune response mice and hamsters to influenza virus subunit vaccine by MDP as a saline solution was recently reported (3, 83). It may be pointed out that despite the use of the partially purified split virus vaccine which may retain "intrinsic" adjuvant in our study, [B30]-MDP in Squalene/PBS or in PBS resulted in better potentiation of the antibody responses than MDP in PBS (data not shown).

BIOLOGICAL ACTIVITIES ASSAYED IN VITRO

Macrophages, and B- and T-lymphocytes

Our studies on stimulation of these immunocompetent cells by bacterial cell walls, their enzymatic digests and synthetic muramyl dipeptides, in terms of increased uptake of [^{14}C]-glucosamine and [^{3}H]-thymidine, were recently published (73, 74), so this subject is not repeated here.

Polymorphonuclear Leukocytes

An assay has been made on stimulating effect of bacterial cell walls, their fragments and synthetic muramyl peptides on surface phagocytosis of polymorphonuclear leukocytes which were obtained from a guinea pig peritoneal cavity irritated by sterile thioglycolate medium. Stimulation of the phagocytosis was determined in terms of increased uptake of [^{3}H]-labelled, heat-killed *Streptococcus pyogenes* (highly virulent strain Sv, type 2) by the polymorphonuclear leukocytes which were incubated with test specimens at 37°C for 2 h, by reference to the method of Midtvedt et al. (49, 78).

Though the study is in a preliminary stage, it was shown that cell walls of *Micrococcus lysodeikticus* (NCTC 2665), *L. Plantarum* (ATCC 8014), *Nocardia corynebacteriodes* (ATCC 14898) and others (data not shown), SEPS from S. epidermidis and [L18]-MDP (Fig. 13) significantly stimulated the polymorphonuclear leukocytes to uptake more of heat-killed cells of *S. pyogenes* than nonstimulated control leukocytes. However, the stimulative activity of MDP itself in this respect was found to be weak, if any (data are not shown).

Complement activation

Table 6 summarizes the assay results on activation of human complement system by cell walls of about 30 gram-positive bacterial species and treponema (S. Inai, M. Matsumoto, K. Nagaki, Y. Watanabe, H. Yamagami, K. Kato, and S. Kotani Abst. 6th Annu. Meet. Jpn. Soc. Immunol., 1976, No. 183, p. 360). The method of determination of complement components and others were described in a previous report (19), and a blocking effect of the classical pathway was examined by addition of EGTA (10 mM) and $MgCl_2$ (3-5 mM) to a test complement serum. Test bacterial cell wall specimens, irrespective of their peptidoglycan type or their immunopotentiating activity, were proved to activate human complement system through the alternative pathway, so far as the EGTA method was adopted, though the activating potency of cell walls of group B peptidoglycan type except *C. insidiosum*, *Arthrobacter* sp. and *Treponema pallidum* all of which lacked the immunoadjuvancy seemed to be weak. A considerable part of test cell walls also consumed human complement by the classical pathway in addition to the alternative one.

Study was then made on whether water-soluble cell wall components prepared by use of either enzymes or chemical means could activate human complement system. Fig. 14 clearly indicates that SEPS (a

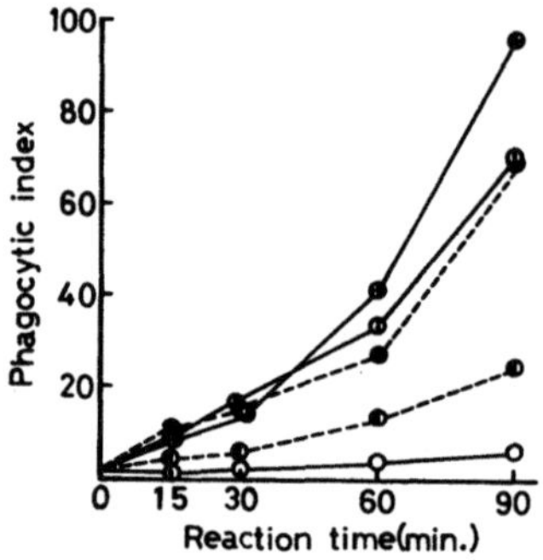

Fig. 13. Stimulation of surface phagocytosis of heat-killed, [^{3}H]-labelled Str. pyogenes by guinea pig peritoneal polymorphonuclear leukocytes by SEPS and [L18]-MDP. ⊕ SEPS 100 μg, ○ SEPS 33 μg, ● [L18]-MDP 154 μg, ◐ [L18]-MDP 51 μg, and ⊖ , 0 μg/ml of the preincubation mixture. Phagocytic index - cpm/ μg protein (an index of leukocyte number) at given time / cpm/ μg protein at 0 time. Reaction time indicates the incubation period after addition of labelled Str. pyogenes.

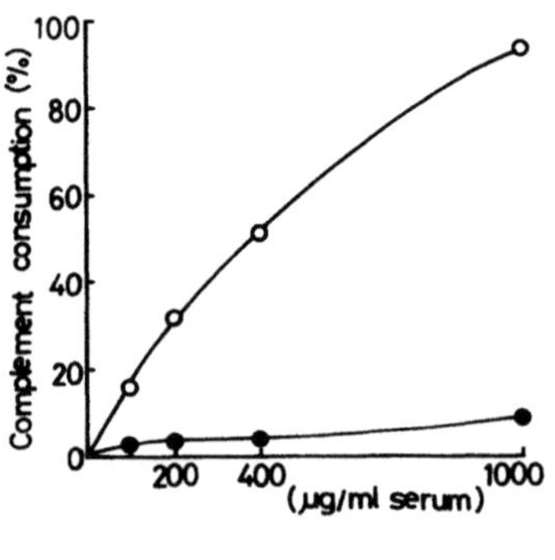

Fig. 14. Activation of human complement system by SEPS and SEPS-M. ○ SEPS, and ● SEPS-M.

polymer of peptidoglycan subunits of S. epidermidis) but not SEPS-M (a monomer), activated the complement system in fresh, pooled human serum. Analyses of complement component consumption profiles and comparison of the consumption in the presence and absence of EGTA (Fig. 15) showed that the complement activation by SEPS mainly went through the alternative pathway.

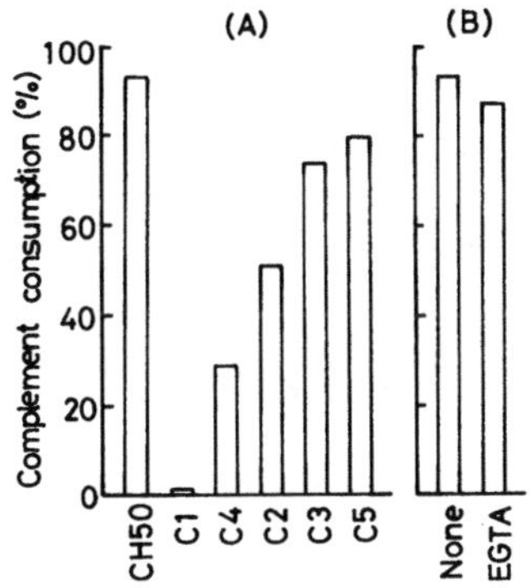

Fig. 15. Complement component consumption profile [A] and the blocking effect EGTA [B] in the complement activation by SEPS. Dose - 1 mg/ml serum.

The assay results with synthetic 6-O-acyl-muramylpeptides are presented in Fig. 16. We can see that [B30]-MDP and [BH48]-MurNAc-L-Ala-D-isoGln-L-Lys-D-Ala cause a definite activation of human complement system, but MDP, [L18]- and [L30]-MDPs do not. An unexpected finding was that a D-isoasparagine analogue of [B30]-MDP which has been shown to be inactive in the immunopotentiation and other biological activities so far as examined, showed a definite complement activation activity comparable to that of [B30]-MDP itself. Fig. 17 indicates that [B30]-MDP, unlike SEPS, activates human complement system by the classical pathway. The D-isoasparagine analogue of [B30]-MDP gave essentially the same results. Further study is needed, but the above finding suggest that [B30]-muramyl dipeptides, either D-isoglutamine or D-isoasparagine type, may activate human complement by a mechanism different from that by antigen-antibody complexes, because the possibility that human serum contains the antibody against [B30]-muramyl dipeptides seems to be small.

[B48]-MurNAc-L-Ala-D-isoGln-L-Lys-D-Ala, on the other hand, was shown to activate human complement, though only partially, mainly by the alternative pathway (Fig. 18).

TABLE VI

Activation of Complement System in Fresh, Pooled Human Serum by Bacterial Cell Walls

Species (strain)	Dose (mg/ml serum)	CH50	C1	C4	C2	C3	C5	EGTA -	EGTA +
M. lysodeikticus (NCTC 2665)[a]	2	94	0	7	0	95	99	90	94
M. lysodeikticus (IFO 3333)[a]	2	94	0	22	17	89	97		
S. epidermidis (ATCC 155) CW[a]	1	45	0	0	26	49	50	97	97 [2 mg/ml][d]
" " " " PG	0.4	95	30	48	73	83	62		
S. aureus (FDA 209P)	0.2	95	53	67	90	91	95	94	99
G. tetragena (ATCC 15292)	2	95	16	26	53	70	96		
Sar. lutea (IFO 3232)	2	94	0	19	33	78	94		
Str. pyogenes (S43/100)	2	94	18	59	91	96	99	98	98
Str. salivarius (HHT)	2	94	15	33	44	86	99	99	99
Str. salivarius (IFO 3350)	2	94	0	52	100	91	99		
Str. faecalis (IFO 12580)	2	94	18	52	96	93	99	99	99
Str. Lactis (IFO 12546)	2	94	9	30	44	89	99		
Str. thermophilus (IFO 3535)	2	95	11	26	62	78	98		
Str. sanguis (ATCC 10556)	2	94	46	52	55	93	97	98	99 [1]
Str. mutans (BHT)	1							98	98
Str. Mutans (KIR)	0.4	95	2	21	46	72	93	98	98
L. plantarum (ATCC 8014) CW	0.1	98	46	47	40	90	94	95	95 [1]
" " " " PG	0.1	98	0	3	10	72	84		
B. megaterium (KM)	2	94	5	26	0	78	99		
Cl. botulinum (190L)	2	72	11	16	52	73	76		
Stm. gardneri (ATCC 23911)	1							88	90
A. viscosus (ATCC 15987)	0.2	98	35	50	53	91	98	99	92
C. diphtheriae (P.W.8)	0.2	94	0	38	56	86	99	90	90
Myc. rhodochrous (ATCC 184)	1							87	75
Myc. tuberculosis (H37Rv)	1							85	85
N. corynebacteriodes (ATCC 14898)	1							89	79

TABLE VI (continued)

Species (strain)	Dose (mg/ml serum)	CH50	C1	C4	C2	C3	C5	EGTA –	EGTA +
N. erythropolis (ATCC 4277)	1							89	77
N. gardneri (IFO 3385)	1							88	85
Arthrobacter sp. (NCIB 9423)[b]	2							34	27
Microb. lacticum (ATCC 8280)[b]	1	54	0	17	54	43	46		
Eub. limosum (ATCC 10825)[b]	2	30							
C. poinsettiae (NCPP 177)[b]	2	33							
C. betae (NCPP 373)[b]	1	21	0	20	3	55	71	34	27 [2]
C. insidiosum (NCPP 1110)[b]	0.2	94	0	38	56	86	99	90	90
Am. regularis[b]	2	30							
T. pallidum (Kazan)[b,c]	1	67	34	45	43	63	43	53	38

[a] These cell walls lacked the immunoadjuvancy by themselves, but their enzymatic digests exhibited a definite immunopotentiating activity (36).

[b] These cell walls lacked the immunoadjuvancy at least by themselves (37).

[c] T. Umemoto, K. Kato, M. Tsujimoto, and S. Kotani, unpublished.

[d] Dose of test specimens used in the EGTA method.

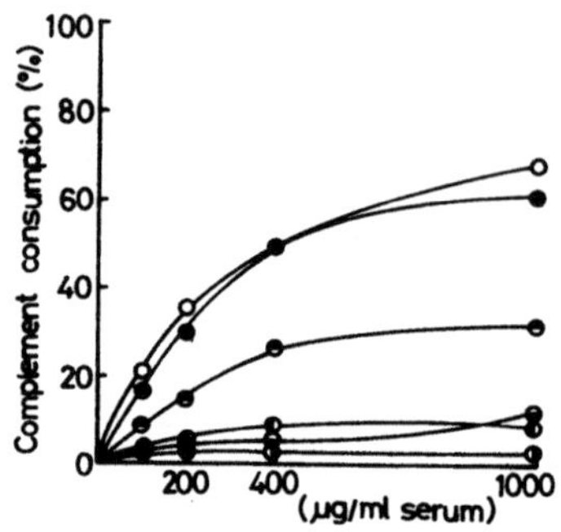

Fig. 16. Activation of human complement system by 6-O-acyl-MDPs. ◐ MDP, ◐ [L18]-MDP, ◒ [L30]-MDP, ○ [B30]-MDP, ● [B30]-MDP (D-isoAsn), ◓ [BH48]-MurNAc-L Ala-D-isogln-L-Lys-D-Ala.

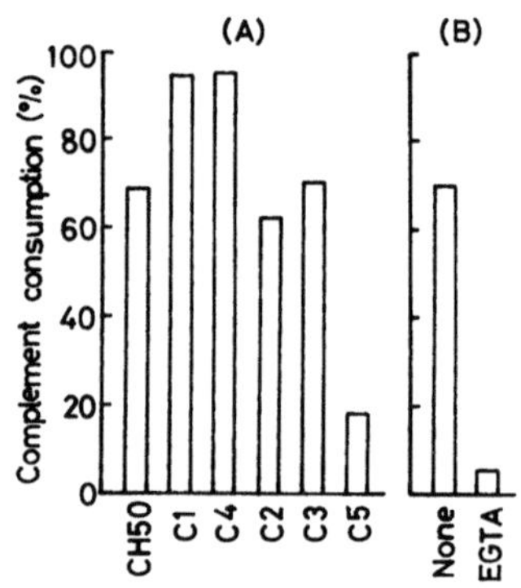

Fig. 17. Complement component consumption profile [A] and the blocking effect of EGTA in the complement activation by [B30]-MDP. Dose - 1 mg/ml serum.

Liberation of Serontonin in Rabbit Blood Platelets

Rotta, Masek and their coworkers (57, 60) reported that peptidoglycans of S. pyogenes, Streptococcus pneumoniae and S. aureus lysed blood platelets of rabbits and rats, liberation of Serotonin from these platelets. By reference to their studies, we have examined the serotonin liberating activity of cell walls of various bacterial species which are different in the peptidoglycan type

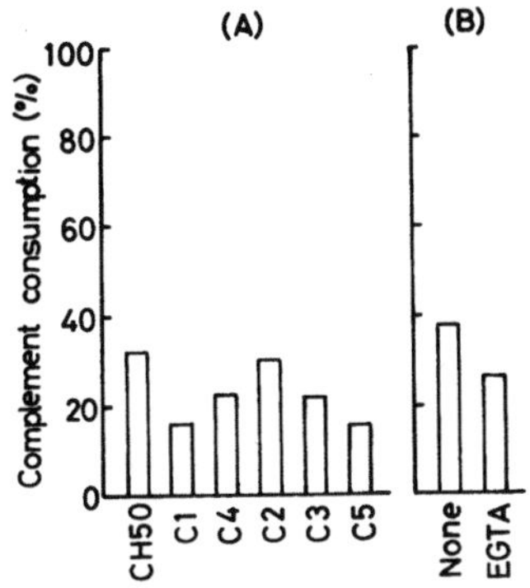

Fig. 18. Complement component consumption profile [A] and the blocking effect of EGTA in the complement activation by [BH48]-MurNAc-L-Ala-D-isoGln-L-Lys-D-Ala. Dose - 1 mg/ml serum.

and immunopotentiating and related biological activities (K. Harada, T. Kitaura, T. Nakajima, and S. Kotani, Abstr. 5th Annu. Meet. Jpn. Soc. Bacteriol., 1979, No. C-I-7, p. 120). Serotonin was estimated by the Snyder method (68). All test cell wall specimens, including the walls of M. lysodeikticus (NCTC 2665, IFO 3333), Arthrobacter sp. (NCIB 9423), Corynebacterium betae (NCPP 373), and Corynebacterium insidiosum (NCPP 1110) that lack the immunoadjuvancy by themselves at least (37), were shown to cause significant release of serotonin (Table 7).

The assay was then made on the serotonin liberating activity of water-soluble fragments of S. epidermidis cell wall peptidoglycan. SEPS was definitely active at a dose of 6.3 μg/ml reaction mixture, but SEPS-M was inactive even at a high dose of 400 μg/ml. The results of assay with synthetic compounds are shown in Table 8, indicating that all of test 6-O-acyl muramyl-dipeptides as well as MDP were inactive, but [BH48]-MurNAc-L-Ala-D-isoGln-L-Lys-D-Ala exhibited a definite serotonin liberating activity. Neither [BH48]-MDP (L-Ala and L-Ser type)nor MurNAc-L-Ala-D-isoGln-L-Lys-D-Ala had the activity. The dose response relationships were examined on representative bacterial cell walls, SEPS and the [BH48]-muramyltetrapeptide, (Table 9). The [BH48]-muramyltetrapeptide was shown to have a definite, serotonin liberating activity comparable to that of S. pyogenes cell walls, and stronger than other cell walls. In this connection, Rotta et al. (59) reported that synthetic MDP and MurNAc-L-Ala-D-isoGln-L-Lys-Ala, but not the di- or tetrapeptide portion, caused morphologically evident lysis of rabbit blood platelets only at an extremely high dose (500 μg/ml).

TABLE VII

Release of Serotonin from Rabbit Blood Platelets by Bacterial Cell Walls, Peptidoglycans and Cytoplasmic Membranes

Species (strain)		% Release of serotonin at 38°C for 1 hr
M. lysodeikticus (NCTC 2665)		75
M. lysodeikticus (IFO 3333)		76
S. epidermidis (ATCC 155)		80
" "	[PG][a]	52
S. aureus (STA-EMP-P)		88
" "	[CM][b]	-6
S. aureus (STA-EMP-L)	[CM][b]	-13
Str. pyogenes (Sv, type 3)		88
Str. pyogenes (Su, type 3)		89
Str. pyogenes (T12, type 12)		86
L. plantarum (ATCC 8014)		82
" "	[PG][a]	74
C. diphtheriae (PW 8)		46
Myc. rhodochrous (ATCC 184)		34
A. viscosus (ATCC 15987)		84
A. viscosus (ATCC 15988)		82
A. viscosus (ATCC 19246)		82
A. naeslundii (ATCC 12104)		81
A. naeslundii (human isolate)		85
N. canicruria (ATCC 17896)		61
N. corynebactriodes (ATCC 14898)		74
N. polychromogenes		47
Stm. gardneri (ATCC 23911)		88
Stm. aureofaciens (IAM 0087)		73
Arth. atrocyaneus (ATCC 13752)		92
Arthrobacter sp. (NCIB 9423)		83
C. betae (NCPP 373)		82
C. insidiosum (NCPP 1110)		84
Am. regularis		69
T. pallidum (Kazan)	[PG][a]	56
None		0

[a] Peptidoglycan

[b] Cytoplasmic membrane

Dose: 100 μg/ml reaction mixture.

TABLE VIII

Assay for Activity of MDP and 6-O-acyl-MDPs to Release Serotonin From Rabbit Blood Platelets

Test Materials	Dose µg(nmole)/ml	% Release of serotonin Experiments I	II	III	IV
MDP	100	-6			
MDP(L-isoGln)	100	-3			
[L18]-MDP	154		1		
[L24]-MDP	171			-11	
[L30]-MDP	188		-7		
[B30]-MDP	188 (202)		-6	-18	
[B46]-MDP	234			- 7	
[BH48]-MDP	243			-26	-6
[BH48]-MDP(L-Ser)	246			-19	-4
[BH48]-MDP-L-Lys-D-Ala	291			53	88
" at 4°C					9
MDP-L-Lys-D-Ala	148			-26	-6

Contractile Effect on Ileum

Fig. 19 illustrates the contraction of a strip (1 cm long) of guinea pig ileum bathed in Tyrode's solution in a Magnus' tube . at 37°C by addition of cell walls of N. corynebacteriodes (ATCC 14898) and Streptomyces gardneri (ATCC 23911) at a concentration of about 6 µg/ml. We can see that the ileum strip shows a long-lasting contraction.

Studies with other cell wall specimens disclosed that the cell walls or peptidoglycans active in the immunopotentiation exhibited a definite contractile effect (Fig. 20), whereas the cell walls lacking the immunoadjuvancy caused no contraction of the ileum strip, and A. atrocyaneus cell walls holding a slight immunoadjuvant activity exhibited a weak, but definite contractile effect (Fig. 21).

TABLE IX

Release of Serotonin from Rabbit Blood Platelets by Cell Walls, Peptidoglycans, a Polymer of Peptidoglycan Subunits and a 6-_O_acyl-muramyltetrapeptide (dose-response)

Test materials		Release of serotonin Dose (μg/ml) 100	25	6.3	1.6	0.4
Str. pyogenes (Sv, type 3)	CW	++	++	++	++	+
S. aureus (STA-EMP-P)	CW	++	++	++	+	-
S. epidermidis (ATCC 155)	CW	++	++	+	-	-
	PG		+	-	-	-
	SEPS	++	++	+	-	
L. plantarum (ATCC 2665)	CW	++	++	+	-	-
	PG			+	-	-
N. corynebacteriodes (ATCC 14898)	CW	++	+	-	-	
Stm. gardneri (ATCC 23911)	CW	++	++	-	-	
C. insidisum (NCPP 1110)	CW	++	++	++	-	
T. pallidum (Kazan)	PG	++	++	+	+	
[BH48]-MDP-L-Lys-D-Ala	Synthetic	++	++	++	++	

Grading: <30% -, 30-60% +, > 60% ++

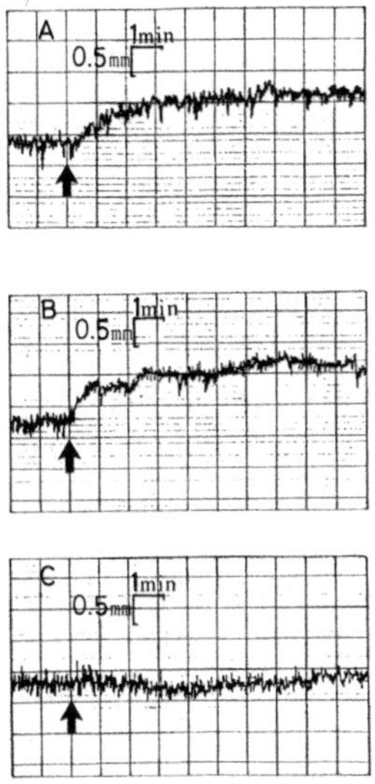

Fig. 19. A contractile effect of cell walls of N. corynebacteriodes [A] and Stm. gardneri [B] on a strip of guinea pig ileum. C - Control. The concentration of test specimens in the bathing medium was adjusted to be 5.56 μg/ml. Point and bracket indicate mean ± standard error.

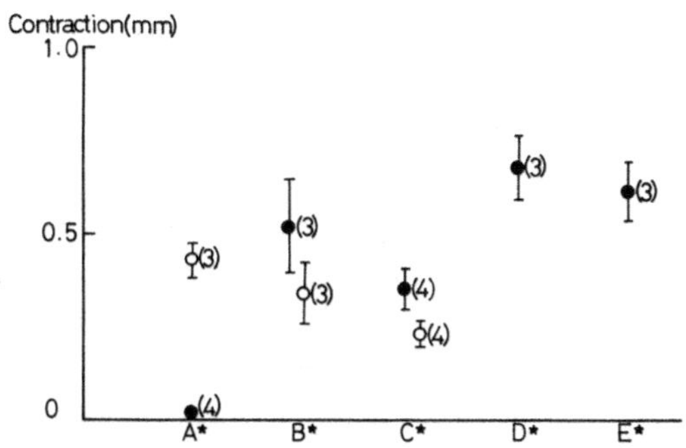

Fig. 20. A contactile effect of cell walls or peptidoglycan having the immunopotentiating activity on a strip of guinea pig ileum. A. - S. epidermids (ATCC 155), B - Str. pyogenes (type 3, 0175), C - L. plantarum)ATCC 8014), D Stm. gardneri)ATCC 23911), and E - N. corynebacteriodes (ATCC 14898). ● Cell walls, ○ peptidoglycan. Legends as in Fig. 19. Number in parenthesis shows the number of strips of guinea pig ileum.

Comparison was made on the ileum contractile effect of water-soluble SEPS and SEPS-M, S. epidermidis cell walls and peptidoglycan (Fig. 22). It was found that the cell walls themselves lacked the

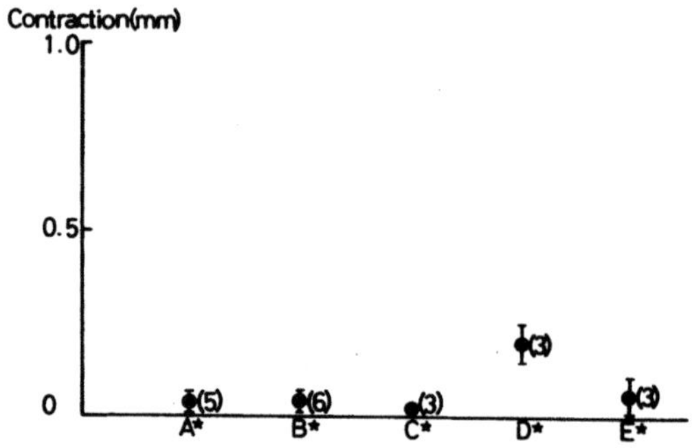

Fig. 21. A contractile effect of cell walls lacking the immuno-potentiating activity on a strip of guinea pig ileum. A - M. lysodeikticus (NCTC 2665), B - S. epdermidis (ATCC 155), C - Arth. atrocyaneus (ATCC 13752), D - C. insidiosum (NCP 1110), and E - Am. reguralis. Legends as in Fig. 20.

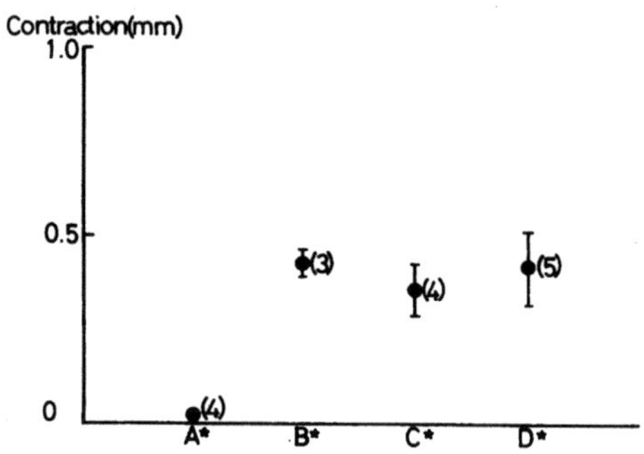

Fig. 22. A contractile effect of S. epidermidis cell walls, the peptidoglycan SEPS, and SEPS-M. A - Cell walls, B - peptidoglycan, C - SEPS, and D - SEPS-M. Legends as in Fig. 20.

contractile activity in accord with their inability in immuno-potentiation, but the peptidoglycan and its water-soluble fragments having the immunopotentiating activity caused a definite contraction of the ileum strip.

With regards synthetic compounds (Fig. 23), strips of the guinea pig ileum showed a definite contractile response to MDP, [L18]- and [B30]-MDPs, but not to their L-isoglutamine and D-iso-asparagine analogues devoid of the immunoadjuvancy. [BH48]-MDP, in contrast with other synthetic specimens, caused relaxation of the ileum strip, and its L-isoglutamine or D-isoasparagine analogue showed no effects, indicating that the observed relaxation was due to a specific action of [BH48]-MDP. There were neat dose-response relationships with the contractile on relaxative activity of SEPS, SEPS-M and the synthetic compounds (data are not shown).

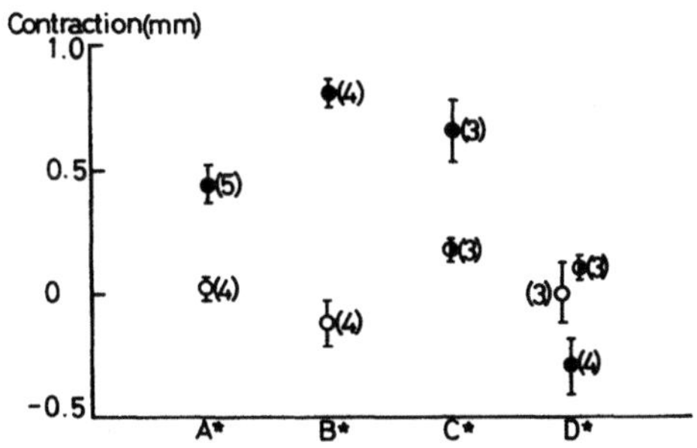

Fig. 23. A contractile effect of MDP and 6-O-acyl-MDPs on a strip of guinea pig ileum. A - MDP, B - [L18]-MDP, C - [B30]-MDP, and D - [BH48]-MDP. ○ L-isoglutamine analogue, and ◐ D-isoasparagine analogue. Dose - 5.56 µg MDP equivalent (each 11.2 nmoles). Other legends as in Fig.

SUMMARY

1. Bacterial cell walls have versatile biological (immunological, pharmacological and pathological) activities, especially those modulating natural and acquired defense mechanisms. Many of these activities seem to be related with each other.

2. Peptidoglycan subunit monomer, particularly N-acetylmuramyl-L-alanyl-D-isoglutamine are the chemical entity responsible for the biological activities of bacterial cell walls. It should be pointed out, however, that though N-acetylmuramyl peptides were the essential minimum structure, they needed some additional structures or physical properties to efficiently exert some of their biological activities.

3. The biological activities of bacterial cell walls, with those of endotoxic lipopolysaccharides, could be involved in maturation, maintenance or aging of host defense mechanisms and other functions, in view of so versatile modulating activities of cell walls and the existence of numerous bacteria as normal flora immediately after the birth, although at the present time we have no experimental evidences supporting this speculation.

4. If we could either utilize or control the biological activities of bacterial cell walls effectively we could do so much to promote our health and to restrain the diseases.

REFERENCES

The following list of references is not comprehensive, but biased to studies of our and related laboratories. For reports from other institutions, please refer to literatures quoted in the reviews and papers listed here.

1. Adam, A., Ellouz, F., Ciorbaru, R., Petit, J. F., and Lederer, E., 1975, Peptidoglycan adjuvants: minimal structure required for activity. Z. Immun.-Forsch. 149(s): 341.

2. Appleyard, G., and Maber, H. B., 1974, Plaque formation by influenza viruses in the presence of trypsin. J. Gen. Virol. 25: 351.

3. Audibert, F., Chedid, L., and Hannoun, C., 1977, Augmentation de la response immunitaire au vaccin grippal par un glycopeptide synthetique adjuvant (N-acetylmuramly-L-alanyl-D-isoglutamine), C. R. Acad. Sc. Paris, Serie D. 285: 467.

4. Azuma, I., Kishimoto, S., Yamamura, Y., and Petit, J. F., 1971, Adjuvanticity of mycobacterial cell walls. Jpn. J. Microbiol. 15: 193.

5. Azuma, I., Sugimura, K., Taniyama, T., Yamawaki, M., Yamamura, Y., Kusumoto, S., Okada, S., and Hiba, T., 1976, Adjuvant activity of mycobacterial fractions: adjuvant activity of synthetic N-acetylmuramyl-dipeptide and the related compounds. Infect. Immun. 14: 18.

6. Azuma, I., Sugimura, K, Yamamura, Y., Kusumoto, S., Tarumi, Y, and Shiba, T., 1976, Adjuvant activity of synthetic cell wall peptidoglycan subunits on monoazobenzenearsonate-N-aceytl-L-tyrosine and bacterial α-amylase in guinea pigs. Jpn. J. Microbiol. 2-: 63.

7. Azuma, I., Sugimura, K., Yamawaki, M., Uemiya, M., Kusumoto, S., Okada, S., Shiba, T., and Yamamura, Y., 1978, Adjuvant activity of synthetic 6-"mycoloyl"-N-acetylmuramyl-L-alanyl-D-isoglutamine and related compounds. Infect. Immun. 20: 600.

8. Azuma, I., Sugimura, K., Yamawaki, M., Uemiya, M., and Yamamura, Y., 1977, Mitogenic activity of cell-wall components in mouse spleen cells. Microbiol. Immunol. 21: 111.

9. Chedid, L., 1978, Past, present and future of the synthetic immunoadjuvant MDP and its analogs. Biochem. Pharmacol. 27: 2183.

10. Chedid, L., 1979, Immunostimulation. Springer Semin. Immunopathol. 2: 1.

11. Chedid, L., Audibert, F., and Johnson, A. G., 1978, Biological activities of muramyl dipeptide, a synthetic glycopeptide analogous to bacterial immunoregulating agents. Prog. Allergy. 25: 63.

12. Chedid, L., Audibert, F., and Parant, M., 1978, Une nouvelle famille d'immunoregulateurs synthetiques: le muramyl dipeptide et ses analogues. Path. Biol. 26: 527.

13. Ellouz, F., Adam, A., Ciorbaru, R., and Lederer, E., 1974, Minimum structural requirements for adjuvant activity of bacterial peptidoglycan derivatives. Biochem. Biophys. Res. Commun. 59: 1317.

14. Emori, K., and Tanaka, A., 1978, Granuloma formation by synthetic bacterial cell wall fragment: Muramyl dipeptide. Infect. Immun. 19: 613.

15. Hamada, S., Narita, T., Kotani, S., and Kato, K., 1971, Studies on cell walls of group A Streptococcus pyogenes, type 12. II. Pyrogenic and related biological activities of the higher molecular weight fraction of an enzymatic digest of the cell walls. Biken J. 14: 217.

16. Heymer, B., 1975, Biological properties of the peptidoglycan, Z. Immun.-Forsch. 149(S): 245.

17. Heymer, B., Finger, H., and Wirsing, C.-H., 1978, Immunoadjuvant effects of the synthetic muramyl-dipeptide (MDP) N-acetylmuramyl-L-alanyl-D-isoglutamine. Z. Immun.-Forsch. 155: 87.

18. Igarashi, T., Okada, M., Azuma, I, and Yamamura, Y., 1977, Adjuvant activity of synthetic N-acetylmuramyl-L-alanyl-D-isoglutamine and related compounds on cell-mediated cytotoxicity in syngeneic mice. Cell. Immunol. 34: 270.

19. Inai, S., Nagai, K., Ebisu, S., Kato, K., Kotani, S., and Misaki, A., 1976, Activation of the alternative complement pathway by water-insoluble glycans of Streptococcus mutans: The relation between their chemical structures and activating potencies. J. Immunol. 117: 1256.

20. Koga, T., Maeda, K., Onoue, K., Kato, K., and Kotani, S., 1979, Chemical structure required for immunoadjuvant and arthritogenic activities of cell wall peptidoglycans. Mol. Immunol. 16: 153.

21. Koga, T., Pearson, C. M., Narita, T., and Kotani, S., 1973, Polyarthritis induced in the rat with cell walls from several bacteria and two Streptomyces sp. Proc. Soc. Exp. Biol. Med. 143: 824.

22. Koga, T., Kotani, S., Narita, T., and Pearson, C. M., 1976, Induction of adjuvant arthritis in the rat by various bacterial cell walls and their water-soluble components. Int. Arch. Allergy Appl. Immun. 51: 206.

23. Kohashi, O., Pearson, C. M., Beck, F. W. J., Narita, T., and Kotani, S., 1976, Arthritogenicity in rats of cell walls from several streptococci, Staphylococci and two other bacteria. Proc. Soc. Exp. Biol. Med.152: 199.

24. Kohashi, O., Pearson, C. M., Shimono, T., and Kotani, S., 1976, Preparation of various fractions from Mycobacterium smegmatis, their arthritogenicity and their preventive effect on adjuvant disease. Int. Arch. Allergy Appl. Immun. 51: 451.

25. Kohashi, O., Pearson, C. M., Watanabe, Y., Kotqni, S., and Koga, T., 1976, Structural requirements for arthritogenicity of peptidoglycans from Staphylococcus aureus and Lactobacillus plantarum and analogous synthetic compounds. J. Immun. 116: 1635.

26. Kotani, S., Harada, K., Kitaura, T., Hashimoto, Y., Matsubara, T., and Chimori, M., 1962, Lysis of isolated BCG cell walls with enzymes. Biken J. 5: 117.

27. Kotani, S., Hashimoto, S., Matsubara, T., Kato, K., Harada, K., Kogami, J., Kitaura, T., and Tanaka, A., 1963, Lysis of isolated BCG cell walls with enzymes II. Demonstration of 'bound wax D' as a component of BCG cell walls. Biken J. 6: 181.

28. Kotani, S., Kinoshita, F., Morisaki, I., Shimono, T., Okunaga, T., Takada, H., Tsuijimoto, M., Watanabe, Y., Kato, K., Shiba, T., Kusumoto, S., and Okada, S., 1977, Immunoadjuvant activities of synthetic 6-O-acyl-N-acetylmuramyl-L-alanyl-D-isoglutamine with special reference to the effect of its administration with liposomes. Biken J. 20: 95.

29. Kotani, S., Kinoshita, F., Watanabe, Y., Morisaki, I., Shimono, T., Kato, K., Shiba, T., Kusumoto, S., Ikenaka, K., and Tarumi,

Y., 1977, Effects of chemical modification of the glutamic acid residue in N-acetylmuramyl peptides on the immunoadjuvancies of the molecules. Biken J. 20: 125.

30. Kotani, S., Kitaura, T., Hashimoto, S., Chimori, M., and Kishida, H., 1964. Influence of extraction of 'bound wax D' of BCG with trichloroacetic acid on its adjuvant activity on development of a delayed type of hypersensitivity. Biken J.6:321.

31. Kotani, S., Kitaura, T., Higashigawa, M., Kato, K., Mori, Y., Matsubara, T., and Tsujimoto, T., 1960, Studies on the immunological properties of the cell wall-, particle- and soluble-fractions of sonicated BCG cells. Biken J.3: 159.

32. Kotani, S., Kitaura, T., Hirano, T., and Tanaka, A., 1959, Preparation and chemical composition of the cell walls of BCG. Biken J. 2: 129.

33. Kotani, S., Matsubara, T., Kitaura, T., Mori, Y., Chimori, M., and Kishida, H., 1963, Adjuvant activity in development of a delayed type of hypersensitivity of a lipid fraction isolated from enzymatically digested cell walls of *Corynebacterium diphtheriae*. Biken J. 6: 211.

34. Kotani, S., Narita, T., Stewart-Tull, D. E. S., Shimono, T., Watanabe, Y., Kato, K., and Iwata, S., 1975, Immunoadjuvant activities of cell walls and their water-soluble fractions prepared from various gram-positive bacteria. Biken J. 18: 77.

35. Kotani, S., Watanabe, Y., Kinoshita, F., Kato, K., Harada, K., Shiba, T., Kusumoto, S., Tarumi, Y., Idenaka, K., and Okada, S., 1977, Gelation of the amoebocyte lysate of *Tachypleus tridentatus*by cell wall digest of several gram-positive bacterial and synthetic peptidoglycan subunits of natural and unnatural configurations. Biken J. 20: 5.

36. Kotani, S., Watanabe, Y., Kinoshita, F., Kato, K., and Perkins, H. R., 1977, Immunoadjuvant activities of the enzymatic digests of bacterial cell walls lacking immunoadjuvancy by themselves. Biken J.20: 87.

37. Kotani, S., Watanabe, Y., Kinoshita, F., Kato, K., Schleifer, K. H., Perkins, H. R., 1977, Inabilities as an immunoadjuvant of cell walls of the group B peptidoglycan types and those of arthrobacters. Biken J. 20: 1.

38. Kotani, S., Watanabe, Y., Kinoshita, F., Morisake, I., Kato, K., Shiba, T., Kusumoto, S., Tarumi, Y., and Ikenaka, K., 1977,

The effect of replacement of L-alanine residue by glycine, L-serine or D-alanine in an N-acetylmuramyl-L-alanyl-D-isoglutamine on immunoadjuvancies of molecules. Biken J. 20: 39.

39. Kotani, S., Watanabe, Y., Kinoshita, F., Shimono, T., Morisaki, I., Shiba, T., Kusumoto, S., Tarumi, Y., and Idenaka, K., 1975, Immunoadjuvant activities of synthetic N-acetylmuramyl-peptides of -amino acids. Biken J. 18: 105.

40. Kotani, S., Watanabe, Y., Narita, T., Shimono, T., Stewart-Tull, D.E.S., Iwata, S., Yamaguchi, H., Iwata, K., Shimizu, T., Mifuchi, I., Nozawa, Y., Ito, Y., Kanetsuna, F., Yano, K., Misaki, A., Matsuoka, T., and Fukui, K., 1975, Immunoadjuvant activities of fungal cell walls. Biken J. 18: 135.

41. Kotani, S., Watanabe, Y., Shimono, T., Harada, K., Shiba, T., Kusumoto, S., Yokogawa, K., and Taniguchi, M., 1976, Correlation between the immunoadjuvant activities and pyrogenicities of synthetic N-acetylmuramly-peptides and -amino acids. Biken J. 19: 9.

42. Kotani, S., Watanabe, Y., Shimono, T., Kinoshita, F., Narita, T., Kato, K., Stewart-Tull, D. E. S., Morisaki, I., Yokogawa, K., and Kawata, S., 1975, Immunoadjuvant activities of peptidoglycan subunits from the cell walls of Staphylococcus aureus and Lactobacillus plantarum. Biken J. 18: 83.

43. Kotani, S., Watanabe, Y., Shimono, T., Narita, T., Kato, K., Stewart-Tull, D. E. S., Kinoshita, F., Yokogawa, K., Kawata, S., Shiba, T., Kusumoto, S., and Tarumi, Y., 1975, Immunoadjuvant activities of cell walls, their water-soluble fractions and peptidoglycan subunits, prepared from various gram-positive bacteria, and of synthetic N-acetylmuramyl peptides. Z. Immun. -Forsch. 149(S): 302.

44. Krause, R. M., 1975, Immunological activity of the peptidoglycan. Z. Immun. -Forsch. 149(S): 136.

45. Kusumoto, S., Inage, M., and Shiba, T., 1978, Synthesis of long chain fatty acid esters of N-acetylmuramyl-L-alanyl-D-isoglutamine in relation to antitumor activity. Tetrahedron Lett. 49: 4899.

46. Kusumoto, S., Okada, S., Yamamoto, K., and Shiba, T., 1978, Synthesis of 6-O-acyl derivatives of immunoadjuvant active N-acetylmuramyl-L-alanyl-D-isoglutamine. Bull. Chem. Soc. Jpn. 51: 2122.

47. Kusumoto, S., Tarumi, Y., Ikenaka, K., Shiba, T., 1976, Chemical synthesis of N-acetylmuramyl peptides with partial structures of bacterial cell wall and their analogs in relation to immunoadjuvant activities. Bull. Chem. Soc. Jpn. 49: 533.

48. Masek, K., Zaoral, M., Jezek, J., and Strake, R., 1978, Immunoadjuvant activity of synthetic N-acetylmuramyl dipeptide. Experientia 34: 1363.

49. Midtvedt, T., and Melby, K., 1978, Phagocytosis of ^{32}P-labelled E. coli by human polymorphonuclear cells (PMN). Acta Path. Microbiol. Scand. Sect. B. 86: 193.

50. Nagai, Y., Akiyama, K., Kotani, S., Watanabe, Y., Shimono, T., Shiba, T., and Kusumoto, S., 1978, Structural specificity of synthetic peptide adjuvant for induction of experimental allergic encephalomyelitis, Cell. Immunol. 35: 168.

51. Nagai, Y., Akiyama, K., Suzuki, K., Kotani, S., Watanabe, Y., Shimono, T., Shiba, T., Kusumoto, S., Ikuta, F., and Takeda, S., 1978, Minimum structural requirements for encephalitogen and for adjuvant in the induction of experimental allergic encephalomyelitis. Cell. Immunol. 35: 158.

52. Nagao, S., Tanaka, A., Yamamoto, Y., Koga, T., Onoue, K., Shiba, T., Kusumoto, S., and Kotani, S., 1979, Inhibition of macrophage migration by muramyl peptides. Infect. Immun. 24: 308.

53. Narita, T., Hamada, S., Kotani, S., Hasegawa, K., and Ishida, T., 1971, Studies on cell walls of group A Streptococcus pyogenes, type 12. III. Cardiac lesions produced in mice by a higher molecular weight fraction isolated from a digest of cell walls, with the L-11 enzyme. Biken J. 14: 233.

54. Ohkuni, H., Norose, Y., Hayama, M., Kimura, Y., Kotani, S., Shiba, T., Kusumoto, S., Yokogawa, K., and Kawata, S., 1977, Adjuvant activities in production of reaginic antibody in mice of bacterial cell wall peptidoglycans or peptidoglycan subunits and of synthetic N-acetylmuramyl-dipeptides. Biken J. 20: 131.

55. Ohkuni, H., Norose, Y., Ohta, M., Hayama, M., Tsujimoto, M., Kotani, S., Shiba, T., Kusumoto, S., Yokogawa, K., and Kawata, S., 1979, Adjuvant activities in production of reaginic antibody by bacterial cell wall peptidoglycan or synthetic N-acetylmuramyl dipeptides in mice. Infect. Immun. 24: 313.

56. Parant, M., 1979, Biological properties of a new synthetic adjuvant, muramyl dipeptide (MDP). Springer Semin. Immunopathol. 2: 101.

57. Raskova, H., Ryc, M., Rotta, J., and Masek, K., 1971, Release of 5-hydroxy-tryptamine and morphological changes in blood platelets induced by mucopeptide of streptococcal cell walls. J. Infec. Dis. 123: 587.

58. Rotta, J., 1975, Endotoxin-like properties of the peptidoglycan. Z. Immun.-Forsch. 149(S): 230.

59. Rotta, J., Rýc, M., Mašek, K., and Azoral, M.,1979, Biological activity of synthetic subunits of streptococcus peptidoglycan. I. Pyrogenic and thrombocytolytic activity. Expt. Cell. Biol. 47: 257.

60. Rýc, M., and Rotta, J., 1975, The thrombocytolytic activity of bacterial peptidoglycan. Z. Immun.-Forsch. 149(S): 265-272.

61. Schleifer, K. H., and Kandler, O., 1972, Peptidoglycan types of bacterial cell walls and their taxonomic implications. Bacteriol. Rev. 36: 407.

62. Schleifer, K. H., and Seidel, P. H., 1974, The immunochemistry of peptidoglycan. Antibodies against a synthetic immunogen crossreacting with peptidoglycan. Eur. J. Biochem. 43: 509.

63. Schwab, J. H., and Smialowicz, R., 1975, Interaction of bacterial cell wall polymers and rat macrophages. Z. Immun.-Forsch.149(S): 283.

64. Seidel, P. H., and Schleifer, K. H., 1977, The immunochemistry of peptidoglycan. Antibodies against a synthetic immunogen crossreacting with an interpeptide bridge of peptidoglycan. Eur. J. Biochem. 74: 353.

65. Shiba, T., Okada, S., Kusumoto, S., Azuma, I., and Yamamura, Y., 1978, Synthesis of 6-O-mycoloyl-N=acetylmuramyl-L-alanyl-D-isoglutamine with antitumor activity. Bull. Chem. Soc. Jpn. 51: 3307.

66. Siddiqui, W. A., Taylor, D. W., Kan, S.-C., Kramer, K., Richmond-Crum, S.M., Kotani, S., Shiba, T., and Kusumoto, S.. 1978, Vaccination of experimental monkeys against Plasmodium falciparum: A possible safe adjuvant. Science. 201: 1237.

67. Smith, S. M., Burrel, R., and Snyder, I. S., 1978, Complement activation by cell wall fractions of Miczopolyspora faeni. Infect. Immun. 22: 568.

68. Snyder, S. H., Axelrod, J., and Zweig, M., 1965, A sensitive and specific fluorescence assay for tissue serotonin. Biochem Pharmacol.14: 831.

69. Stewart-Tull, D. E. S., Shimono, T., Kotani, S., Kato, M., Ogawa, Y., Yamamura, Y., Koga, T., and Pearson, C. M., 1975, The adjuvant activity of a non-toxic water-soluble glycopeptide present in large quantities in the culture filtrate of Mycobacterium tuberculosis strain DT. Immunology 29: 1.

70. Stewart-Tull, D. E. S., Shimono, T., Kotani, S., and Knights, B. K., 1976, Immunosuppressive effect in mycobacterial adjuvant emulsions of mineral oils containing low molecular weight hydrocarbons. Int. Arch. Allergy Appl. Immun. 52: 118.

71. Sugimura, K., Uemiya, M., Saiki, I., Azuma, I., and Yamamura, Y., 1979, The adjuvant activity of synthetic N-acetylmuramly-dipeptide: Evidence of initial target cells for the adjuvant activity. Cell. Immunol. 43: 137.

72. Takada, H., Kotani, S., Kusumoto, S.,Tarumi, Y., Ikenaka, K., and Shiba,T., 1977, Mitogenic activity of adjuvant-active N-acetylmuramyl-L-alanyl-D-isoglutamine and its analogues. Biken J. 20: 81

73. Takada, H., Tsugimoto, M., Kato, K., Kotani, S., Kusumoto, S., Inage, M., Shiba, T., Yano, I., Kawata, S., and Yokogawa, K., 1979, Macrophage activation by bacterial cell walls and related synthetic compounds. Infect. Immun. 25: 48.

74. Takada, H., Tsujimoto, M., Kotani, S., Kusumoto, S., Inage, M., Shiba, T., Nagao, S., Yano, I., Kawata, S., and Yokogawa, K., 1979, Mitogenic effects of bacterial cell walls, their fragments, and related synthetic compounds on thymocytes and splenocytes of guinea pigs. Infect. Immun. 25: 645.

75. Tanaka, A., Nagao, S., Nagao(Saito), R., Kotani, S., Kusumoto, S., and Shiba, T., 1979, Stimulation of the reticuloendothelial system of mice by muramyl dipeptide. Infect. Immun. 24: 302.

76. Tanaka, A., Nagao, S., Saito, R., Kotani, S., Kusumoto, S., and Shiba, T., 1977, Correlation of stereochemically specific structure in muramyl dipeptide between macrophage activation and adjuvant activity. Biochem. Biophys. Res. Commun. 77: 621.

77. Tanaka, A., Saito, R., Sugiyama, S., Morisaki, I., Kotani, S., Kusumoto, S., and Shiba, T., 1977, Adjuvant activity of synthetic N-acetlmuyramyl peptides in rats. Infect. Immun. 15: 332.

78. Trippestad, A., and Midtvedt, T., 1968, Phagocytosis of ^{32}P-labelled E. coli by rat peritoneal polymorphonuclear leukocytes. Evaluation of a method. Acta Path. Microbiol. Scand. 74: 259.

79. Tsujimoto, M., Kinoshita, F., Okunaga, T., Kotani, S., Kusumoto, S., Yamamoto, K., and Shiba, T., 1979, Higher immunoadjuvant activities of N-acetyl-β-D-glutaminyl-(1-4)-N-acetylmuramyl-L-alanyl-D-isoglutamine in comparison with N-acetylmuramyl-L-alanyl-D-isoglutamine. Microbiol. Immunol. 23: 933.

80. Uemiya, M., Saiki, I., Kusama, T., Azuma, I., and Yamamura, Y., 1979, Adjuvant activity of mycoloyl derivatives of N-acetylmuramyl-L-alanyl-D-isoglutamine in mice and guinea pigs. Microbiol. Immunol. 23: 821.

81. Uemiya, M., Sugimura, K., Kusama, T., Saiki, I., Yamawaki, M., Azuma, I., and Yamamura, Y., 1979, Adjuvant activity of 6-O-mycoloyl derivatives of N-acetylmuramyl-L-seryl-D-isoglutamine and related compounds in mice and guinea pigs. Infect. Immun. 24: 83.

82. Wahl, S. M., Wahl, L. M., McCarthy, B., Chedid, L., and Mergenhagen, S. E., 1979, Macrophage activation by mycobacterial water soluble compounds and synthetic muramyl dipeptide. J. Immunol. 122: 2226.

83. Webster, R. G., Glezen, W. P., Hannoun, G., and Laver, W. G., 1977, Potentiation of the immune response to influenza virus subunit vaccines. J. Immunol. 119: 2073.

84. Wildfener, A., Heymer, B., Spliker, D., Schleifer, K. H., Vanek, E., and Haferkamp, O., 1975, Use of Limulus assay to compare the biological activity of peptidoglycan and endotoxin. Z. Immun.-Forsch. 149(S): 258.

85. Yamamoto, Y., Nagao, S., Tanaka, A., Koga, T., and Onoue, K., 1978, Inhibition of macrophage migration by synthetic muramyl dipeptide. Biochem. Biophys. Res. Commun. 80: 923.

86. Yamamura, Y., Azuma, I., Sugimura, K., Kusumoto, S., and Shiba, T., 1976, Immunological activity of synthetic cell-wall peptidoglycan subunits. Proc. Jpn. Acad. 52: 58.

87. Yamamura, Y., Azuma, I., Sugimura, K., Yamawakim, M., Uemiya, M., Kusumoto, S., Okada, S., and Shiba, T., 1976, Adjuvant activity of 6-O-mycoloyl-N-acetylmuramyl-L-alanyl-D-isoglutamine Gann 67: 867.

88. Yamamura, Y., Azuma, I., Sugimura, K., Yamawaki, M., Uemiya, M., Kusumoto, S., Okada, S., and Shiba, T., 1977, Immunological and antitumor activities of synthetic 6O-mycoloyl-N-acetylmuramyl-dipeptides. Proc. Jpn. Acad. 53: 63.

89. Yamamura, Y., Azuma, I., Taniyama, T., Sugimura, K., Hirao, F., Tokuzen, R., Okabe, M., Nakahara, W., Yasumoto, K., and Ohta, M., 1977, Immunotherapy of cancer with cell wall skeleton of Mycobacterium bovis-Bacillus Calmette-Guerin: Experimental and clinical results. Ann. N.Y. Acad. Sci. 277: 209.

90. Yokogawa, K., Kawata, S., Takemura, T., and Yoshimura, Y., 1975, Purification and properties of lytic enzymes from Streptomyces globisporus 1829. Agr. Biol. Chem. 29: 1533.

PERTUSSIS INDUCED IMMUNOMODULATION

Thomas Klein, William Benjamin, Alvin Winters
and Herman Friedman

Department of Medical Microbiology and Immunology
University of South Florida College of Medicine
Tampa, FL 33612

INTRODUCTION

Bordetella pertussis (pertussis) is a gram negative coccobacillus and was identified to be the etiological agent of "whooping cough" by Bordet and Gengou in 1906 (7). Much of the early work on pertussis was concerned with identifying the protective antigens so that an effective vaccine could be produced for humans. A whole cell vaccine was introduced in the 1940's and today is administered world-wide to millions of infants (31). The present vaccine appears to be of major benefit in preventing infant whooping cough, but because of its associated toxicity recent emphasis has been placed on developing a non-whole cell, more highly purified vaccine (40).

Beginning in the 1940's, whole-cell vaccine preparations of pertussis were observed to alter biological systems in man and experimental annimals including the induction of a state of histamine hypersensitivity (34). In addition, pertussis was observed to alter immune function. Greenberg and Fleming (18) were the first to demonstrate that pertussis vaccine (PV) acted as an adjuvant. They showed that mixtures of PV and diphtheria toxoid resulted in enhanced levels of antitoxin antibody. The adjuvant effect has subsequently been observed for other antigens, both T dependent and T independent, and is thought to be due to both heat-labile (pertussis toxin) and heat-stable (endotoxin) components. Dresser et al. and others have shown that pertussis induced augmentation of antibody formation is greatest for immunoglobulins of the IgG and IgE classes (12, 25, 30, 35). On an immune cell basis, the adjuvant effect of pertussis has been shown to involve influences on helper T cell function (11, 19, 35). However, direct effects on precursors of antibody forming cells have been indicated in *in vitro* systems (32) and under conditions of high antigen dose (11).

Pertussis also induces a lymphocytosis in man and experimental animals (28). Morse et al. have demonstrated that this effect is due to a heat-labile component of the bacteria termed lymphocytosis-promoting factor (LPF). Lymphocytosis appears to occur because of a failure of lymphocytes to emigrate from the blood into the lymph nodes at a normal rate (29). In addition, it has been shown that LPF is a mitogen for mouse T cells *in vitro* and that the proliferative response requires the presence of a surface-immunoglobulin positive accessory cell (21).

The involvement of macrophages in immunomodulation by pertussis has been repeatedly suggested but only rarely demonstrated. Unanue et al. (36) demonstrated that antigen containing macrophages treated with PV *in vitro* elicited a much higher antibody response when injected into mice than did antigen containing macrophages not treated with PV. Levine and Sowinski (26) demonstrated that PV injection inhibited the outpouring of macrophages into a zone of thermal coagglutination necrosis in the brain. Finger et al. (14) showed that PV injection resulted in significant alteration of the phagocytic cells of the RES. Additional indirect evidence has suggested that the PV induced enhanced resistance to the lethal effects of intracellular bacteria (22) and viruses (23) is mediated by macrophages. From this and other evidence demonstrating an effect on macrophage function of certain other bacterial products (this publication), it seems reasonable to expect that pertussis may significantly alter macrophage function.

Accordingly, we have begun an examination of the ways in which PV and its biologically active components might alter macrophage function. Our results demonstrate that PV injection can significantly alter murine peritoneal macrophage phagocytosis, spreading, migration, lysosomal enzyme production, and viral growth inhibitory activity, and that both heat-labile and heat-stable components of PV are involved. Furthermore, it appears that T lymphocytes are only partially responsible for the expression of the PV effects. These results suggest that pertussis like other bacterial adjuvants can significantly alter basic macrophage function and may therefore exert some of its biological effects through macrophage mechanisms.

MATERIALS AND METHODS

Two strains of mice were used for these studies. Female mice, strain BDF_1/Cox (C57BL/6 Cox X DBA/2 Cox), weighing 17-20 g, were obtained from Laboratory Supply, Indianapolis, IN. Athymic nude (nu/nu) and heterozygous (nu/+) mice of both sexes were from a colony maintained at our institution. This colony was developed from a C3H/HeN background by the NIH. Nude and heterozygous mice were maintained in isolated quarters using aseptic procedures (16).

B. pertussis was furnished by Connaught Laboratories, Inc., Swiftwater, PA, as an inactivated suspension of organisms adjusted to a concentration of 4 mg/ml (dry weight). Vaccine diluent consisted of physiological saline containing 0.02% thimerosal as preservative. This vaccine injected intravenously into mice at a dose of 40 μg/ml/gram body weight caused a leukocytosis 4 days later of $10^5/mm^3$ of blood and 100% mortality following injection of 5 mg histamine diphosphate.

The culture medium used in this study was Dulbecco's Modified Eagle Medium containing 10% heat-inactivated fetal calf serum, antibiotics and heparin (10 units/ml). Peritoneal leukocytes were obtained by lavage. Mice were sacrificed by cervical dislocation, the abdomen swabbed with alcohol, and the skin removed to expose the peritoneum. Culture medium (4.0 ml) was injected into the peritoneal cavity, mixed by gentle massage, and the peritoneal leukocytes withdrawn by means of a sterile needle and syringe. The peritoneal cells were washed by centrifugation, counted in a hemocytometer, and adjusted to specified numbers for plating. Culturing of peritoneal cells was accomplished in 35 mm plastic dishes (Falcon, Oxnard, CA) and incubations were performed at 37°C in a humidified atmosphere of 5% CO_2 and air. To facilitate studies involving phagocytosis and spreading, glass cover-slips (12 mm) were incubated in the 35 mm culture dishes as previously described (4).

Sheep red blood cells (SRBC) in Alsever's Solution were obtained from Lee Labs, Inc., Grayson, GA and used in the phagocytosis assay (5). Erythrocytes (3) were prepared by washing 3 times in Hanks Balanced Salt Solution and resuspending to 5 percent. Erythrocyte-antibody (EA) complexes were prepared by incubating E's with a 1:5000 dilution of Difco hemolysin for 30 min at 37°C. Following incubation EA's were washed by centrifugation and resuspended to 5 percent. Erythrocyte-antibody-complement (EAC) complexes were prepared by incubating EA's with 5% mouse serum for 10 min at 37°C. EAC's were washed and resuspended as above.

RESULTS

Mouse peritoneal macrophages do not readily bind (rosette) or ingest SRBC's *in vitro*. However, these cells do bind EAC's *in vitro* and will ingest or phagocytize such complexes if obtained from animals previously injected intraperitoneally with various substances (3). We have previously reported that intraperitoneal injection of PF result-d in enhanced phagocytosis of yeast particles by peritoneal cells (15). To extend these observations, the present series of studies was designed to examine the E and EAC phagocytic ability of peritoneal macrophages from animals injected intravenously with PV.

Groups of mice were injected via lateral tail vein with varying doses of PV or vaccine diluent and the peritoneal cells harvested by lavage at varying times after injection. Peritoneal leukocytes were adjusted to 1.5×10^6/ml in culture medium, plated, and incubated for 0.5 hours. Non-adherent leukocytes were removed by rinsing with medium and adherent cells incubated for an additional hour. Subsequently, E's or EAC's suspended in culture medium was added to adherent cell cultures and the preparations were incubated at 37°C for 1 hr to allow for phagocytosis by adherent cells. Following incubation, cover-slips containing adherent cells were removed from the culture dishes, dipped in hypotonic medium to lyse external erythrocytes and stained. Three hundred mononuclear cells per cover-slip were examined at random microscopically. Cells containing one or more erythrocyte were scored as positive for phagocytosis. The results show (Table 1) that in uninjected animals the extent of E phagocytosis by peritoneal cells is much lower than EAC phagocytosis. However, EAC phagocytosis by peritoneal mononuclear cells is significantly enhanced on Day 6 following an intravenous injection of PV.

TABLE I

Phagocytosis by Peritoneal Mononuclear Leukocytes of Erythrocyte-Antibody-Complement (EAC) Complexes and Erythrocytes (E) Following Intravenous Administration of Either Pertussis Vaccine (PV) or Vaccine Diluent (SM)

Dose of Vaccine (μg/gram body wt)	Time after injection (days)	% EAC phagocytosis		% E phagocytosis	
		SM	PV	SM	PV
Uninjected	-	21 ± 3[a]		5 ± 3	
40	2	14 ± 3	19 ± 2	3 ± 1	2 ± 1
	4	20 ± 4	22 ± 5	8 ± 2	3 ± 1
	6	19 ± 4	45 ± 5[b]	5 ± 1	6 ± 2
	10	28 ± 5	40 ± 6	9 ± 3	6 ± 1
	14	18 ± 3	24 ± 5	7 ± 2	4 ± 1
	18	14 ± 1	19 ± 4	3 ± 1	3 ± 1

[a] Mean ± S.E., four to eleven determinations per point.

[b] $p < 0.01$ when compared to SM.

The injection of microbial and non-microbial substances into experimental animals has been demonstrated to significantly enhance the spreading ability of peritoneal macrophages (17) and to enhance the activity of certain lysosomal enzymes such as acid phosphatase (8, 27, 39). These changes in macrophage function have been suggested to precede or accompany significant changes in the macrophages capability to participate in immune response or resistance to infection. It was of interest, therefore, to examine the influence of intravenous PV administration on these parameters of macrophage function.

The extent of peritoneal macrophage spreading was determined with modification according to the method of Bianco et al. (4). Briefly peritoneal cells in medium were applied to 13 mm glass cover-slips in culture dishes and were allowed to adhere for 30 min. Non-adherent cells were subsequently removed by rinsing and the cover-slip preparations transferred to fresh medium and incubated for an additional hour. Cell preparations were fixed and stained. The extent of cell spreading was estimated by projecting the cells onto the screen of a microscope projection attachment and randomly selecting and transcribing 100 monocytes per cover-slip. The total area of 100 cells was determined by means of an electronic plainimeter (Model 9864A Digitizer, Hewlett Packard, Loveland, CO). The intracellular acid phosphatase activity of peritoneal macrophages was determined following lysis of adherent cell cultures with 0.1% Triton X-100 (2). Cell lysate preparations were mixed with B-glycerophosphate and the enzyme activity determined by measuring the amount of inorganic phosphate released from the substrate during a 2 hour incubation. The results (Table II) demonstrate that there is little effect of PV on the rapid spreading of peritoneal macrophages. In contrast, intravenous administration of PV significantly enhances the acid phosphatase activity of the monocyte/macrophage system as early as Day 2 following injection. Of the four parameters studied so far, PV injection appears to significantly alter both EAC phagocytosis and acid phosphatase enzyme activity. Because the pertussis organism is composed of both heat-labile and heat-stable biologically active components it was of interest to examine which group of components was responsible for the alteration of macrophage function.

Groups of mice were injected i.v. with vaccine diluent, PV, PV heated to 56°C to destroy heat labile toxin, and PV heated to 80°C to destroy pertussis toxin. Six days following injection of the mice, peritoneal cells were removed by lavage and tested for EAC phagocytosis and acid phosphatase activity. The results (Table III) demonstrate that heating the vaccine to 56°C did not diminish the PV induced enhancement of EAC phagocytosis and lysosomal enzyme activity, suggesting that heat-labile toxin is not involved. However, heating the vaccine to 80°C ablated the PV effects, suggesting that pertussis toxin may be involved in the PV induced alteration of macrophage function.

The effect of microbial products on macrophage function has in some systems been demonstrated to require T lymphocytes (10). With

TABLE II

Adherent Mononuclear Leukocyte Spreading and Lysosomal Enzyme Activity Following Intravenous Administration of Either Pertussis Vaccine (PV) or Vaccine Diluent (SM)

Dose of Vaccine (μg/gram body wt.)	Time after injection	Spreading[a] ($\mu^2 \times 10^{-2}$)		Acid phosphatase[b] (nmoles PO_4 released/min/mg protein)	
		SM	PV	SM	PV
Uninjected	-	94 ± 2		8.0 ± 0.6	
20	2	-	-	9.4 ± 0.8	16.5 ± 1.0[c]
	6	-	-	8.8 ± 0.6	10.9 ± 0.9
	14	-	-	9.5 ± 0.4	11.3 ± 0.3
40	2	91 ± 2	97 ± 2	10.3 ± 0.8	18.4 ± 0.9[c]
	4	92 ± 3	89 ± 5	8.6 ± 1.0	13.9 ± 0.6[c]
	6	96 ± 3	97 ± 4	9.8 ± 0.6	14.3 ± 1.2[c]
	10	89 ± 4	101 ± 4	7.7 ± 0.8	15.0 ± 1.2[c]
	14	105 ± 3	124 ± 5[c]	8.5 ± 0.4	16.1 ± 1.4[c]
	18	99 ± 4	104 ± 3	7.7 ± 0.7	11.6 ± 1.6[c]

a Average area of 100 adherent cells. Mean ± SE, four to eight determinations per data point.

b Acid phosphatase activity of adherent mononuclear cells. Mean ± SE, three to five determinations per data point.

c $p \leq 0.01$ when compared to SM

this in mind, we examined for the requirement of T cell function in PV-induced alteration of macrophage acid phosphatase activity. Thymic (Nu/+) and athymic (Nu/Nu) C3H/HeN mice were injected as before with either PV or diluent. The results (Table IV) demonstrate that PV injection into C3H/HeN mice possessing an intact thymus produces an enhancement of peritoneal macrophage acid phosphatase activity through Day 14 following injection. However, PV injection into nude mice causes an early increase in enzyme activity, but this effect is not sustained with time after injection as in animals possessing intact T cell function.

Resident peritoneal macrophages when placed in culture gradually spread and display long cytoplasmic projections (9). We have already demonstrated that PV injection does not substantially enhance the early spreading ability of macrophages incubated for less than two hours. However, when peritoneal cells were cultured for twenty-

TABLE III

Phagocytosis and Lysosomal Enzyme Activity of Adherent Mononuclear Leukocytes Following Intravenous Administration of Pertussis Vaccine (PV), Heated Pertussis Vaccine (HPV) or Vaccine Diluent (SM)

Treatment	%EAC Phagocytosis	p[a]	Acid Phosphatase (nmole PO_4 released/min/mg protein)	p[a]
SM	11.2 ± 1.5[b]	-	7.7 ± 0.9[c]	-
PV	40.9 ± 4.7	<0.001	12.6 ± 1.3	<0.01
HPV (56°C, 25 min)	49.8 ± 6.2[d]	<0.001	12.5 ± 1.1	<0.01
HPV (80°C, 30 min)	14.8 ± 1.9	<0.2	8.0 ± 0.4	<0.9

a Comparison of PV versus SM injected animals.

b Mean ± S.E., six to twelve determinations per data point.

c Mean ± S.E., four to seven determinations per data point.

TABLE IV

Lysosomal Enzyme Activity of Adherent Mononuclear Leukocytes Obtained from Either C3H/HeN Heterozygous (Nu/+) or Nude (Nu/Nu) Mice Following Intravenous Injection of Pertussis Vaccine (PV) or Vaccine Diluent (SM)

Dose of Vaccine (µg/gram body wt)	Time After Injection (Days)	Acid Phosphatase[a] Activity in Nu/+		Acid Phosphatase Activity in Nu/Nu	
		SM	PV	SM	PV
Uninjected	-	10.3 ± 0.3[b]		10.1 ± 0.5	
20	2	10.1 ± 0.7	18.3 ± 1.1	12.4 ± 1.7	20.6 ± 0.6
20	6	9.4 ± 0.7	15.1 ± 0.2	8.4 ± 0.1	11.1 ± 0.9
20	14	7.6 ± 0.4	18.2 ± 0.9	9.8 ± 1.6	11.6 ± 1.0[c]

a Acid Phosphatase Activity - nmoles PO_4 released/min/mg protein.

b Mean ± S.E., three to seven determinations per data point.

c Not significantly different from SM, $t = 0.906$.

four hours, it was observed that those from PV treated animals did not display the elongated appearance of normal peritoneal cells. This is illustrated in Figure 1. Figure 1a and 1b are mouse peritoneal cells obtained from SM injected and PV injected mice, respectively. The cells had been removed 6 days following injection of the stimuli, incubated for 2 hr on glass cover-slips, and subsequently fixed and stained. No obvious difference can be seen between the two groups, with both displaying a rounded morphology. However, if identical preparations are allowed to incubate for 24 hr an obvious difference can be noted. Figure 1c is representative of cells obtained from SM injected animals and incubated for 24 hrs. The cells from PV treated animals (Figure 1d) appear very similar to cells incubated for only 2 hr in that they are more rounded than elongated. The extent of elongation was estimated in similar preparations with the aid of any eye-piece micrometer and cells stretching 20 μm or more were considered as being elongated. Table V demonstrates that following a two hour cultivation there is no

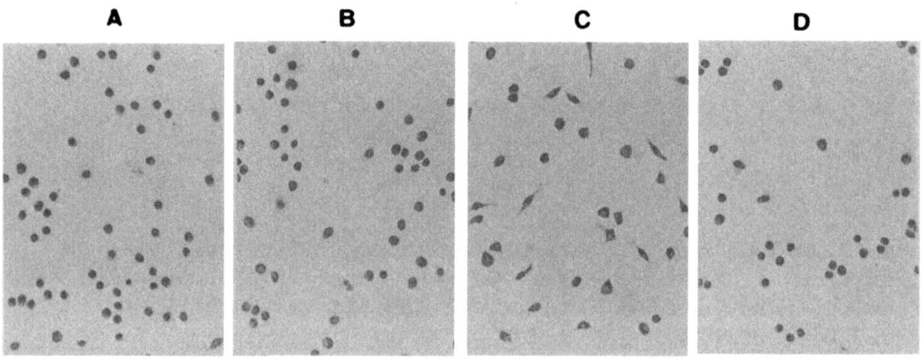

Fig. 1. Spreading ability of cultured adherent peritoneal leukocytes. Cells removed from mice 6 days following either (A) SM or (B) PV injection and cultured 2 hrs. Cells removed from either (C) SM or (D) PV and cultured for 24 hrs. (Magnification x 174).

difference between cells from control or PV injected animals, with elongation in both groups at a minimum. However, following a 24 hr cultivation 40-60% of adherent mononuclear cells from control animals had elongated while those from PV injected animals failed to display this response suggesting a PV induced suppression of this macrophage functional parameter. In studies not shown, both groups of cells readily ingested carbon particles.

TABLE V

Elongation of Adherent Peritoneal Leukocytes Following the Intravenous Administration of Pertussis Vaccine (PV) or Saline-Merthiolate (SM)

Days Following Injection	Percent of Adherent Cells Elongated				P^b
	PV	SM	PV	SM	
	2h[a]		2h		
2	2 $\pm$ 1[c]	6 $\pm$ 1	8 $\pm$ 1	59 $\pm$ 8	<0.001
6	4 $\pm$ 1	5 $\pm$ 1	6 $\pm$ 1	40 $\pm$ 4	<0.001
14	6 $\pm$ 1	7 $\pm$ 2	20 $\pm$ 2	56 $\pm$ 7	<0.001

[a] Incubation time of adherent cell cultures *in vitro*.

[b] P value comparing 24 h PV to SM by Student's *t* test.

[c] Mean $\pm$ S.E. three to five determinations per point.

The spreading of phagocytic cells appears to involve the action of contractile elements (microfilaments and microtubules) located near the cell surface (20, 37). Because macrophage migration also appears to rely on these contractile events (38), it seemed likely that random migration of peritoneal macrophages might also be suppressed by PV treatment. To examine this possibility, we studied the random migration of these cell populations by means of the agarose microdroplet technique. In this procedure, peritoneal leukocytes are suspended in 0.2% agarose and 2 µl droplets are dispensed into the wells of microtiter plates and allowed to solidify. Subsequently, the cell-containing droplets are covered with culture medium and incubated for 48 hours at 37°C. The extent of migration is determined by microscopically measuring the diameter of the cell button at 0, 24, 48 hours. The results are reported in terms of migration index which is the ratio of PV cell migration over control cell migration. The results in Table VI demonstrate that by Day 2 following injection of PV a significant decrease in random migration is observed and that by Day 6 post injection an even greater inhibition of migration is observed.

Finally, we would like to present some information relative to the ability of PV to enhance the resistance of the host to the lethal effects of viral infection. In the case of other microbial adjuvants, enhanced non-specific resistance to infection has been attributed to the adjuvant's ability to enhance macrophage function. The following evidence suggests that a similar mechanism is operating in the PV induced resistance to virus challenge.

TABLE VI

Random Migration of Peritoneal Leukocytes Following Intravenous Administration of Either Pertussis Vaccine (PV) or Saline-Merthiolate (SM)

Expt. No.	Days Following Injection	Migration Index[a] 24 h	48 h
1	2	0.71	0.70
2	2	0.72	0.67
1	6	0.52	0.35
2	6	0.39	0.21

[a] Migration index = PV/SM.

The intraperitoneal injection of a plaque type variant of MAdl adenovirus (American Type Culture Collection) into C3H/HeN (nu/+) mice which are heterozygous for the nude trait results in a lethal pneumonia only at relatively high virus dose. However, virus injection into C3H/HeN (Nu/Nu) nude mice is uniformly more lethal suggesting an involvement of T lymphocytes in resistance to this virus (Table VII). We wanted to see in this system if administration of PV prior to virus challenge could in some way ameliorate the lethal effects of the virus. Working with the heterozygotes first, we divided the animals into two groups. The first group received an intraperitoneal injection of 250 μg of PV, while the second group received only vaccine diluent. Seven days later, both groups received 1×10^8 pfus (20 LD_{50s}) of virus and the animal survival rates

TABLE VII

Survival of C3H/HeN Heterozygous (Nu/+) and Nude (Nu/Nu) Mice Following Intraperitoneal Injection of Mouse Adenovirus

Group	Number of Mice Inoculated	Virus dose (pfu)	Percent mortality at 30 days
	10	1×10^6	10
Nu/+	10	1×10^7	80
	10	1×10^8	100
	5	1×10^6	100
Nu/Nu	5	1×10^7	100
	5	1×10^8	100

were followed for 65 days. The results (Table VIII) demonstrate that under these conditions PV provided complete protection against the lethal effects of the virus. Furthermore, heating the vaccine to 80°C prior to injection did not diminish its protective capability, suggesting a role of PV endotoxin or other heat-stable components in the resistance effect.

Our next question concerned the relative contribution of T lymphocytes in the enhanced resistance following PV injection. Groups of C3H/HeN nude mice were injected either intravenously or intraperitoneally with PV and challenged seven days later with 1×10^8pfu of virus. Figure 2 demonstrates that intraperitoneal injection of PV into nude mice delayed, but did not prevent the lethal effects of virus challenge. These results differed from those obtained in heterozygous animals, wherein, PV afforded a complete and sustained resistance to virus. Figure 2 also demonstrates that intravenous injection of PV failed to provide protection in these animals.

TABLE VIII

Effect of Intraperitoneal Injection of Pertussis Vaccine (PV), Heated Pertussis Vaccine (HPV), or Vaccine Diluent (SM) Seven Days Prior to Intraperitoneal Challenge with Mouse Adenovirus on Survival of C3H/HeN Heterozygous (Nu/+) Mice

Treatment	Number of Mice Inoculated	Virus Dose (pfu)	Percent Mortality at 65 Days
SM	10	1×10^8	100
PV	10	1×10^8	0
HPV (80°C, 30 min)	10	1×10^8	0

DISCUSSION

Previously, we had demonstrated (15) that within 3 days following the intraperitoneal injection of PV, mouse peritoneal cells displayed enhanced phagocytosis of yeast. In the present study, we have extended these observations to EAC phagocytosis by peritoneal cells following intravenous injection of PV. These results (Table I) demonstrate that PV administered systemically can significantly stimulate the monocyte/macrophage system of the mouse as evidenced by enhanced EAC phagocytosis of peritoneal cells. Although other investigators have demonstrated a similar enhancement of EAC phagocytosis following intraperitoneal injection of bacteria and other

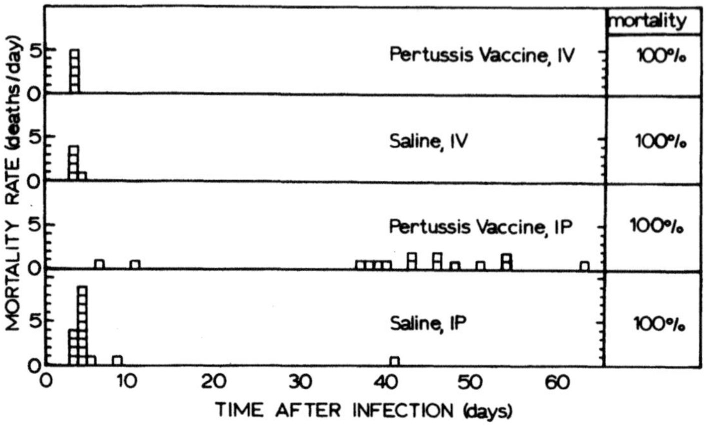

Fig. 2. Effect of Intravenous or Intraperitoneal Injection of Pertussis Vaccine (PV) or Vaccine Diluent (SM) Seven Days Prior to Intraperitoneal Challenge with Mouse Adenovirus on Survival of C3H/HeN Nude (Nu/Nu) Mice.

stimuli (3, 5, 13), the present results appear unique in that PV induced enhancement of macrophage EAC phagocytosis was accomplished following intravenous injection. The PV effect appears to be related to the mechanism of phagocytosis as opposed to C3b receptor expression, for in control experiments EAC rosetting ability of cells from control and PV injected animals was equivalent (>90%) at a time when phagocytosis of PV cells was enhanced.

Peritoneal macrophages obtained from animals injected either intraperitoneally or intravenously with various stimuli spread more rapidly when placed in culture than cells from non-injected animals (9, 33). This rapid spreading ability has been related to other functional alterations of macrophages (6). The results in Table II, however, demonstrate that the intravenous injection of PV has little effect on macrophage spreading during the first few hours in culture. It was demonstrated, however, that macrophages from PV injected animals failed to spread and elongate like the cells from control animals following incubation for 24 hrs (Figure 1 and Table V). In addition, random migration of explanted macrophages was inhibited on days 2 and 6 following PV injection (Table VI). Since plasma membrane associated microfilaments appear to be involved in endocytosis and cell motility (1, 37), enhancement of EAC phagocytosis coupled with reduced cell spreading and motility may reflect a PV induced gradual commitment of the macrophage microfilament system and/or membrane to the former process at the expense of the latter function. This suggests a functional limitation of the macrophage at a given point in time following stimulation. Clearly, further studies are needed using PV and other stimuli which are designed to examine a variety of macrophage functions simultaneously to obtain a better understanding of the relationship between the various parameters of macrophage function.

Table II demonstrates that as early as 2 days following PV injection the lysosomal enzyme activity of peritoneal macrophages is increased at least two-fold over controls and stays significantly elevated through day 18 following PV injection. Further studies (Table III) suggested that a heat-labile component of the vaccine was responsible for the enhanced lysosomal enzyme activity of macrophages obtained 6 days following PV injection. However, preliminary data in our laboratory suggest that although the heat-labile component may be responsible for the day 6 effects on lysosomal enzyme activity, the day 2 enhancement of enzyme function may be related to a heat-stable component, possibly endotoxin. This derives from our findings that macrophage enzyme activity is not enhanced in C3H/HeJ mice on day 2 following PV injection and that 80°C heated vaccine enhances enzyme function on day 2 in conventional mice.

The results in Table IV demonstrate that PV injection can exert a significant effect on macrophage lysosomal enzyme function in nude, athymic mice. However, it appears that competent T cells are required for a sustained PV induced enhancement of macrophage function because in nude animals acid phosphatase activity had returned to control values by day 6 following PV while in animals containing a thymus the PV effect persisted through day 14. These results suggest two mechanisms involved in the PV effects on macrophage, the first one being relatively T cell independent and occurring immediately following PV injection, and the second requiring competent T cell function and contributing to a persistent effect on peritoneal macrophages. It will be of interest in future studies to examine the role of the various biologically active components of PV in these mechanisms to obtain a clearer understanding of these complex PV induced effects.

Finally, concerning the viral resistance promoting effect of PV (Table VIII and Figure 2) our present interpretation suggests the following. Intraperitoneal PV injection causes an inflammatory exudate in the peritoneal cavity altering its cellular and humoral content (24), and possibly the functioning of the peritoneal cells. When virus is introduced into this milieu a substantial portion is eliminated by the exudate components. In the heterozygot mouse, the small amount of virus that escapes this initial destruction is finally eliminated by T dependent immune mechanisms. However, in the nude mouse such mechanisms are deficient, and the small amount of virus that escapes initial destruction eventually kills the host. Studies are currently in progress in our laboratory to define the cellular and/or humoral basis for the PV induced resistance to viral infection.

SUMMARY

Current evidence suggests that pertussis and its biologically active components alter immune responsiveness primarily by influencing T lymphocyte function. In addition, influences on macrophage and B lymphocyte function have been suggested. However, little information exists on the specific ways in which pertussis and its active components alter macrophage function. We have investigated the effect of intact and heated pertussis vaccine (PV) on macrophage phagocytosis, spreading, lysosomal enzyme production, and viral growth inhibitory activity in normal and thymus deficient mice. These studies demonstrate that peritoneal macrophages removed from mice following intravenous injection of PV display enhanced EAC phagocytosis and lysosomal enzyme activity. Both effects of PV treatment appear to be dependent upon heat-labile components in the vaccine. The *in vitro* spreading ability of macrophage explanted from PV injected mice is unaltered at 1.5 hours in culture but is inhibited following a 24 hour culture period. In addition, *in vitro* leukocyte migration of peritoneal cells obtained from PV treated animals is inhibited. Studies examining the effect of PV on the lethal effects of virus challenge demonstrate that intraperitoneal administration of PV can induce an enhanced resistance to subsequent virus challenge and that this effect of PV is independent of heat-labile components in the vaccine. Studies in nude mice suggest that although PV induced increases in lysosomal enzyme activity and viral resistance are observed in these animals, these responses are not sustained in the absence of T lymphocytes. Our results suggest that PV injection can significantly alter macrophage function, and that both heat-labile and heat-stable components of PV are involved. Furthermore, it appears that T lymphocytes are only partially involved in the expression of PV effects.

REFERENCES

1. Axline, S., and Reaven, E., 1974, Inhibition of phagocytosis and plasma membrane mobility of the cultivated macrophage by cytochalasin B. J. Cell Biol. 62: 647.

2. Barrett, A., and Heath, M., 1977, Lysosomal Enzymes, p. 19-145. *In* J. Dingle (ed.), Lysosomes a laboratory handbook. North Holland Publishing Co., New York.

3. Bianco, C., 1976, Methods for the study of macrophage Fc and C3 receptors, p. 407-415. *In* B.R. Bloom and J. R. David (eds.), *In vitro* methods in cell-mediated and tumor immunity. Academic Press Inc., New York.

4. Bianco, C., Eden, A., and Cohn, Z., 1976, The induction of macrophage spreading: role of coagulation factors and the complement system. J. Exp. Med. 144: 1531.

5. Bianco, C., Griffin, F., and Silverstein, S., 1975, Studies of the macrophage complement receptor. J. Exp. Med. 141: 1278.

6. Blanden, R., 1968, Modification of macrophage function. J. Reticuloendothel. Soc. 5: 179.

7. Bordet, J., and Genous, O., 1906, Le microbe de la coqueluche. Ann. Inst. Pasteur 20: 731.

8. Burley-Rosset, M., Florentin, I., Khalil, A., and Mathe, G.,1976, Nonspecific macrophage activation by systemic adjuvants. Int. Archs. Allergy Appl. Immun. 51: 594.

9. Cohn, Z., and Benson, B., 1965, The differentiation of mononuclear phagocytes. J. Exp. Med. 121: 153.

10. David, J., and Remold, H., 1976, Macrophage activation by lymphocyte mediators and studies on the interaction of macrophage inhibition factor (MIF) with its target cell, p. 401-426. In D. S. Nelson (ed.) Immunobiology of the Macrophage. Academic Press, Inc., New York.

11. Dresser, D., 1972, The role of T cells and adjuvant in the immune response of mice to foreign erythrocytes. Eur. J. Immunol. 2: 50.

12. Dresser, D., Wortis, H., and Anderson, H., 1970, The effect of pertussis vaccine on the immune response of mice to sheep red blood cells. Clin. Exp. Immunol. 7: 817.

13. Edelson, P., and Erb, C., 1978, Biochemical and functional characteristics of the plasma membrane of macrophages from BCG-infected mice. J. Immunol. 120: 1532.

14. Finger, H., Heymer, B., Wirsing, C., Emmerling, P., and Hof, H., 1978, Riversion of dextran sulfate-induced loss of antibacterial resistance by Bordetella pertussis. Infect. Immun. 19: 950.

15. Fishel, C., Halkias, D., Klein, T., and Szentivanyi, A., 1976, Characteristics of cells present in peritoneal fluids of mice injected intraperitoneally with Bordetella pertussis. Infect. Immun. 13: 263.

16. Giovanella, B., and Stehlin, J., 1973, Heterotransplantation of human malignant tumors in "nude" thymusless mice. I. Breeding and mainteance of "nude" mice. J. Nat. Cancer Inst. 51: 615.

17. Gotze, O., Bianco, C., and Cohn, Z., 1979, The induction of macrophage spreading by factor B of the properdin system. J. Exp. Med. 149: 372.

18. Greenberg, L., and Fleming, D., 1947, Increased efficiency of diptheria toxoid when combined with pertussis vaccine. Cand. J. Pub. Health. 38: 279.

19. Hamaoka, T., and Katz, D., 1973, Cellular site of action of various adjuvants in antibody responses to hapten-carrier conjugates. J. Immunol. 111: 1554.

20. Halentjaris, T., Lombardi, P., and Glasgow, L., 1976, Effect of cytochalasin B on the adhesion of mouse peritoneal macrophages. J. Cell Biol. 69: 407.

21. Ho, M., Kong, A., and Morse, S., 1979, The in vitro effects of Bordetella pertussislymphocytosis-promoting factor on murine lymphocytes. J. Exp. Med. 149: 1001.

22. Hof, H., Emmerling, P., Finger, H., and Wirsing, C., 1978, Influence of killed Bordetella pertussis cells on the resistance against infection with Listeria monocytogenes. 261. Bakt. Hyg. I. Abt. Orig. A 240: 208.

23. Kirchner, H., Scott, M., Hirt, H., and Munk, K., 1978, Protection of mice against viral infection by Corynebacterium parvum and Bordetella pertussis. J. Gen. Virol. 41: 97.

24. Klein, T., Pross, S., and Benjamin, W., 1978, Characterization of mouse peritoneal exudate and associated leukocyte adherence inhibitory activity after intraperitoneal injection of either Bordetella pertussis or Corynebacterium parvum vaccines. Infect. Immun. 22: 778.

25. Kong, A., and Morse, S., 1976, The effect of Bordetella pertussis on the antibody response in mice to type III pneumococcal polysaccharide. J. Immunol. 116: 989.

26. Levine, S., and Sowinski, R., 1972, Inhibition of macrophage response to brain injury. Am. J. Pathol. 67: 349.

27. Morland, B., and Morland, J., 1978, Selective induction of lysosomal enzyme activities in mouse peritoneal macrophages. J. Reticuloendothel. Soc. 23: 469.

28. Morse, S., 1965, Studies on the lymphocytosis induced in mice by Bordetella pertussis. J. Exp. Med. 121: 49.

29. Morse, S., 1976, Biologically active components and properties of Bordetella pertussis. Adv. Appl. Microbiol. 20: 9.

30. Mota, I., and Peixoto, J., 1966, A skin-sensitizing and thermolabile antibody in the mouse. Life Sciences 5: 1723.

31. Munoz, J., and Bergman- R., 1977, Bordetella pertussis immunological and other biological activities. Marcel Dekker, Inc. New York.

32. Murgo, A., and Athanassiades, T., 1975, Studies on the adjuvant effect of Bordetella pertussis vaccine to sheep erythrocytes in the mouse. J. Immunol. 115: 928.

33. North, R., 1969, Cellular kinetics associated with the development of acquired cellular resistance. J. Exp. Med. 130: 299.

34. Parfentjev, I., and Goodline, M., 1948, Histamine shock in mice sensitized with Hemophilus pertussis vaccine. J. Pharmacol. Exptl. Therap. 92: 411.

35. Suko, M., Ogita, T., Okudaira, H., and Horiuchi, Y., 1977, Preferential enhancement of IgE antibody formation by Bordetella pertussis. Int. Archs. Allergy Appl. Immun. 54: 329.

36. Unanue, E., Askonas, B., and Allison, A., 1969, A role of macrophages in the stimulation of immune responses by adjuvants. J. Immunol. 103: 71.

37. Wilkinson, P., 1976, Cell-membrane activation of macrophage function, p. 41-48. In G. Mathe, I. Florentin, M. Simmler (eds.), Recent results in cancer research, vol. 56. Springer-Verlag, New York.

38. Wilkinson, P., 1976, Cellular and molecular aspects of chemotaxis of macrophages and monocytes, p. 349-365. In D. Nelson (ed.), Immunobiology of the macrophage. Academic Press, New York.

39. Yagel, S., Gallily, R., and Weiss, D., 1975, Effect of treatment with the MER fraction of tubercle bacilli on hydrolytic lysosomal enzyme activity of mouse peritoneal macrophages. Cell. Immunol. 19: 381.

40. Zakharova, M., 1979, Theortetical outlines on the preparation of a noncellular pertussis vaccine. In C. R. Manclark and J. C. Hill (eds.), International Symposium on Pertussis, pp. 320. DHEW Publication No. (NIH) 79-1830. Washington, DC.

ACKNOWLEDGMENTS

We would like to acknowledge the technical assistance of Carole Guzzaldo. This study was supported in part by Public Health Service Grant AI 15108-01 from the National Institute of Allergy and Infectious Diseases.

ROLE OF ACTIVATED MACROPHAGE SUPEROXIDE ANIONS AND HYDROGEN PEROXIDE IN IMMUNE SUPPRESSION

J. Terrell Hoffeld, Zvi Metzger and Joost J. Oppenheim

Laboratory of Microbiology and Immunology
Cellular Immunology Section
NIH, NIDR
Bethesda, MD 20205

Bacterial cells and their products are among the most potent inducers of macrophage activation (2). In turn, activated macrophages can be both stimulators and suppressors of lymphocyte functions. Dr. Oppenheim has already detailed what we believe to be the stimulatory macrophage mechanisms (22). The suppression of lymphocyte function *in vitro* and/or *in vivo* has been attributed to a growing list of macrophage-derived materials (Table I) (1). Despite the longevity of most of the macrophage products which are suppressive, it is difficult to reproduce, with culture supernatants, the full extent of suppression observed in the original cultures. This suggested that the suppressive activity of activated macrophages might be mediated by short-lived products and/or required close macrophage-lymphocyte contact. Since the complement fractions and prostaglandins are relatively labile and difficult to isolate from supernatants of lymphocyte cultures suppressed by activated macrophages, they remained reasonable candidates as mediators of the suppression. An additional group of short-lived, potentially-suppressive substances released by activated macrophages is the group of oxygen metabolites, including the superoxide anion and hydrogen peroxide. Since these bactericidal molecules had not been previously considered in the context of lymphocytostasis, we have investigated their involvement in several *in vitro* models of the immune response. In this paper, we will first consider the mechanism of the production of superoxide by macrophages and the mode of its toxic action on other cells. We will then present data implicating superoxide as having a damping effect on the normal antibody response, *in vitro*. Finally, we will show that the overwhelming suppressive effect of macrophages activated by exposure to *Corynebacterium parvum* (*C. parvum*; *Propionibacterium acnis*) cells is mediated by both hydrogen peroxide and prostaglandins, together.

TABLE I

Products of Activated Macrophages Suppressing Lymphocyte Responses(1):

1. Thymidine
2. Arginase
3. Polyamine Oxidase
4. Complement Fragments
5. Prostaglandins
6. Cyclic AMP
7. Interferon

The events of the activation of macrophages include what is normally referred to as the "oxidative metabolic burst" (24). During the process of phagocytosis of bacteria, there is an enhancement of the activity of the hexose monophosphate shunt (HMPS; pentose pathway) which provides the cell with reduced nicotinamide adenine dinucleotide phosphate (NADPH) (2). This compound can then be oxidized by either of two pathways (Figure 1): a) in the presence of oxidized glutathione (GSSG), the NADPH will be oxidized, thus reducing the GSSG to two molecules of reduced glutathione (GSH); or b) in the presence of oxygen and the enzyme, NADPH oxidase, the direct oxidation of NADPH frequently "leaks" molecules of the oxygen radical, superoxide anion ($O_2^{\cdot}$) (6). This oxygen-derived metabolite reacts readily with any available organic substrate (e.g., bacterial cells) or can interact with water or itself to yield several other highly reactive oxygen metabolites (8):

hydrogen peroxide: $O_2^{\cdot} + O_2^{\cdot} + 2H^+ \text{-----------} H_2O_2 + O_2$

hydroxyl radical: $O_2^{\cdot} + H_2O_2 \text{-----------} OH^{\cdot} + O_2 + OH^-$

singlet oxygen: $O_2^{\cdot} + OH^{\cdot} \text{-----------} {}^1O_2 + OH^-$

Each of these molecules can also interact with organic substrates and lead to bacterial cell destruction. In the presence of an halide ion, these molecules can contribute to the myeloperoxidase reaction, which provides another powerful bactericidal mechanism in the phagosome (24). If these reactions were limited to the phagosome, alone, there would be no potential danger to nearby eukaryotic cells; however, the NADPH oxidase is distributed over the entire cell membrane and is directed outward, resulting in a constant "spillage" of oxygen metabolites to the activated macrophage's surroundings (14). This excess of oxygen metabolites is measurable in the aqueous medium as H_2O_2, which is thought to mediate the tumoricidal capacity of activated macrophages (14). The lethal action of oxygen metabolites on the eukaryotic target cell is apparently due to a peroxidation of unsaturated membrane lipids which is initiated by the hydroxyl radical (Figure 2) (8). This peroxidation

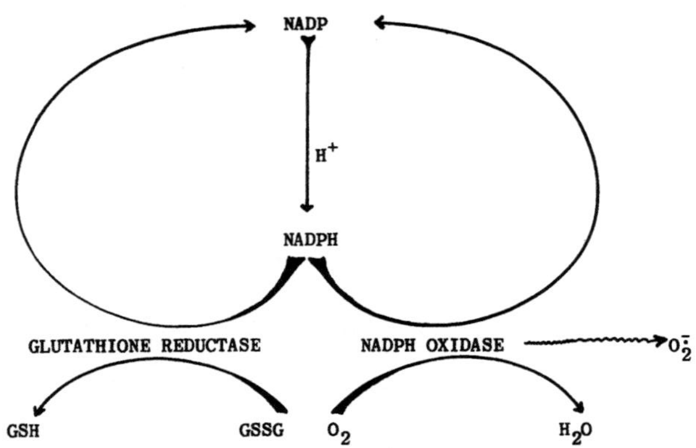

Fig. 1. NADPH-dependent pathways for the reduction of glutathione and the generation of superoxide anions: NADP=nicotinamide adenine dinucleotide phosphate (oxidized), NADPH=nicotinamide adenine dinucleo phosphate (reduced), GSSG=disulfide (oxidized) glutathione, GSH=sulfhydryl (reduced) glutathione. NADP is reduced to NADPH by hydrogen donated from the glucose-6-phosphate dehydrogenase reaction of the hexose monophosphate shunt. NADPH can be reoxidized either by the glutathione reductase reaction of the NADPH oxidase reaction. During the NADPH oxidase reaction, superoxide anions (O_2^-) are commonly released.

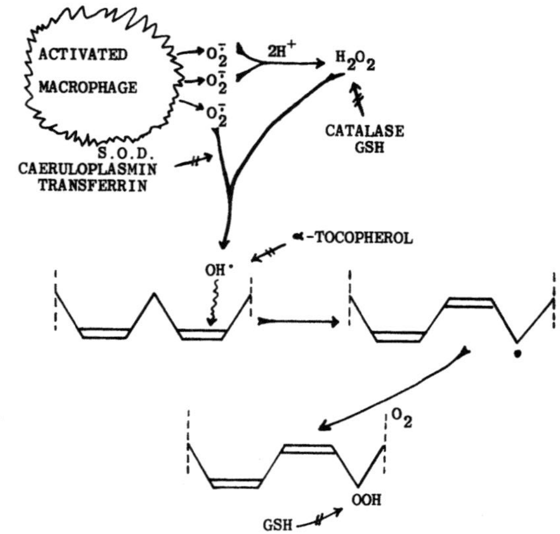

Fig. 2. Pathways of peroxidation of unsaturated fatty acids by oxygen metabolites: Hydroxyl radical attacks a segment of unsaturated fatty acid chain, shifting the double bond and setting up a radical center. This radical center can then react with oxygen to yield a fatty acid hydroperoxide (-OOH). Commonly, the fatty acid chain will cleave at the site of the hydroperoxide, releasing short chain fragments and disrupting the lipid from which it is derived.

process sets up a chain reaction which causes the release of fatty acid chains of varying lengths, culminating in the disruption of membrane architecture (5). Arachidonate chains released in this manner can serve as substrates for prostaglandin synthesis (23) and the lipid hydroperoxides produced by membrane peroxidation have been shown to enhance cyclooxygenase activity (9). Thus, macrophage activaction can result in the release of a shower of potentially suppressive and relatively short-lived substances.

Under the conditions of a "normal" immune response, either in vivo or in vitro, oxygen radicals and lipid hydroperoxides are produced, without a noticeable suppressive effect. Activated macrophages generate superoxide anions and the membrane lipids of dying cells autoxidize, yet the neighboring lymphocytes continue to respond (7). In vivo, the constitutive and induced release by macrophages of superoxide dismutase and catalase, as well as their constitutive regeneration of reduced glutathione will protect macrophages and neighboring cells from peroxidative damage. Additionally, serum levels of those radical scavengers as well as transferrin, caeruloplasmin, and α-tocopherol are very portective of cells challenged by peroxidative insult (7). Since serum is such an important variable in most in vitro models of the immune response, we considered the possibility that an important serum variable might be its capacity to function as a radical scavenger in vitro.

In order to test this possibility, we adopted the murine primary antibody response (25) as an in vitro model of a "normal" immune response. Since this experimental system has been shown to be critically dependent on particular commerical lots of fetal calf serum (FCS) (18), and since glutathione had been shown to occur in certain lots of FCS, but not adult sera (3), we investigated the possibility that the presence of the radical-scavenging tri-peptide, glutathione (15) might be the important variable in different lots of FCS. We found that the reduced glutathione (GSH) content of multiple lots of FCS correlated directly with the capacity of those lots to support a primary antibody response, in vitro (10). Additionally, if the GSH content of the FCS was oxidized by heating, the response supported by that FCS was greatly diminished, but was fully restorable by the addition of fresh GSH (10). Thus, the survival and activity of the murine spleen cells, in culture, was critically dependent upon the presence and function of glutathione.

Another sulfhydryl-containing compound, the presence of which has been shown to enhance the survival and activity of murine spleen cells in culture, is 2-mercaptoethanol (2-ME) (4). We investigated the possibility that the enhancing capacity of 2-ME might be mediated by glutathione in the FCS. There was a precedent for the assumption that 2-ME acted upon a component of FCS, since Opitz et al. (20) had reported that pulsing of FCS with 2-ME and removing the unreacted 2-ME by lyophilization produced an FCS which supported the same enhanced antibody response as an untreated FCS in the presence of 2-ME. They identified the FCS component which reacted with 2-ME as a 46,000 dalton protein (21) further supporting the plausibility of an assumed relationship of 2-ME and glutathione, since the serum carrier for glutathione, ligandin, has the same molecular weight (12). In order to distinguish whether the FCS component which reacted with 2-ME was the large carrier (46,000 dalton) or the carrier-borne small GSH molecule (307 daltons), we exhaustively dialyzed FCS. Removal of the low molecular weight fraction of FCS prevented it from supporting an enhanced antibody response, either in the presence of 2-ME or when it had been pulsed with 2-ME either before or after dialysis (11). 2-ME treatment of either FCS dialysate or GSH restored the ability of either a dialyzed or a heated FCS, respectively, to support an enhanced antibody response (Figure 3). These data showed that 2-ME interacted with glutathione, presumably by the formation of a mixed disulfide, which could easily dissociate to relase GSH (13). That enhancement of GSH availability apparently enhanced the antibody response, in vitro.

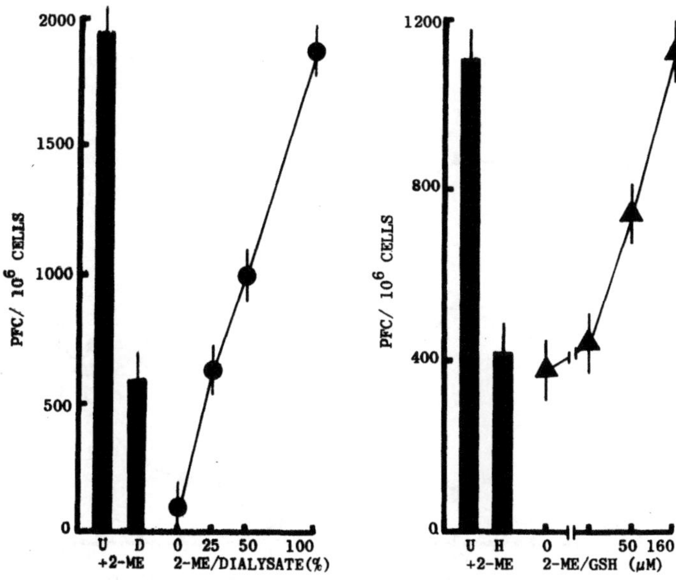

Fig. 3. Effect of 2-ME-pulsed dialysate or 2-ME-pulsed GSH on the antibody response of cultures containing dialyzed or heated FCS: Histograms represent the anti-sheep erythrocyte primary antibody response of cultures containing untreated (U) FCS and 50 μM 2-ME, dialyzed (D) FCS and 50 μM 2-ME or heated (H) FCS and 50 μM 2-ME. Graded doses of the appropriate additive were added to cultures containing no 2-ME. Direct (IgM) plaque forming cells (PFC) were measured after 96 hours of culture. Error bars represent one standard error.

We could then ask the question of whether the 2-ME/GSH was enhancing *via* the radical-scavenging function of glutathione, or by some other of the many known functions of glutathione (16). We tested a number of radical scavengers and antioxidants in the absence of 2-ME, or in the presence of either suboptimal (5 μM) or optimal (50 μM) doses of 2-ME, to see if there was any additive or synergistic effect of the agents tested. We found that scavengers specific for H_2O_2, $OH^{\cdot}$, or $^1O_2$ had little effect on the system. In contrast, superoxide dismutase (S.O.D.) enhanced the antibody response in the presence of suboptimal or no 2-ME and did not affect the response in the presence of the optimal concentration of 2-ME (Figure 4). Additionally, an equimolar solution of the lipid antioxidants, n-propyl gallate (nPrG), butylated hydroxyanisole (BHA) and butylated hydroxytoluene (BHT) had an effect qualitatively similar to that seen with S.O.D. (Figure 4). We conclude that the enhancement of the antibody response *in vitro*, by the GSH in FCS, especially in the presence of 2-ME, is mediated by the radical-scavenging capacity of GSH. Thus as is the case *in vivo*

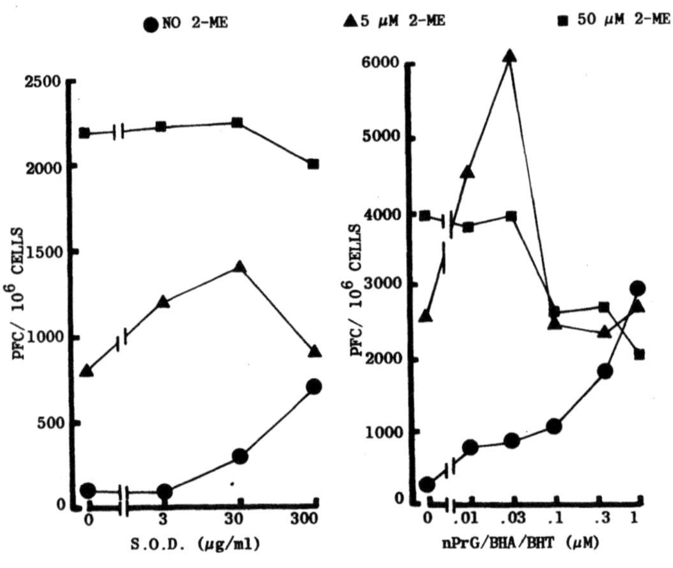

Fig. 4. Effect of a superoxid scavenger or lipid antioxidants on the antibody response in cultures containing various concentrations of 2-ME. Graded doses of superoxide dismutase (S.O.D.) or an equimolar solution of n-propyl gallate, butylated hydroxyanisole and butylated hydroxytoluene (nPrG/BHA/BHT) were added to cultures containing 0,5 or 50 μM 2-ME. Direct (IgM) anti-sheep erythrocyte plaque-forming cells (PFC) were measured after 96 hr of culture. Standard errors were <10%.

(7), in the course of a "normal" antibody response, in vitro, the responding cells must be protected from peroxidative insult initiated by metabolically active macrophages and/or propagated by auto-oxidation of dead cells.

In a number of chronic bacterial infections in which the bacteria are poorly degraded by macrophages, and hence, serve as continual stimuli for macrophage activation, the lymphocytes become hyporeactive. Since we already had evidence that the oxygen metabolites produced by activated macrophages could damp a normal immune response, we investigated the possibility that macrophages hyperactivated by exposure, in vivo, to formalin-killed C. parvum cells might suppress lymphocyte response, in vitro. Ten to thirteen days after mice were injected intraperitoneally with C. parvum, the peritoneal cells (PC) were collected by saline lavage. This cell population consisted of 81% macrophages, 6% lymphocytes, 13% neutrophils, and <1% basophils (17). Results of experiments using only the adherent fraction of this population did not differ significantly from those in which the entire population had been used, so the mixed population was used for the sake of convenience. The addition of graded doses of the C. parvum-activated PC caused a

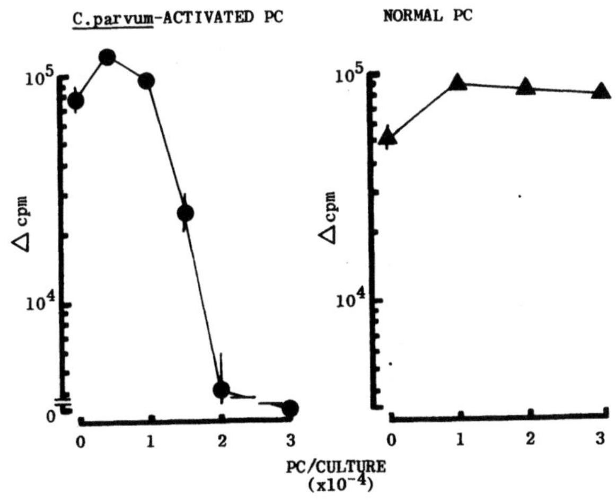

Fig. 5. Effects of C. parvum-activated or normal peritoneal cells on Concanavalin A-induced lymphocyte proliferation: 10^5 normal spleen cells were cultured with various numbers of peritoneal cells, as designated by the abscissae. Uptake of tritiated thymidine was measured after 72 hours of culture. Net cpm (Δcpm) of identical cultures with and withour Concanavalin A are plotted on the ordinate. Standard errors, where not designated by bars, were smaller than the symbols.

significant depression of the tritiated-thymidine incorporation by concanavalin A-stimulated normal spleen cells (Figure 5). In contrast, unstimulated PC caused no suppression. Supernatant-mixing experiments and counting of lymphocytes ruled out the possibility that this suppression was due to the release of non-labelled thymidine by the macrophages and suggested that the suppression was due to a direct action on cell proliferation by some agent(s) which were relatively short-lived. Additionally, the fact that this suppression occurred even in the presence of 2-ME and FCS with a high glutathione content suggested that C. parvum-activated macrophages could overwhelm those protective mechanisms. As a consequence, additional mediators besides superoxide had to be considered.

Since the production of prostaglandins had been shown to be one sequela of the oxidative metabolic burst (9), we investigated the involvement of this group of potentially suppressive materials as well as the oxygen metabolites in the suppression of lymphocyte proliferation by C. parvum-activated PC. The addition of even excessively high doses of PGE_1, PGE_2, or $PGE_{2\alpha}$ could not duplicate the suppression seen in the cultures (17). The addition of either catalase or indomethacin, over wide dose ranges could not completely reverse the suppression in the cell cultures. In contrast, the addition of doses of both indomethacin and catalase was able to totally reverse the suppression produced by C. parvum-activated PC (Figure 6). These data implicated a combined effect of prostaglandins and the oxygen metabolites (specifically, H_2O_2) in the suppression by bacterially-activated macrophages of lymphocyte proliferation.

We have presented data which show that when a normal spleen cell population responds to an easily degradable antigen, the production of oxygen metabolites produces a damping of the response. This damping can be kept relatively in check both by serum factors (*viz.*, S.O.D., GSH) which scavenge radicals and by agents which enhance the action of any of these scavenging mechanisms (*viz.*, 2-ME by its effect on GSH). In contrast, macrophages which have been exposed to poorly-degradable C. parvum cells and are hyperactivated both by phagocytosis and by T cell signals, can totally suppress a mitogen-driven proliferation response. The excessive production of superoxide leads to the accumulation of hydrogen peroxide in the aqueous medium and the resultant production of prostaglandins (9). Thus, under the conditions of a chronic bacterial infection, the macrophage can suppress the response of lymphocytes over a range from a minor decrease to a total suppression with major cell damage. This hierarchy of suppression, proportional to the types of antigenic challenge presented to the macrophage, presents the other side of the macrophage's "personality" to contrast the characteristics presented by Dr. Oppenheim. In combination, these data show how macrophages can be the ultimate regulators of immune responses initiated by bacterial challenge.

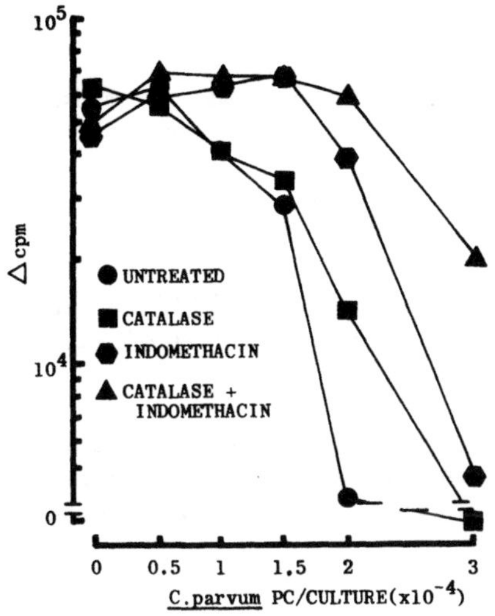

Fig. 6. Effects of indomethacin, catalase or both on suppression of lymphocyte proliferation produced by C. parvum-activated peritoneal cells: Doses of 10 μg/ml indomethacin, 10,000 U/ml catalase, or the combination of these were added to cultures of 10^5 Concanavalin A-stimulated spleen cells to which various numbers of C. parvum-activated peritoneal cells had been added. Uptake of tritiated thymidine was measured after 72 hours of culture. Net cpm (Δ cpm) of identical cultures with and without Concanavalin A are plotted on the ordinate. Standard errors were all <10%.

ABBREVIATIONS

C. parvum	- Corynebacterium parvum
FCS	- Fetal Calf Serum
GSH	- Reduced (Sulfhydryl) Glutathione
GSSG	- Oxidized (Disulfide) Glutathione
H_2O_2	- Hydrogen Peroxide
NADPH	- Reduced Nicotinamide Adenine Dinucleotide
$^1O_2$	- Singlet Oxygen
O_2^-	- Superoxide Anion
$OH^\cdot$	- Hydroxyl Radical
PC	- Peritoneal Cells
2-ME	- 2-mercaptoethanol

REFERENCES

1. Allison, A. C., 1978, Mechanisms by which activated macrophages inhibit lymphocyte responses. Immunol. Rev., 40: 3.

2. Babior, B. M., 1978, Oxygen-dependent microbial killing by phagocytes. N. Engl. J. Med. 298: 659.

3. Bump, E. A., and Reed, D. J., 1977, A unique property of fetal bovine serum: High levels of protein-glutathione mixed disulfides. In Vitro. 13: 115.

4. Chen, C., and Hirsch, J. G., 1972, The effects of mercaptoethanol and of peritoneal macrophages on the antibody-forming capacity of nonadherent mouse spleen cells in vitro. J. Exp. Med. 136: 604.

5. Dianzani, M. U., and Ugazio, G., 1978, Lipid peroxidation. pp 669-707. In T. F. Slater (ed.), Biochemical mechanisms of liver injury. Academic Press. New York.

6. Dewald, B., Bagglioni, M., Curnutte, J. T., and Babior, B. M., 1979, Subcellular localization of the superoxide-forming enzyme in human neutrophils. J. Clin. Invest. 63: 21.

7. Dormandy, T.L., 1978, Free-radical oxidation and antioxidants. Lancet, I: 647.

8. Halliwell, B., 1978, Biochemical mechanisms accounting for the toxic action of oxygen on living organisms: The key role of superoxide dismutase. Cell Biol. Int. Rpts. 2: 113.

9. Hemler, M. E., Cook, H. W., and Lands, W. E. M., 1979, Prostaglandin biosynthesis can be triggered by lipid peroxides. Arch. Biochem. Biophys. 193: 340.

10. Hoffeld, J. T., and Oppenheim, J. J., 1980, The capacity of fetal calf serum to support a primary antibody response, in vitro, is determined in part by its reduced glutathione content. Cell. Immunol. (in press).

11. Hoffeld, J. T., and Oppenheim, J. J., 1980, Enhancement of the primary antibody response by 2-mercaptoethanol is mediated by its action on glutathione in serum. (Submitted).

12. Jakoby, W. B., 1978, The glutathione S-transferases: A group of multifunctional detoxification proteins. Adv. Enzymol. 46: 383.

13. Jocelyn, P. C., 1967, The standard redox potential of cysteine-cystine from the thiol-disulphide exchange reaction with glutathione and lipoic acid. Eur. J. Biochem. 2: 327.

14. Johnston, R. B., Jr., Godzik, C. A., and Cohn, Z. A., 1978, Increased superoxide anion production by immunologically activated and chemically elicited macrophages. J. Exp. Med.148: 115.

15. Kosower, N. S., and Kosower, E. M., 1976, The glutathione-glutathione disulfide system. pp. 55-84. In Free radicals in biology, vol. II. W. A. Pryor (ed.). Academic Press, New York.

16. Kosower, N. S., and Kosower, E. M., 1978, The glutathione status of cells. Int. Rev. Cytol. 54: 109.

17. Metzger, Z., Hoffeld, J. T., and Oppenheim, J. J., 1980, Macrophage-mediated suppression: I. Evidence for participation of both hydrogen peroxide and prostaglandins in suppression of murine lymphocyte proliferation. J. Immunol. (in press).

18. Mishell, R. I., and Dutton, R. W., 1967, Immunization of disociated spleen cell cultures from normal mice. J. Exp. Med. 126: 423.

19. Nathan, C. F., Silverstein, S. C., Brukner, L. H., Cohn, Z. A., 1979, Extracellular cytolysis by activated macrophages and granulocytes: II. Hydrogen peroxide as a mediator of cytotoxicity. J. Exp. Med. 149: 100.

20. Opitz, H. G., Opitz, U., Lemke, H., Hewlett, G., Schreml, W., and Flad, H. D., 1977, The role of fetal calf serum in the primary immune response in vitro. J. Exp. Med., 145: 1029.

21. Opitz, H. G., Opitz, U., Lemke, H., Flad, H. D., Hewlett, G., and Schlumberger, H. D., 1977, Humoral primary immune response in vitro in a homologous mouse system: Replacement of fetal calf serum by a 2-mercaptoethanol or macrophage-activated fraction of mouse serum. J. Immunol. 119: 2089.

22. Oppenheim, J. J., Steeg, P. S., and Moore, R. N., 1980, Bidirectional macrophage-lymphocyte interactions modulate immune responses. (this volume).

23. Pryor, W. A., and Stanley, J. P., 1975, A suggested mechanism for the production of malonaldehyde during the autoxidation of polyunsaturated fatty acids. Nonenzymatic production of

prostaglandin endoperoxides during autoxidation. J. Org. Chem. 24: 3615.

24. Quie, P. G., Mills, E. L., and Holmes, B., 1977, Molecular events during phagocytosis by human neutrophils. Prog. Haemotol. X: 193.

25. Schreier, M. H., and Nordin, A. A., 1977, An evaluation of the immune response in vitro. pp. 127-162. In B and T cells in immune recognition. F. Loor and G. E. Roelants (eds.). J. Wiley and Sons, New York.

INDEX